PET/CT and Patient Outcomes, Part I

Editor

RATHAN M. SUBRAMANIAM

PET CLINICS

www.pet.theclinics.com

Consulting Editor
ABASS ALAVI

April 2015 • Volume 10 • Number 2

ELSEVIER

1600 John F. Kennedy Boulevard • Suite 1800 • Philadelphia, Pennsylvania, 19103-2899

http://www.pet.theclinics.com

PET CLINICS Volume 10, Number 2
April 2015 ISSN 1556-8598, ISBN-13: 978-0-323-35982-5

Editor: John Vassallo (j.vassallo@elsevier.com)
Developmental Editor: Meredith Clinton

PET Clinics (ISSN 1556-8598) is published quarterly by Elsevier Inc., 360 Park Avenue South, New York, NY 10010-1710. Months of issue are January, April, July, and October. Periodicals postage paid at New York, NY, and additional mailing offices. Subscription prices per year are $225.00 (US individuals), $327.00 (US institutions), $115.00 (US students), $255.00 (Canadian individuals), $369.00 (Canadian institutions), $140.00 (Canadian students), $275.00 (foreign individuals), $369.00 (foreign institutions), and $140.00 (foreign students). To receive student and resident rate, orders must be accompanied by name of affiliated institution, date of term, and the signature of program/residency coordinator on institution letterhead. Orders will be billed at individual rate until proof of status is received. Foreign air speed delivery is included in all Clinics subscription prices. All prices are subject to change without notice. POSTMASTER: Send address changes to PET Clinics, Elsevier Health Sciences Division, Subscription Customer Service, 3251 Riverport Lane, Maryland Heights, MO 63043. **Customer Service: 1-800-654-2452 (U.S. and Canada); 314-447-8871 (outside U.S. and Canada). Fax: 314-447-8029. E-mail: journalscustomerservice-usa@elsevier.com (for print support); journalsonlinesupport-usa@elsevier.com (for online support).**

Reprints. For copies of 100 or more of articles in this publication, please contact the Commercial Reprints Department, Elsevier Inc., 360 Park Avenue South, New York, NY 10010-1710. Tel.: 212-633-3874; Fax: 212-633-3820; E-mail: reprints@elsevier.com.

PET Clinics is covered in MEDLINE/PubMed (Index Medicus).

Contributors

CONSULTING EDITOR

ABASS ALAVI, MD, PhD (Hon), Dsc (Hon)
Professor of Radiology, Division of Nuclear
Medicine, Department of Radiology, University
of Pennsylvania School of Medicine, Hospital
of the University of Pennsylvania, Philadelphia,
Pennsylvania

EDITOR

RATHAN M. SUBRAMANIAM, MD, PhD, MPH
Associate Professor of Radiology, Oncology, Head and Neck Surgery, Health Policy and
Management, Russell H. Morgan Department of Radiology and Radiological Sciences, Sidney
Kimmel Comprehensive Cancer Center, Johns Hopkins School of Medicine; Department of Health
Policy and Management, Johns Hopkins Bloomberg School of Public Health, Johns Hopkins
University, Baltimore, Maryland

AUTHORS

TIM AKHURST, MD, FRACP
Associate Professor, Division of Radiation
Oncology and Cancer Imaging, Centre for
Molecular Imaging, Peter MacCallum Cancer
Centre, East Melbourne; The Sir Peter
MacCallum Department of Oncology, The
University of Melbourne, Melbourne, Victoria,
Australia

ANTHONY CIARALLO, MD
PET/CT Clinical Fellow, Russell H. Morgan
Department of Radiology and Radiological
Sciences, Johns Hopkins School of
Medicine, Baltimore, Maryland

DANIEL GREENSPAN, MD
Department of Radiology, Memorial Sloan
Kettering Cancer Center, New York, New York

RODNEY J. HICKS, MD, FRACP
Professor, Division of Radiation
Oncology and Cancer Imaging, Centre
for Molecular Imaging, Peter MacCallum
Cancer Centre, East Melbourne; The Sir Peter
MacCallum Department of Oncology, The
University of Melbourne, Melbourne, Victoria,
Australia

HEATHER A. JACENE, MD
Department of Imaging, Dana-Farber Cancer
Institute; Department of Radiology, Brigham
and Women's Hospital, Harvard Medical
School, Boston, Massachusetts

HOSSEIN JADVAR, MD, PhD, MPH, MBA
Department of Radiology, Keck School of
Medicine of USC, University of Southern
California, Los Angeles, California

NATALIYA KOVALCHUK, PhD
Medical Physicist, Department of Radiation
Oncology, Boston Medical Center, Boston,
Massachusetts

ROBERT M. KWEE, MD, PhD
Radiology Resident, Department of Radiology,
Maastricht University Medical Center,
Maastricht, The Netherlands

ANN S. LACASCE, MD
Lymphoma Program, Dana-Farber Cancer
Institute; Department of Medicine, Brigham
and Women's Hospital, Harvard Medical
School, Boston, Massachusetts

LIZZA LEBRON, MD
Department of Radiology, Memorial Sloan Kettering Cancer Center, New York, New York

MICHAEL MACMANUS, MD, FRANZCR
Professor, The Sir Peter MacCallum Department of Oncology, The University of Melbourne; Division of Radiation Oncology and Cancer Imaging, Department of Radiation Oncology, Peter MacCallum Cancer Centre, East Melbourne, Victoria, Australia

CHARLES MARCUS, MD
Postdoctoral Research Fellow, Russell H. Morgan Department of Radiology and Radiological Sciences, Johns Hopkins School of Medicine, Johns Hopkins University, Baltimore, Maryland

NEETA PANDIT-TASKAR, MD
Molecular Imaging and Therapy Service, Department of Radiology, Memorial Sloan Kettering Cancer Center, New York, New York

PATRICK J. PELLER, MD
Chief Medical Officer, Eka Medical Center - Jakarta, BSD City, Tangerang, Indonesia

ERIC M. ROHREN, MD, PhD
Professor, Department of Radiology and Nuclear Medicine; Section Chief, PET/CT, The University of Texas MD Anderson Cancer Center, Houston, Texas

SARA SHEIKHBAHAEI, MD, MPH
Postdoctoral Research Fellow, Russell H. Morgan Department of Radiology and Radiological Sciences, Johns Hopkins School of Medicine, Johns Hopkins University, Baltimore, Maryland

RATHAN M. SUBRAMANIAM, MD, PhD, MPH
Associate Professor of Radiology, Oncology, Head and Neck Surgery, Health Policy and Management, Russell H. Morgan Department of Radiology and Radiological Sciences, Sidney Kimmel Comprehensive Cancer Center, Johns Hopkins School of Medicine; Department of Health Policy and Management, Johns Hopkins Bloomberg School of Public Health, Johns Hopkins University, Baltimore, Maryland

MEHDI TAGHIPOUR, MD
Post Doctoral Research Fellow, Russell H. Morgan Department of Radiology and Radiological Sciences, Johns Hopkins School of Medicine, Baltimore, Maryland

SREE HARSHA TIRUMANI, MD
Department of Imaging, Dana-Farber Cancer Institute; Department of Radiology, Brigham and Women's Hospital, Harvard Medical School, Boston, Massachusetts

MINH TAM TRUONG, MD
Associate Professor and Clinical Director, Department of Radiation Oncology, Boston Medical Center, Boston University School of Medicine, Boston, Massachusetts

Contents

There is a growing body of evidence that point to the value of 18F fluoro-deoxyglucose-PET/CT in the management of head and neck cancer (HNC) patients and predicting patient-related outcomes. FDG-PET/CT changes the baseline staging (compared with CT or MR imaging), guides appropriate therapy selection, separates the responders and non-responders for therapy assessment, adds value to clinical assessment in follow-up, and predicts patient survival outcomes. FDG-PET/CT can identify the recurrences in earlier stages and individualize follow-up regimens in HNC patients. This article reviews the value of FDG-PET/CT in management strategy and survival outcome of HNC patients.

^{18}F-fluorodeoxyglucose–positron emission tomography/computed tomography (FDG-PET/CT) plays a key role in the evaluation of undiagnosed lung nodules, when primary lung cancer is strongly suspected, or when it has already been diagnosed by other techniques. Although technical factors may compromise characterization of small or highly mobile lesions, lesions without apparent FDG uptake can generally be safely observed, whereas FDG-avid lung nodules almost always need further evaluation. FDG-PET/CT is now the primary staging imaging modality for patients with lung cancer who are being considered for curative therapy with either surgery or definitive radiation therapy.

Breast cancer is the most common malignancy in females. Imaging plays a critical role in diagnosis, staging and surveillance, and management of disease. Fluoro-deoxyglucose (FDG) PET the imaging is indicated in specific clinical setting. Sensitivity of detection depends on tumor histology and size. Whole body FDG PET can change staging and management. In recurrent disease, distant metastasis can be detected. FDG PET imaging has prognostic and predictive value. PET/MR is evolving rapidly and may play a role management, assessment of metastatic lesions, and treatment monitoring. This review discusses current PET modalities, focusing on of FDG PET imaging and novel tracers.

PET with fluorodeoxyglucose F 18/computed tomography (^{18}F-FDG PET/CT) has evolved into an indispensable imaging technique in the management of patients with esophageal cancer. Staging with ^{18}F-FDG PET/CT is strongly associated with overall survival and certain ^{18}F-FDG PET/CT parameters predict patient survival. Current evidence supporting the validity of the use of ^{18}F-FDG PET/CT in the tumor delineation process for radiation treatment planning in patients with esophageal cancer is still limited. It is useful in determining treatment response after neoadjuvant therapy and thereby has an impact on management. ^{18}F-FDG PET/CT plays a role in the diagnosis of recurrent disease in patients with a background of clinical suspicion.

The role of PET and PET/computed tomography (CT) has evolved significantly in the last few decades. 2-Deoxy-2-[18F]-fluoro-ᴅ-glucose (FDG)-PET/CT is now an integral part of the management of patients with lymphoma. FDG-PET/CT at the time of initial staging can help in appropriate staging of the patients. Both interim and end-of-therapy PETs have significant prognostic value in patients with Hodgkin lymphoma and aggressive non-Hodgkin lymphoma and more accurately assess for the presence of residual malignancy than anatomic imaging. The impact of interim FDG-PET/CT on risk-adapted strategies is an area of active investigation and the results of ongoing clinical trials will be informative.

This article presents a review of multiple myeloma, precursor states, and related plasma cell disorders. The clinical roles of fluorodeoxyglucose PET/computed tomography (CT) and the potential to improve the management of patients with multiple myeloma are discussed. The clinical and research data supporting the utility of PET/CT use in evaluating myeloma and other plasma cell dyscrasias continues to grow.

The performance of fludeoxyglucose F 18 (FDG)–PET/computed tomography (CT) in the initial and follow-up evaluation of patients with melanoma is well established. Groups are beginning to investigate whether the inclusion of FDG-PET/CT into a staging or surveillance algorithm results in an improvement in patient outcome and whether such an imaging program would be cost-effective.

Many standard nonimaging-based prediction tools exist for prostate cancer. However, these tools may be limited in individual cases and need updating based on the improved understanding of the underlying complex biology of the disease and the emergence of the novel targeted molecular imaging methods. A new platform of automated predictive tools that combines the independent molecular, imaging, and clinical information can contribute significantly to patient care. Such a platform will also be of interest to regulatory agencies and payers as more emphasis is placed on supporting those interventions that have quantifiable and significant beneficial impact on patient outcome.

Fluorodeoxyglucose (FDG) PET/computed tomography (CT) is used most frequently in the surveillance of iodine-refractory differentiated thyroid cancer with increased thyroglobulin level after therapy. This article evaluates the impact of FDG-PET/CT on clinical management and the prognostic implications of a positive scan. In the studies reviewed, FDG-PET/CT changed the course of management in 14% to 78% of patients with suspected recurrence, and a positive scan was associated with poorer survival. Similar conclusions are supported in the literature for anaplastic and medullary thyroid cancers, although these are based on fewer studies on account of the lower prevalence of these subtypes.

Incorporation of PET/computed tomography (CT) in radiotherapy planning plays a critical role in assisting gross tumor volume delineation for radiotherapy planning and delivery. As radiotherapy techniques evolve to become more conformal with the increasing use of intensity-modulated radiotherapy and stereotactic body radiotherapy, whereby sharp dose gradients exist between the target and adjacent normal tissue, accurate contouring of tumor targets is vital for the success of radiotherapy to achieve cure and locoregional control. This article outlines the integration of PET/CT into radiotherapy planning for head and neck, lung, and other solid tumors.

PET CLINICS

PROGRAM OBJECTIVE

The goal of the *PET Clinics* is to keep practicing radiologists and radiology residents up to date with current clinical practice in positron emission tomography by providing timely articles reviewing the state of the art in patient care.

TARGET AUDIENCE

Practicing radiologists, radiology residents, and other health care professionals who provide patient care utilizing radiologic findings.

LEARNING OBJECTIVES

Upon completion of this activity, participants will be able to:
1. Review the role of PET imaging in lymphoma and multiple myeloma.
2. Discuss the role of PET imaging in the management of breast cancer, melanoma, and thyroid cancer.
3. Describe radiotherapy planning.

ACCREDITATION

The Elsevier Office of Continuing Medical Education (EOCME) is accredited by the Accreditation Council for Continuing Medical Education (ACCME) to provide continuing medical education for physicians.

The EOCME designates this enduring material for a maximum of 15 *AMA PRA Category 1 Credit*(s)™. Physicians should claim only the credit commensurate with the extent of their participation in the activity.

All other health care professionals requesting continuing education credit for this enduring material will be issued a certificate of participation.

DISCLOSURE OF CONFLICTS OF INTEREST

The EOCME assesses conflict of interest with its instructors, faculty, planners, and other individuals who are in a position to control the content of CME activities. All relevant conflicts of interest that are identified are thoroughly vetted by EOCME for fair balance, scientific objectivity, and patient care recommendations. EOCME is committed to providing its learners with CME activities that promote improvements or quality in healthcare and not a specific proprietary business or a commercial interest.

The planning committee, staff, authors and editors listed below have identified no financial relationships or relationships to products or devices they or their spouse/life partner have with commercial interest related to the content of this CME activity:

Tim Akhurst, MD, FRACP; Anthony Ciarallo, MD; Anjali Fortna; Daniel Greenspan, MD; Kristen Helm; Rodney J. Hicks, MD, FRACP; Brynne Hunter; Heather A. Jacene, MD; Hossein Jadvar, MD, PhD, MPH, MBA; Robert M. Kwee, MD, PhD; Ann S. LaCasce, MD; Sandy Lavery; Lizza Lebron, MD; Michael MacManus, MD, FRANZCR; Charles Marcus, MD; Mahalakshmi Narayanan; Neeta Pandit-Taskar, MD; Eric M. Rohren, MD, PhD; Sara Sheikhbahaei, MD, MPH; Rathan M. Subramaniam, MD, PhD, MPH; Mehdi Taghipour, MD; Sree Harsha Tirumani, MD; Minh Tam Truong, MD; John Vassallo.

The planning committee, staff, authors and editors listed below have identified financial relationships or relationships to products or devices they or their spouse/life partner have with commercial interest related to the content of this CME activity:

Patrick J. Peller, MD is on the speakers bureau for General Electric Company doing business as GE Healthcare.

UNAPPROVED/OFF-LABEL USE DISCLOSURE

The EOCME requires CME faculty to disclose to the participants:
1. When products or procedures being discussed are off-label, unlabelled, experimental, and/or investigational (not US Food and Drug Administration [FDA] approved); and
2. Any limitations on the information presented, such as data that are preliminary or that represent ongoing research, interim analyses, and/or unsupported opinions. Faculty may discuss information about pharmaceutical agents that is outside of FDA-approved labelling. This information is intended solely for CME and is not intended to promote off-label use of these medications. If you have any questions, contact the medical affairs department of the manufacturer for the most recent prescribing information.

TO ENROLL

To enroll in the *PET Clinics* Continuing Medical Education program, call customer service at 1-800-654-2452 or sign up online at http://www.theclinics.com/home/cme. The CME program is available to subscribers for an additional annual fee of USD $235

METHOD OF PARTICIPATION

In order to claim credit, participants must complete the following:
1. Complete enrolment as indicated above.
2. Read the activity.
3. Complete the CME Test and Evaluation. Participants must achieve a score of 70% on the test. All CME Tests and Evaluations must be completed online.

CME INQUIRIES/SPECIAL NEEDS

For all CME inquiries or special needs, please contact elsevierCME@elsevier.com.

Preface
PET/CT: Adding Value to Patient Outcomes and Health Care Delivery

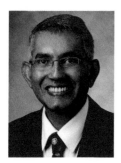

Rathan M. Subramaniam, MD, PhD, MPH
Editor

This is the first issue in the two-part *PET Clinic* series of "PET/CT and Patient Outcomes." Adding value to patients and patient outcomes at reasonable cost, which a society can afford, is the founding principle for providing an affordable health care delivery. Advanced imaging tests, such as CT, PET/CT, and MRI, are expensive, and their utilization and benefit must be justified for the clinical context, benefit the patients, and reduce the unnecessary waste of resources in providing care. The cost of PET/CT is entirely justifiable, if the information provided by PET/CT leads to cost saving by avoiding delays in therapy decision-making and starting therapies, by avoiding very expensive and inappropriate therapies, and by identifying therapy failures early so that appropriate therapy can be commenced sooner, improves patient quality of life, and predicts patient outcomes.

PET/CT provides value to patients by providing additional information to clinicians in assessing the disease stage, deciding on appropriate therapy, assessing the therapy success or failure, predicting patient outcomes, and providing additional information about disease status in follow-up, if a patient has symptoms or signs suspicious of recurrence. As carefully put together by an international group of authors in this issue, PET/CT provides added value to patients and their outcomes in head and neck cancer, lung cancer, breast cancer, esophageal cancer, lymphoma, multiple myeloma, melanoma, prostate cancer, thyroid cancer, and radiation therapy planning.

Depending on the tumor type, the strength of evidence for the added value and patient outcome varies, in the appropriate clinical context.

It is also important to recognize that PET/CT has pitfalls. Lack of standardization in reporting can lead to harmful effects, such as unnecessary biopsies, and inappropriate utilization, such as surveillance imaging, which result in patient anxieties and drive up the cost of health care delivery. As a professional community, it is our responsibility to mitigate these harmful effects and provide the best care to our patients at the right time, in the right setting, and by the right teamwork. We should be careful and thoughtful before recommending biopsies and additional imaging tests and strongly discourage performing surveillance PET/CT imaging without symptoms or signs suggestive of recurrence in follow-up. Our collaborative teamwork with our clinicians would enhance our service to our patients and reduce many of the harmful effects. This will truly magnify the benefits and added value of PET/CT to all of our patients.

Rathan M. Subramaniam, MD, PhD, MPH
Russell H. Morgan Department of Radiology and
Radiology Science
Johns Hopkins Medical Institutions
601 North Caroline Street/JHOC 3235
Baltimore, MD 21287, USA

E-mail address:
rsubram4@jhmi.edu

PET Clin 10 (2015) xi
http://dx.doi.org/10.1016/j.cpet.2015.01.001
1556-8598/15/$ – see front matter © 2015 Published by Elsevier Inc.

CrossMark

pet.theclinics.com

Preface

PET/CT: Adding Value to Patient Outcomes and Health Care Delivery

PET Clin 10 (2015) xi
http://dx.doi.org/10.1016/j.cpet.2015.07.001
1556-8598/15/$ – see front matter © 2015 Published by Elsevier Inc.

18F FDG PET/CT and Head and Neck Cancer
Patient Management and Outcomes

Sara Sheikhbahaei, MD, MPH[a], Charles Marcus, MD[a],
Rathan M. Subramaniam, MD, PhD, MPH[a,b,c,*]

KEYWORDS

- Head and neck squamous cell cancer • Survival outcome • Management change • Prognosis
- Therapy response

KEY POINTS

- 18F-Fluoro-deoxyglucose (FDG)-PET/computed tomography (CT) is considered a cost-effective imaging for the diagnosis and staging of head and neck cancer (HNC) and provides more accurate staging compared with conventional work-up; accurate staging improves therapy selection.
- High negative predictive value (NPV) of FDG-PET/CT in therapy assessment and follow-up can be used to individualize follow-up regimens in patients who have been treated for HNC.
- Patients with negative post-therapy or follow-up FDG-PET/CT have significantly longer survival than those with a positive post-therapy or follow-up FDG-PET/CT.
- The optimal timing for performing the first follow-up FDG-PET/CT scan could be approximately 6 months post-treatment; subsequent follow-up FDG-PET/CT can be tailored based on the findings and clinical context.
- The use of FDG-PET/CT during follow-up adds value to clinical assessment, detects recurrence, could alter patient management for salvage or palliative treatment, and could predict survival.

INTRODUCTION

HNC accounts for 650,000 cases annually worldwide.[1] The incidence of HNC has remained relatively stable over the past decade, with a decrease in the average age at diagnosis mostly due to a rise in disease associated with human papillomavirus (HPV).[2,3] In the United States, there is an estimate of 55,000 new HNC cases every year and approximately 12,000 deaths each year.[2] Head and neck squamous cell carcinoma (HNSCC) accounts for 90% of HNCs and is known

to have high rates of recurrence.[4] The 5-year locoregional and distant failure rates in patients treated with induction chemotherapy (ICT) and chemoradiotherapy (CRT) are found to be 31% and 13%, respectively.[5] The overall 5-year survival rate for all stages is approximately 60%.[6] The survival depends on several factors, the most important of which is disease staging.[4,7,8] The 5-year survival varies widely from 91% in stage I to less than 4% in metastatic stage IV patients.[8]

Moreover, follow-up and surveillance of patients with treated HNSCC is especially important,

The authors have nothing to disclose.
[a] Russell H. Morgan Department of Radiology and Radiological Sciences, Johns Hopkins School of Medicine, JHOC 3230, 601 North Caroline Street, Baltimore, MD 21287, USA; [b] Sidney Kimmel Comprehensive Cancer Center, Johns Hopkins School of Medicine, 601 North Caroline Street, Baltimore, MD, USA; [c] Department of Health Policy and Management, Johns Hopkins Bloomberg School of Public Health, Johns Hopkins University, 624 North Broadway, Baltimore, MD 21205, USA
* Corresponding author. Russel H. Morgan Department of Radiology and Radiological Sciences, Johns Hopkins University, 601 North Caroline Street/JHOC 3235, Baltimore, MD 21287.
E-mail address: rsubram4@jhmi.edu

pet.theclinics.com

because significant morbidity and mortality in these cases are associated with recurrent disease.[9] This underscores the need for better imaging modalities for staging, therapy selection, assessing response, and predicting outcome. FDG-PET/CT is a valuable imaging test for management of many human solid tumors.[10–14] There is a growing body of evidence that indicates FDG-PET/CT has a significant impact on HNC staging, on therapeutic assessment, and during surveillance.[6,7,9,15–25] The objective of this article is to review the value of FDG-PET/CT for patient management and outcome.

VALUE OF FDG PET/CT – INITIAL TREATMENT STRATEGY
Impact on Staging and Therapeutic Planning

FDG-PET/CT has been rapidly adopted for diagnosis and staging purposes of HNC since 2001.[7] In a cohort of 436 HNC patients from 4 integrated health systems, VanderWalde and colleagues[26] report an increasing trend in performing pretreatment FDG-PET/CT scan, from 12.5% in 2005 to 34% in 2008. The use of FDG-PET/CT in detecting

occult primary tumors, tumor size and stage, locoregional nodal spread, and distant nodal/ organ metastases has been well established.[7,17,27]

National Comprehensive Center Network (NCCN) clinical practice guidelines in HNC (updated version 2013) recommend performing PET/ CT in initial staging of patients who seem to have stages III and IV disease of oral cavity, oropharynx, hypopharynx, and larynx.[28] They also suggest using PET/CT in evaluation of distant metastasis in nasopharyngeal carcinoma and mucosal melanoma as well as evaluation of occult primary tumors, particularly in patients presenting with a neck mass (**Fig. 1**).[28]

Furthermore, treatment protocols for HNCs depend mainly on primary tumor location and staging.[4,7,27] The goal of HNC therapy is either cure or palliation, depending on disease severity or progression. The mainstay of treatment has evolved gradually from surgery to radiation therapy (RT)/CRT. Recommended treatment in early or localized disease (stages I–II) of oral cavity, pharyngeal, and laryngeal cancer is surgical resection or definitive RT. Patients with locally advanced disease (stages III–IV) are typically

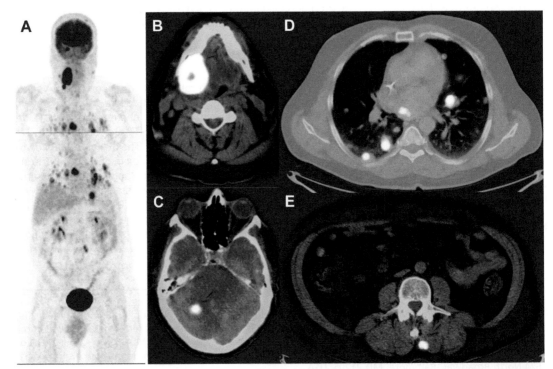

Fig. 1. Impact of FDG-PET/CT on staging: anterior maximum-intensity projection (MIP) (*A*), axial fused FDG-PET. CT (*B–E*) images of a 57-year-old man who underwent a staging FDG-PET/CT study for a T4N2aM1, HPV-positive, SCC of the right tongue base. The staging PET/CT study revealed metabolically active (SUVmax 17.3) right tongue base mass (*red arrow, B*) with additional metastatic lesions in the brain (*red arrow, C*) (SUVmax 10.4), lungs (SUVmax 11.2), and paraspinal soft tissue (*red arrow, E*) (SUVmax 9.2).

treated with concurrent CRT. Some patients with stages III to IVB disease can be treated with ICT to shrink a primary tumor in preparation for future surgery or RT. Current standard of treatment of patients with metastasis or recurrent disease is single-agent or combination palliative chemotherapy.[8,27–30] The cost of treatment constitutes a large percentage of the overall expenses of care in patients with HNC.[3] Therefore, an accurate staging improves decision making and helps in avoiding unnecessary interventions.[3,17,31] FDG-PET/CT provides more accurate staging in HNCs compared with conventional work-up and may alter management (**Fig. 2**). Several studies have corroborated this functionality.[7,32–36]

Studies by Wang and colleagues[32] and Deantonio and colleagues[33] showed that FDG-PET/CT scan results in staging changes in 57% (16 of 28) and 22% (5 of 22) of patients, respectively, compared with neck CT. Similarly, Abramyuk and colleagues[34] conducted a retrospective study on 102 untreated HNC patients to evaluate the effect of FDG-PET/CT on stage modification and patients' management compared with conventional staging. Histopathology confirmation considered as reference standard. Implementation of FDG-PET/CT led to a significant change in tumor (T), nodal (N), metastasis (M), and clinical staging. In T staging, inclusion of FDG-PET/CT resulted in downstaging of 36 patients and upstaging of 10

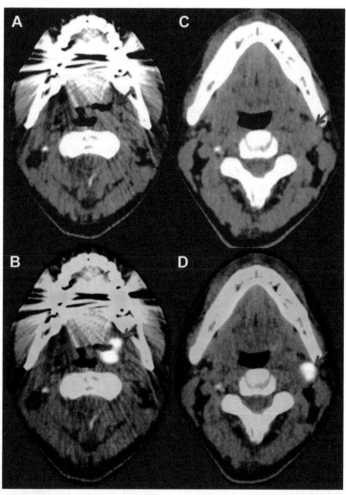

Fig. 2. Change in stage and impact on treatment planning: axial CT (*A, C*) and fused FDG-PET/CT (*B, D*) images of a 56-year-old man who was clinically diagnosed with a T1N0M0 left tonsillar SCC, who underwent a staging FDG-PET/CT study. The study revealed an intensely FDG avid (SUVmax 11.3) mass in the left tonsillar fossa (*red arrows, A, B*) and a metabolically active (SUVmax 8.7), metastatic, left level 2 cervical lymph node (*red arrows, C, D*), thereby changing the stage to T1N2bM0 and changing the treatment plan from single modality therapy to combined chemoradiation.

patients compared with conventional imaging. In N staging, 27 patients were downstaged whereas 8 were upstaged. In M staging, FDG-PET/CT shifted 13 of 102 patients from M0 to M1. Overall, by using FDG-PET/CT, 9 patients were upstaged and 18 patients were downstaged. The implementation of FDG-PET/CT also resulted in treatment change—RT modification—in 14 patients.

Furthermore, in a multicenter prospective study on 233 newly diagnosed HNSCC patients, Lonneux and colleagues[35] showed that FDG-PET/CT scan altered the staging in 43% of patients, 30% of whom were classified to a more advanced stage and 13% were classified as having a less advanced stage. In addition, FDG-PET/CT imaging altered the therapeutic plan in 32 (13.7%) patients. In another study conducted by Ha and colleagues,[36] among 36 untreated HNSCC patients, FDG-PET/CT changed the treatment plan in 11 (31%) of cases.

A recent systematic review evaluates the cost and economic burden associated with HNSCC.[3] Although using a combined hybrid PET/CT scan seems expensive as an initial screening test, Wissinger and colleagues[3] have indicated that the resultant reduction of unnecessary additional procedures or treatments offset the cost of FDG-PET/CT for the health service. Thus FDG-PET/CT is considered a cost-effective screening imaging for the diagnosis and staging of HNSCC. Also, a prospective cost minimization analysis study in Australia showed that assessing nodal response with incorporation of FDG-PET/CT helped avoid the need for many unnecessary neck dissections, resulting in a considerable cost reduction for health service.[31] These results suggest that implementation of FDG-PET/CT before treatment allows optimization of therapeutic goals in further management.

In a recent study, however, VanderWalde and colleagues[26] described the stage migration phenomenon during the PET era. In this retrospective cohort, a total of 958 patients diagnosed with HNC, identified via tumor registries, were included. Patients were categorized into pre-PET era (2000–2004, n = 522) and PET era (2005–2008, n = 436). Based on the results, within the PET era, FDG-PET/CT implementation was significantly associated with increased diagnosis of locally advanced disease (odds ratio [OR] 2.86). Although use of PET was significantly associated with stage-specific survival benefit in patients with locally advanced disease (2-year survival in PET vs no PET: 52.2% vs 32.1%), there was no difference in overall survival (OS) in all patients (2-year survival in PET vs no PET: 53.2% vs 55.5%). They suggest that the improved survival in patients with locally advanced disease could

be a reflection of a selection bias or stage migration. Although the retrospective nature of the study, unknown intention and timing of PET scan, and nonrepresentative study population could have confounded the results, further research needs to be performed to determine whether the use of PET scan improves the OS in all patients with HNC.

Impact on Detection of Unknown Primary Tumors

Cancer of unknown primary (CUP) is defined as the presence of histologic proved metastatic disease, with no identified primary tumor at presentation after a thorough conventional work-up.[7,37] Several studies indicated the usefulness of FDG-PET/CT scan in detection of unknown primary tumors (**Fig. 3**).[37–39] In a meta-analysis of 16 studies comprising a total of 302 patients, Rusthoven and colleagues[37] reported an overall sensitivity of 88.3%, specificity of 74.9%, and accuracy of 78.8% for FDG-PET/CT in the detection of primary tumors in patients with cervical metastases. FDG-PET detected 24.5% of tumors that were not apparent after comprehensive diagnostic work-up. Kwee and Kwee[39] in another meta-analysis estimated the tumor detection rate and pooled sensitivity and specificity of FDG-PET/CT as 34%, 84%, and 84%, respectively, considering patients with cervical and extracervical metastatic CUP. The heterogeneity in the extent of subsequent diagnostic work-up among the included studies might overestimate their result.

The detection of primary tumors in patients with CUP could be a decisive criterion in further management of patients and leads to RT planning modification, target volume delineation, and reduction in treatment-associated morbidities.[7] Patients with known primaries in the head and neck receive site-specific treatment, whereas patients with persistent unknown primaries are treated with panmucosal RT or empirical chemotherapy.[38]

Impact on Detection of Second Primary Tumors

Patients with HNSCC often harbor synchronous multiple primary cancers due to smoking and drinking habits.[7,40,41] The most frequent site of secondary tumors is aerodigestive tract and head and neck (**Fig. 4**). Distant metastasis and second primary tumors are among the leading cause of treatment failure and death in patients with HNSCC.[17,41] FDG-PET/CT has been increasingly used for the detection of synchronous tumors and considered to have a good diagnostic performance. A review of 12 studies published between

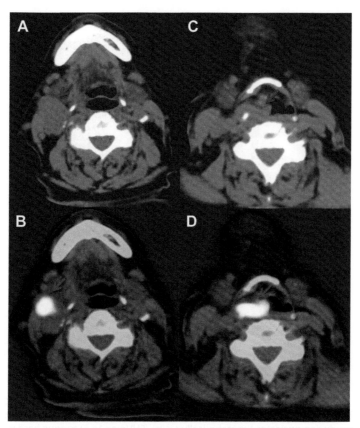

Fig. 3. Localization of primary tumor: axial CT (*A, C*) and fused FDG-PET/CT (*B, D*) images of an 80-year-old man who presented with a neck mass. Clinical evaluation revealed asymmetric appearance of the right hemilarynx. He underwent an FDG-PET/CT study for further evaluation. The study revealed an intensely FDG avid (SUVmax 12.6) right supraglottic mass (*red arrow, C, D*) with metabolically active (SUVmax 11.5), metastatic cervical lymphadenopathy (*red arrow, A, B*).

2000 and 2011 evaluated the utility of FDG-PET/CT in detecting distant metastasis/second primary tumors in patients with HNC at initial staging, reporting pooled sensitivity and specificity of 88% (83–93%) and 95% (94–96%) for FDG-PET/CT, respectively.[40]

The ability of detection of malignancies by FDG-PET/CT depends on the site and type of malignancies.[17] Himeno and colleagues[42] discussed the limitation of FDG-PET/CT in detection of Tis and T1a esophageal cancers. Hanamoto and colleagues[43] conducted a study on 347 untreated HNSCC patients to evaluate the utility of FDG-PET/CT in detection of synchronous tumors at initial staging. The sensitivities of FDG-PET/CT for detection of synchronous esophageal cancers were 0% in T1a, 60% in T1b, 0% in T2, 100% in T3, and 100% in T4, respectively. Similar studies also indicated the lower diagnostic sensitivity of FDG-PET/CT in early detection of synchronus tumors of upper gatrointestinal tract, especially esophageal cancer in patients with HNSCC.[42,44]

Overall, FDG-PET/CT has a good sensitivity and specificity compared with MR imaging or CT alone in HNC imaging (**Fig. 5**).[45] Studies comparing the utility of FDG-PET/CT versus other conventional anatomic imaging in the staging of HNC suggest that FDG-PET/CT is often superior in detecting small regional lymph node metastases (<10 mm) that seem morphologically normal in locating primary tumors, particularly in patients presenting with a neck mass and in detection of distant metastasis (**Fig. 6**).[7,45,46] FDG-PET/CT can also better evaluate HPV-correlated necrotic lymph nodes, particularly in combination with contrast CT (**Fig. 7**).[47]

Nevertheless, FDG-PET/CT is shown to have limited usefulness in staging T1 tumors, predominantly when performed with low-dose unenhanced CT, and low specificity in osteomandibular lesions.[17] A prospective study on 314 newly diagnosed HNSCC patients showed that false-negative results of FDG-PET/CT were obtained for 22.3% of T1 tumors and 2.2% T2 tumors (*P*<.001).[48] In contrast, MR imaging was found

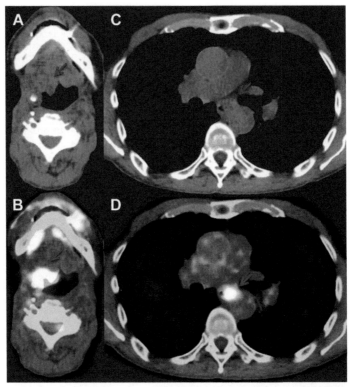

Fig. 4. Detection of synchronous second primary cancer: axial CT (*A, C*) and fused FDG-PET/CT (*B, D*) images of a 65-year-old man with a recent diagnosis of SCC of the tongue base (T3N0M0) who underwent a staging FDG-PET/CT study. The PET/CT study demonstrates a metabolically active (SUVmax 14.8) tongue base mass (*red arrows, A, B*) and another hypermetabolic (SUVmax 10.8) lesion in the midesophagus (*red arrows, C, D*), suggestive of a synchronous second primary esophageal cancer. Biopsy of the lesion revealed SCC of the esophagus.

more accurate in detection of T1 tumors and highly accurate in evaluating the primary and osteomandibular tumoral invasion.[45]

Recent studies proposed the evolving role of fused PET/MR imaging in staging of HNC.[17] A retrospective study on 30 patients with oral cavity and hypopharynx carcinoma indicated that in T staging, PET/MR imaging (87%) and MR imaging (90%) were significantly more accurate than PET/CT (67%). In N staging, the sensitivity (77%), specificity (96%), and accuracy (93%) in both PET/MR imaging and PET/CT were the same.[49] PET/MR

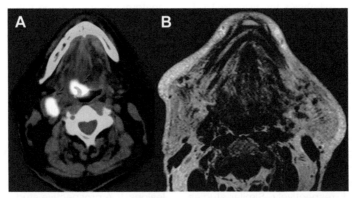

Fig. 5. Image artifacts: axial fused FDG-PET/CT (*A*) and T1-weighted axial MR imaging (*B*) images of a 67-year-old man with a recent diagnosis of SCC of the tongue base, who underwent a staging FDG-PET/CT study. The study demonstrates metabolically active (SUVmax 13.1), tongue base mass (*midline arrow, A*) with hypermetabolic (SUVmax 13.7), metastatic, cervical lymphadenopathy (*right arrow, A*). The staging MR imaging study, however, has been significantly degraded by motion artifact, making it difficult to clearly appreciate the lesions.

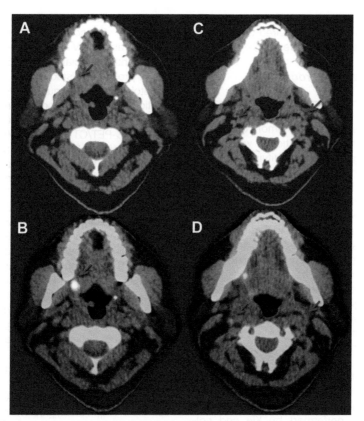

Fig. 6. Detection of subcentimeter metastatic lymphadenopathy: axial CT (*A, C*) and fused FDG-PET/CT (*B, D*) images of a 63-year-old man with a recently diagnosed SCC of the oral cavity. The staging FDG-PET/CT study demonstrates an intensely FDG avid (SUVmax 14.1) soft tissue thickening in the right retromolar trigone (*red arrows, A, B*), compatible with the primary malignancy and metabolically active (SUVmax 5.4), subcentimeter, morphologically normal, metastatic cervical lymphadenopathy (*red arrows, C, D*), bilaterally.

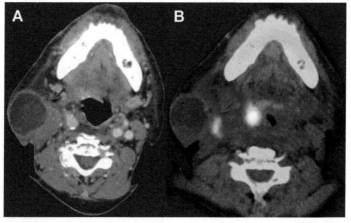

Fig. 7. Cystic nodes in HPV-positive disease: axial CT (*A*) and fused FDG-PET/CT (*B*) images of a 65-year-old man with a history of HPV-positive, SCC, post-CRT, who underwent a post-treatment FDG-PET/CT study. The study reveals a large, cystic neck mass (*red arrows, A, B*) with peripheral FDG uptake (SUVmax 4.8), consistent with viable disease within a cystic residual node.

imaging seems highly accurate in T staging of HNC; however, further studies are required to verify the clinical value of this modality over FDG-PET/CT.

Impact on Survival and Prognostic Stratification

Identifying further prognostic factors along with TNM staging and synchronous tumors could help in distinguishing high-risk patients who might benefit from strengthening or modifying treatment modality.[17] There has been an increasing interest in the use of FDG-PET/CT imaging biomarkers to assess treatment response and survival outcome in patients with HNC.[6,17] Maximum standard uptake value (SUVmax), metabolic tumor volume (MTV), and total lesion glycolysis (TLG) are quantitative biomarkers that are commonly used in patients' risk assessment.[6] Suzuki and colleagues[50] studied 31 patients with newly diagnosed resectable hypopharyngeal squamous cell carcinoma (SCC) and suggested that SUVmax greater than or equal to 13 was a significant prognostic factor for survival independent of clinical T and N staging classification and treatment group. In another study on 49 patients with pharyngeal SCC, Suzuki and colleagues[51] suggested that SUVmax greater than 8 was significantly associated with shorter OS.

A meta-analysis performed by Xie and colleagues[16] reviewed 26 studies to evaluate the prognostic value of FDG-PET/CT in patients with HNC. Pooled survival data depict that patients with lower pretreatment SUVmax have significantly better disease-free survival (DFS), OS, and local control (LC), with ORs of 0.23, 0.24, and 0.27, respectively. In another meta-analysis of 13 studies comprising 1180 patients, Pak and colleagues[52] suggested MTV, TLG, and SUVmax are prognostic predictors of outcome in patients with HNC. Patients with higher MTV showed a 3.06-fold (2.33–4.01) higher risk of adverse events and 3.51-fold (2.62–4.72) higher risk of death than patients with a low MTV. Patients with a high TLG had a 3.10-fold (2.27–4.24) higher risk of events or a 3.14-fold (2.24–4.40) higher risk of death than patients with a low TLG. Regarding the SUVmax, the pooled hazard ratios (HRs) were 1.83 (1.39–2.42) and 2.36 (1.48–3.77) for event-free survival and OS, respectively.

Koyasu and colleagues[53] conducted a study on 108 patients with HNSCC who underwent PET/CT before treatment, with a median follow-up period of 36 months (2.5–73 months). The estimated 2-year disease-specific survival rate was 86.5%. They showed that high SUVmax (>10 g/mL), MTV (>20 cm^3), TLG (>70 g), and ring-shaped uptake pattern significantly predicted patient outcome in

terms of disease-specific survival (DSS) and DFS. Even after correction for the stage and definitive therapy, MTV and uptake pattern remained significantly associated with DSS.

In a prospective study on 52 patients with HNC, Apostolova and colleagues[54] revealed that pretherapeutic SUVmax, MTV, and TLG are significant predictors of disease progression and OS. They propose a novel FDG-PET/CT marker, asphericity—the spatial heterogeneity of FGD uptake, as an independent prognostic factor in HNC survival. The combination of high MTV and asphericity showed a high HR for progression-free survival (HR 22.7) and OS (HR 13.2).

Furthermore, Abd El-Hafez and colleagues[55] prospectively studied 126 patients with oral cavity SCC who underwent pretreatment FDG-PET/CT scan. Patients were followed-up at least 24 months after surgery. Results showed that tumor TLG and nodal SUVmax are independently associated with 2-year DSS. In addition, they proposed a 3-point prognostic scoring system based on presence of neck node, high tumor TLG, and high nodal SUVmax. Patients with score-3 showed a 32-fold increased risk of cancer death compared with those without risk factors (2-year DSS: 26% vs 97%).

There is strong evidence for the potential function of pretreatment FDG-PET/CT quantitative parameters in predicting survival and prognosis of patients with HNC. It is difficult, however, to determine an optimal cutoff value for each variable to risk stratification of patients, because different definitions (cutpoints) are proposed in determining high and low volumetric parameters among the studies.

VALUE OF FDG PET/CT – SUBSEQUENT TREATMENT STRATEGY
Impact on Evaluation of Treatment Response

Treatment monitoring with FDG-PET/CT imaging during early follow-up allows predicting the efficacy of treatments and outcome (**Fig. 8**). Recently, Marcus and colleagues[23] proposed new interpretation criteria for therapy response assessment of HNCs based on the result of post-therapy FDG-PET/CT scan (Hopkins criteria). Therapy response is assessed based on the intensity (compared with the internal jugular vein [IJV] and liver activity) and pattern (focal or diffuse) of FDG-PET uptake in primary tumor and neck nodes and categorized into 5 scores as follows: score 1 (complete metabolic response, FDG uptake less than IJV), score 2 (likely complete metabolic response, focal FDG uptake greater than IJV and lesser than liver), score 3 (likely postradiation inflammation, diffuse uptake greater than IJV or liver), score 4 (likely residual tumor, focal uptake greater than liver), and score 5 (residual tumor, focal and intense FDG uptake). Scores 1, 2, and 3 are

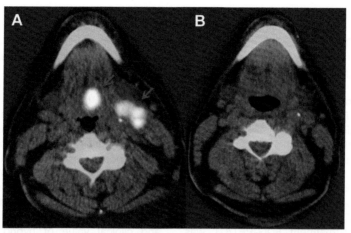

Fig. 8. Therapy response assessment: axial fused FDG-PET/CT (*A*) image of a 48-year-old man with a recent diagnosis of a T2N2bM0, HPV-positive, SCC of the left tongue base, who underwent a staging FDG-PET/CT study. The study demonstrates metabolically active (SUVmax 9.9) left tongue base mass (*midline arrow, A*) and hypermetabolic (SUVmax 9.4), metastatic, cervical lymphadenopathy (*left arrow, A*). After the study he underwent CRT. The axial fused FDG-PET/CT image (*B*) of the study performed 2 months after treatment completion reveals no evidence of FDG avid residual or recurrent disease, consistent with complete response to treatment.

considered negative and scores 4 and 5 are considered positive for residual tumor. This qualitative assessment scoring system was shown to have substantial inter-rater reliability ($\kappa = 0.69$–0.79) and high specificity (92.2%) and NPV (91.1%).[23]

Studies suggest that FDG-PET/CT findings in post-therapy assessment of HNCs are time and therapy dependent. An increase in FDG uptake occurs in recently radiated tissues, which may last 12 to 16 weeks after RT or CRT (**Fig. 9**).[4,7,56] To ensure a balance between the disadvantages of early and late imaging, the first post-treatment

FDG-PET/CT scan to assess response to treatment is generally recommended at approximately 12 weeks post-RT. A significant number of recurrences, however, occur later.

According to the 2013 NCCN clinical practice guidelines,[28] after either RT/or CRT, if clinical assessment is suspicious of a persistent disease or progression, CT scan needs to be performed within 4 to 8 weeks post-treatment as a guide to salvage surgery or neck dissection. If clinical assessment were negative for suspicion of a persistent cancer, PET/CT scan is suggested to

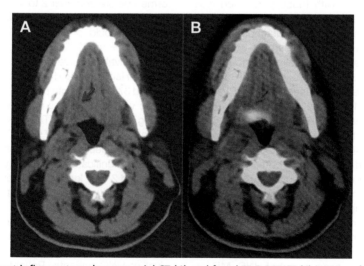

Fig. 9. Post-treatment inflammatory changes: axial CT (*A*) and fused FDG-PET/CT (*B*) images of a 42-year-old man with history of T4N2bMo SCC of the supraglottic larynx, post-total laryngectomy and CRT. The post-treatment PET/CT study, performed 7 weeks after treatment completion, demonstrates diffuse FDG uptake (SUVmax 4.0) in the right vallecula (*red arrow, A, B*), consistent with postradiation changes (Hopkins score 3).

be performed at minimum of 12 weeks after treatment for follow-up, and further management relies on the result of PET/CT scan.[28] This guideline may help identify those patients who can be observed safely without surgery to the neck.

Diagnostic performance of post-treatment FDG-PET/CT scan in early follow-up

In post-therapeutic assessment, the diagnostic accuracy of functional imaging mostly depends on the time interval between the end of treatment and imaging scan. In a meta-analysis of 51 studies comprising 2335 patients, Gupta and colleagues[15] evaluated the diagnostic performance of post-treatment FDG-PET/CT scan in HNC. The impact of timing of post-treatment FDG-PET/CT was also assessed before and after 12 weeks. The pooled sensitivity (79.9% and 72.7%), specificity (87.5% and 87.6%), NPV (95.1% and 94.5%), and positive predictive value (PPV) (58.6% and 52.1%) of FDG-PET/CT were reported for the primary site and the neck nodes, respectively. Sensitivity was higher in both primary tumor (91.9% vs 73.6%, P-value 0.12) and neck nodes (90.4% vs 62.5%, P-value <0.001) in scans performed greater than or equal to 12 weeks compared those less than 12 weeks. Similarly, Isles and colleagues[9] performed a meta-analysis of 27 studies to evaluate the effectiveness of PET in detection of recurrence or residual HNSCC after CRT. They reported pooled sensitivity, specificity, PPV, and NPV of 94%, 82%, 75%, and 95%, respectively. Considering the effect of the timing of scans, they indicated that the sensitivity is significantly higher for scans performed greater than 10 weeks after CRT compared with those performed less than 10 weeks (P-value 0.002).

Another study evaluated the diagnostic accuracy of delayed response assessment with FDG-PET/CT in 44 patients with locally advanced HNC who underwent scan at approximately 16 weeks after CRT. The sensitivity, specificity, PPV, and NPV of primary (100%, 89%, 43%, and 100%) and nodal disease (100%, 92%, 63%, and 100%) were reported. The high NPV of complete metabolic response highly suggested the absence of viable residual disease in both primary and neck nodes in cases of negative result.[57]

Moreover, several studies suggested that FDG-PET/CT scan is superior to other conventional imaging (MRI and/or CT) during early follow-up of HNC patients, particularly before 3 to 6 months post-treatment.[58–61] Studies suggested that in the post-therapeutic assessment of HNC, MR imaging cannot distinguish well between presence of fibrosis/necrosis and residual/recurrent cancer tissue. Thus, FDG-PET/CT is found more accurate than MR imaging for the identification of nonviable tumor and residual cancer.[45,61]

Recent studies proposed that the combination of PET and MR imaging scanners can provide better anatomic delineation.[62] In a study aimed at comparing the diagnostic value of PET/MR imaging with PET/CT, MR imaging, and CT in patients with advanced buccal SCC, Huang and colleagues[63] revealed that PET/MR imaging has the highest sensitivity, specificity, likelihood ratio, and level of confidence in assessing surrounding tissue invasion among 4 modalities. PET/MR imaging could be more beneficial in evaluation of focal invasion, recurrence, and potential metastatic lymph nodes.[62] Studies evaluating the cost-effectiveness and clinical value of hybrid PET/MR imaging compared with PET/CT scan are, however, scarce.

Early post-treatment FDG-PET/CT scan and patient outcome

Recent studies suggested that changes occurring in volumetric FDG-PET/CT parameters before and after treatment could be a prognostic factor for outcome and survival.[6,64,65] In a retrospective study by Yu and colleagues,[64] 28 patients with advanced HNSCC (stages III and IV) who underwent PET/CT before and after ICT were included. They suggested that a reduction in primary tumor metabolic tumor volume (MTV) of at least 42% or in total lesion glycolysis (TLG) of at least 55% after ICT could predict event-free survival with an HR of 6.25. Similarly, Yoon and colleagues[66] showed that a metabolic response during ICT could also predict clinical outcome in patients with advanced HNSCC who received sequential ICT followed by CRT. In 21 patients, FDG-PET was performed before and after 2 to 4 weeks after ICT. Results indicated that a 65% decrease in SUVmax after ICT could predict complete response after CRT (100% vs 33%, P-value 0.003), progression-free survival (P-value <0.001), and OS (P-value 0.001). Hentschel and colleagues[65] prospectively studied 37 patients with HNSCC to assess the prognostic value of changes in primary tumor SUVmax during therapy. FDG-PET/CT was performed before and after 1 to 2 weeks of CRT. Patients with greater than 50% decrease in primary tumor SUVmax showed significantly better 2-year OS (88% vs 38%) and 2-year locoregional control (88% vs 40%) compared with those with less than 50% decrease in primary tumor SUVmax.

Overall, a meta-analysis by Xie and colleagues[16] suggested that the tumor metabolic response after treatment is valuable for predicting long-term survival of HNC patients. Patients with low SUV of post-treatment FDG-PET/CT showed significantly better DFS (OR 0.17) and OS (OR 0.28) compared with those with high SUV. Furthermore, Ceulemans and colleagues[67] conducted a study to evaluate whether FDG-PET scan performed during RT could replace post-therapy scanning in detection of tumor response. In 40 patients with HNC, FDG-PET was performed at the end of the week 4 and 4 months after RT. The 2-year OS rates of patients having complete response compared with those without complete response were determined at 4 weeks (90% vs 71.8%, P-value 0.5) and 4 months (91.8% vs 49.9%, P-value 0.005). This study indicated that evaluation of the tumor response with FDG-PET at 4 months after RT cannot be replaced by scans performed during RT.

Impact on Detection of Recurrence and Surveillance

New treatments might provide important advantages for early detection of recurrence in HNCs. Delayed diagnosis of recurrences was associated with lower cure rates and more expensive salvage treatments at higher costs.

Beswick and colleagues[68] conducted a study to determine patterns of HNC recurrence after concurrent CRT using FDG-PET/CT. Recurrence was detected in 110 of 388 patients, of whom 66% were asymptomatic and 34% had clinical manifestations at the time of imaging. Among the cases that were asymptomatic at presentation, 45% occurred within 6 months, 79% within 12 months, 92% within 18 months, and 95% within 24 months of CRT. Among the cases that presented with clinical manifestation, 51% occurred within 6 months, 62% within 12 months, 76% within 24 months, and 89% within 36 months of RT. Because many of patients with recurrences are asymptomatic, there is a possibility of missing early detection if further regular imaging has not been performed.[28,68]

In nonsurgically treated HNC patients, regular clinical examination and post-treatment imaging evaluation (ie, CT and/or MR imaging with contrast or PET-CT) are recommended for early detection of any local or regional recurrences.[28] In addition, patients with HPV-positive HNC showed a pattern of delayed and disseminated recurrences and distant metastases.[63] Huang and colleagues[63] described that among patients with oropharyngeal carcinoma who developed distant metastasis, approximately 80% of HPV-positive patients developed it after 2 years after completion of RT/CRT compared with less than 5% of HPV-negative patients. Moreover, approximately one-third of HPV-positive patients

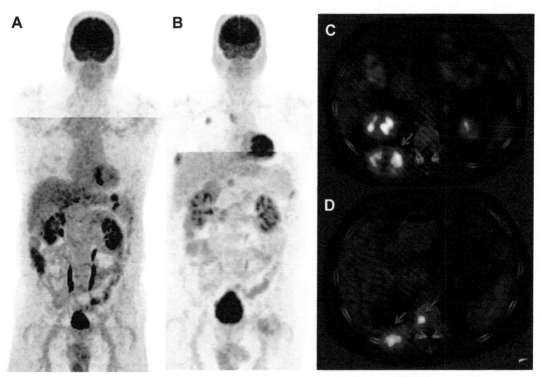

Fig. 10. Detection of recurrent disease: anterior maximum-intensity projection (MIP) images (*A*) of a 79-year-old man with a history of HPV-positive T1N1M0 SCC of the base of tongue, post-CRT, who underwent a restaging FDG-PET/CT study. The study showed no evidence of malignancy. The anterior MIP (*B*), axial fused FDG-PET/CT (*C*, *D*) images of a follow-up PET/CT study performed 10 months after the former study revealed metabolically active (SUVmax 6.8), multiple, metastatic, skeletal lesions (*red arrows, C, D*), consistent with recurrent, metastatic disease.

developed widespread dissemination with spreading to more than 2 organs. This unique pattern of delayed recurrence in HPV-positive HNC also highlights the potential value of FDG-PET/CT incorporation into long-term surveillance of HNCs (**Fig. 10**).

Diagnostic performance of post-treatment FDG-PET/CT scans in long-term follow-up

There are several studies that provide details on accuracy of FDG-PET/CT in long-term follow-up and surveillance of treated HNC patients (**Table 1**).[59,60,69–78] These studies generally report a high accuracy that emphasizes the potential of FDG-PET/CT to be incorporated into the standard guidelines on long-term follow-up of HNSCC.

As elucidated in **Table 1**, most studies assessing FDG-PET greater than 4 months after RT/CRT had consistently high NPV often greater than 90%. The other accuracy values displayed heterogeneity across the studies but sensitivity and NPV distribution seem reasonably homogenous. This suggests that negative PET/CT scans are highly reliable for the absence of recurrence or distant metastasis. On the other hand, the PPV values are more heterogeneous and seem considerably lower than NPV. These findings can translate into significant impact in clinical practice during surveillance of HNC.

Post-treatment FDG-PET/CT scan and management strategy

FDG-PET examinations may be performed after an interval of at least 4 to 6 months after therapy, and those with negative scans may be assumed to have low likelihood of having disease or developing recurrence or death in the short term.[79] As such, these patients may be subjected to less intense follow-up with history and physical examinations and performing imaging surveillance only if there is a suspicion for recurrent or unexplained symptoms.

Moreover, patients with positive FDG-PET during follow-up, regardless of biopsy-proved recurrence, have been shown to have poorer survival outcomes.[75,77,80,81] Therefore, these patients require biopsy or closer follow-up for confirmation and a more intensive surveillance.

The use of FDG-PET/CT during surveillance can detect cases of recurrence, when performed with

Table 1
Summary of studies describing accuracy of FDG-PET/CT in the surveillance of head and neck squamous cell carcinoma

Study	No. Scans	Time Interval (mo)	Sensitivity (%)	Specificity (%)	PPV (%)	NPV (%)	Accuracy (%)	Recurrence
Krabbe et al,[69] 2009	40	6	100	72	47	100	78	Locoregional, DM, SP
	35	9	100	68	29	100	71	
	33	12	100	76	36	100	79	
Abgral et al,[70] 2009	91	7–16	100	85	77	100	90	Locoregional, DM
Ng et al,[71] 2010	179	3–56	87	90	80	94	89	Locoregional, DM
Ghanooni et al,[59] 2011	32	4	92	81	55	98	—	Locoregional, DM, SP
		12	100	86	27	100	—	
Wierzbicka et al,[72] 2011	83	5–22	86	82	79	89	84	Regional
Zundel et al,[73] 2011	52	4–6	100	65	19	100	—	Locoregional, DM
Ho et al,[74] 2013	248	2–8	80	92	35	99	91	Locoregional, DM, SP
	175	7–21	100	96	71	100	96	
	77	17–35	100	99	75	100	99	
Paidpally et al,[75] 2013	134	4–24	85	91	54	98	90	Locoregional, DM, SP
Uzel,[76] 2013	46	2.4–9.4	91	81	64.	96	—	locoregional
Kim et al,[77] 2013	133	3–6	96	91	72	99	92	Locoregional, DM, SP
	119	12	93	95	83	98	94	
Mukundan et al,[60] 2014	50	6	96	92	85	96	—	Recurrence
Robin et al,[78] 2014	116	5.6	96	87	65	99	89	Locoregional, DM

Note, histopathology and/or minimum of 6 months clinical/imaging follow-up were considered gold standard across these studies.

Abbreviations: DM, distant metastasis; locoregional, local and regional recurrences; mo, months; SP, second primary tumor; time interval, time interval between completion of treatment and scans.

Data from Refs.[59,60,69–78]

or without any clinical suspicion, and could alter patient management for salvage or palliative treatment.

Value of FDG PET/CT with clinical suspicion In a recent meta-analysis, Gao and colleagues[82] suggested that a negative FDG-PET/CT scan could be used alone as a justification to rule out distant metastases in suspected recurrent HNC patients after definitive treatment. In this study, 10 FDG-PET/CT studies, comprising 797 imaging examinations, were included. The pooled sensitivity (92% [83–96%]), specificity (95% [91–97%]), positive likelihood ratio (16.7 [9.9–28.4]), and negative likelihood ratio (0.09 [0.04–0.18]) of post-therapy FDG-PET/CT scan in the diagnosis of distant metastasis in suspected recurrent HNC patients were estimated. The investigators suggested that high sensitivity and accuracy of FDG-PET/CT for screening of distant metastasis in suspected patients help in careful selection of eligible patients before salvage treatment.

In a retrospective study, Paidpally and colleagues[75] assessed the impact and added value of follow-up FDG-PET/CT in HNC patients with clinically suspected recurrence. FDG-PET/CT detected recurrence in 42% (13/31) of patients and correctly ruled out the disease in 48.4% (15/31) of clinically suspected patients. In another study, Farber and colleagues[83] evaluated the utility of FDG-PET in detecting recurrent disease in cases that were equivocal on clinical examination and conventional imaging. A total of 28 patients with treated HNSCC was included, all of whom had clinical suspicion of local recurrence by history and physical examination or conventional imaging techniques, such as MR imaging and CT. FDG-PET was performed a median of 13.5 months after treatment, with 25 patients having scan at least 4 months after therapy (4–52 months). All the scans were interpreted visually. FDG-PET provided correct results in 5 of 6 patients with equivocal CT and MR imaging findings (3 negative and 2 positive), which were confirmed by biopsy and clinical follow-up of at least 6 months. Overall, of 12 patients with positive FDG-PET scans, 8 patients underwent further therapy, including surgical salvage (2 patients), re-irradiation/chemotherapy (2 patients), and palliative combination chemotherapy (4 patients). The remaining 4 patients were given supportive care due to lack of toleration for further therapy. FDG-PET/CT has an advantage of providing functional information and leads to a lesser number of equivocal reports compared to other forms of conventional imaging.

Value of FDG PET/CT performed without clinical suspicion FDG-PET/CT scan considered a useful tool in routine surveillance for detection of recurrence in subclinical HNC patients due to its high sensitivity and NPV.[79] Several studies suggested that performing FDG-PET/CT during follow-up could add value to clinical assessment.

Krabbe and colleagues[69] studied the way the FDG-PET affected further management and compared that with regular follow-up. They enrolled a total of 48 patients with SCC of the oral cavity or oropharynx who underwent regular follow-up (history and physical examination) and serial FDG-PET scans at 3, 6, 9 and 12 months after treatment, and 18 were detected to have recurrences. Findings were validated by histopathology or 18 months of clinical follow-up and imaging after initial treatment. FDG-PET induced changes in diagnostic procedures or treatment in 63% of the patients compared with 25% in regular follow-up. Superfluous diagnostic procedures due to false-positive results were performed in 40% of patients in FDG-PET and 100% of them in regular follow-up. This illustrates how using FDG-PET during surveillance may alter the management of the patient.

There is evidence that FDG-PET has significantly higher accuracy compared with regular follow-up. Kim and colleagues[77] conducted a prospective study with 143 patients with HNSCC. These patients underwent curative therapy and assessed with regular follow-up (physical and endoscopic examination) and FDG-PET/CT at 3 to 6 months and 12 months. All surviving patients were followed-up for a median of 30 months (18–45). The sensitivity and NPV of FDG-PET/CT performed in 133 patients at 3 to 6 months was 96% and 99% compared with 11% and 80% on regular clinical follow-up, respectively (P<.001 and P<.05). The sensitivity and NPV of FDG-PET/CT performed in 119 patients at 12 months was 93% and 98% compared with 19% and 80% on regular clinical follow-up, respectively (P<.001 and P<.05). The specificity and PPV were not statistically different. Results were also not significantly different when stratification was made based on locoregional and distant metastases. Thus, FDG-PET/CT surveillance has the potential to detect recurrence that may be missed by regular physical and endoscopic examination of the head and neck.

Value of a subsequent FDG-PET/CT after a negative scan Lee and colleagues[79] suggested that in routine surveillance the initial PET scan should be performed within 6 months after treatment. In subclinical patients with initial negative PET result, next routine PET scan might be performed after 1 year. In a long-term follow-up of 106 true negative HNC patients in initial PET scan, they showed that locoregional recurrence is unlikely for at least 1 year after the initial negative PET scan.

McDermott and colleagues[84] conducted a study to assess the utility of NPV of FDG-PET/CT in surveillance of HNSCC. A total of 512 patients with HNSCC who underwent FDG-PET/CT examinations were included in their study, of whom 214 patients had at least 1 negative scan. They adopted a surveillance protocol in which FDG-PET/CT was performed at 2, 5, 8, and 14 months after therapy. There were recurrences in 19 patients of the 214 who had at least 1 negative scan, leading to an NPV of 91%. The earliest recurrence occurred 3 months after the initial negative scan whereas the latest was 37.3 months after the first negative scan. Of these 214 patients, 114 had 2 consecutive negative FDG-PET/CT scans within 6 months. Recurrence in this subgroup of patients occurred in only 2, resulting in an NPV of 98%. Of the 2 recurrences, 1 occurred 9 months after the first negative FDG-PET/CT and the other occurred 37 months later. They postulated that radiologic surveillance may be terminated in patients with 2 negative FDG-PET/CT scans within 6 months, thus reducing the number of expensive investigations in these patients.

In a retrospective study with long-term follow-up (1–8 years), Ho and colleagues,[74] assessed the value of subsequent surveillance in patients with negative post-treatment PET/CT scan at 3 months. FDG-PET/CT scan was performed at 3 months (248 patients), 12 months (175 patients), and 24 months (77 patients) post-treatment. FDG-PET/CT scans at 12 and 24 months were evaluated only if preceding interval scans were negative. In clinically occult patients, FDG-PET/CT recurrence detection rates were 4% (9/284) at 3 months, 9% (15 of 175) at 12 months, and 4% (3 of 77) at 24 months. Clinically detected recurrence in patients with negative 3-month FDG-PET/CT scan was 6 within 3 to 12 months and 7 within 12 to 24 months. No difference in survival was identified between FDG-PET/CT detected and clinically detected recurrence. They suggest that HNC patients with negative 3-month imaging and low clinical suspicion seem to have limited benefit from further FDG-PET/CT surveillance, although higher-risk groups may still gain from serial FDG-PET/CT scan.

These studies warrant the need for further prospective trials to evaluate the survival benefits of long-term FDG-PET/CT surveillance after a negative FDG-PET/CT result.

Impact on Survival, and Prognostic Stratification

FDG-PET can provide valuable predictive and prognostic information when performed in follow-up and surveillance of HNC patients.[9,16,30,33,85] The prognostic information is useful in tailoring the follow-up surveillance strategy and individualizing patient care. In addition, rehabilitation after primary treatment of some HNC requires multiple surgical procedures, which are usually delayed until it is ensured that lasting tumor control has been established. Prognostic information of FDG-PET in predicting DFS could be justified to start reconstructive procedures early in patients with negative scans in the follow-up period.[85]

A summary of studies assessing the impact of post-treatment FDG-PET/CT on survival outcome of HNC patients is shown in **Table 2**.[74–77,80,81,86–89] Overall, these studies support the usefulness of post-therapy FDG-PET/CT assessment in patients' management and outcome and indicate that FDG-PET/CT positivity was associated with lower DFS and OS rates during the follow-up. In addition to the association between FDG-PET/CT positivity and survival rates, correlation between high SUVmax, high MTV of follow-up FDG-PET scan, and survival was also suggested. Whether performing FDG-PET/CT scan has improved the OS of HNC patients compared with those not did not undergo FDG-PET/CT scan remains, however, uncertain.

Sherriff and colleagues[89] conducted a retrospective study on 301 HNC patients receiving CRT treatment, of whom 92 had FDG-PET/CT scan at a median of 3 (2–8) months post-CRT. Patients were followed for a median of 19 and 25 months in FDG-PET/CT versus non–FDG-PET/CT groups, respectively. Positive FDG-PET/CT scan was defined as presence of any uptake with SUVmax greater than or equal to 3 within the head and neck area. Patients with a negative post-CRT FDG-PET/CT scan had a 91.8% chance of remaining free of local recurrence 19 months post-treatment. In all, patients in the FDG-PET/CT group showed significantly lower 2-year LC rate compared with the non–FDG-PET/CT group, whereas 2-year OS was not significantly different between the 2 groups (see **Table 2**). Similarly, in a cohort of 958 HNC patients, VanderWalde and colleagues[26] compared the survival of patients during the pre-PET era and the PET era. They point to a lack of improved survival over these eras, because no significant differences in 2-year OS rates were found between patients in the pre-PET era via the PET era (75.5 vs 74%). These results could be explained by the effect of lead time bias. The earlier detection of recurrence, using a highly sensitive screening test, might lead to an overestimation of the efficacy of treatment and survival. This highlights the need for high-quality prospective studies to evaluate whether

Table 2
Description of studies assessing the impact of post-treatment FDG-PET on survival in head and neck squamous cell carcinoma

Study	Country	Study Type	No. Patients	Follow-up (mo)	Time Interval (mo)	Patients, Treatment	Description
Studies comparing survival in PET/CT-positive and -negative HNC patients							
Wong et al,[81] 2002	USA	R	143	24	Mean 6.9	HNSCC, surgery, RT, or CRT	2-y DFS and OS rates were higher in patients with negative FDG-PET compared those with positive scans (82% vs 23% for DFS and 97% vs 48% for OS, respectively) FDG-PET positivity was a significant independent risk factor for RFS (multivarate analysis: RR = 3.7, $P<.0003$) and OS (multivariate analysis: RR = 6.9, $P<.0011$) A positive PET interpretation increased the RR of relapse by 4-fold and the RR of death by 7-fold.
Kunkel et al,[80] 2003	Germany	R	97	36	6–9	Oral cavity SCC, curative surgery, and RT	Kaplan-Meier analysis revealed that 3-y survival rates were significantly higher in patients with negative FDG-PET compared those with positive scans (86% vs 44%, P-value <0.0001). Pathologic glucose uptake had an HR of 6.47 (P-value <0.0001) in predicting OS.
Kim et al,[86] 2012[a]	Korea	R	81	35 (4–180)	Median ≈ 6	HNSCC (stages III and IV), surgery, RT, or CRT	Postradiation SUVmax was significantly correlated with locoregional recurrence (HR 1.812; 95% CI [1.361–2.413]; $P<.001$) Patients with MTV >41 mL showed shorter DFS and 2.4-fold higher risk of recurrence/death than those with MTV <41. High MTV (>41 mL) is negative prognostic factor for DFS (P-value 0.04).
Kim et al,[77] 2013	Korea	R	143	30 (15–45)	3–6 and 12	HNSCC, surgery, RT, or CRT	A positive interpretation of PET/CT was significantly associated with poor OS (log-rank test, $P<.001$). A positive FDG-PET/CT during 3–6 mo and 12 mo after treatment together was associated with an 8-fold increase in relative risk of death (8.60; 95% CI, 3.32–22.29; P-value <0.05).

(continued on next page)

Table 2
(continued)

Study	Country	Study Type	No. Patients	Follow-up (mo)	Time Interval (mo)	Patients, Treatment	Description
Uzel et al,[76] 2013	Turkey	R	46	20 (7–36)	Median 3.5 (2–9)	HNSCC, RT, or CRT	Complete metabolic response was observed in 63% of patients. Suspicious residual uptake was present in 10.9% and residual metabolic uptake in 26.0% of patients. Two-year locoregional control (LRC) was 95% in complete responders whereas it was 34% in noncomplete responders (have suspicious or residual FDG uptake)
Paidpally et al,[75] 2013	USA	R	134	40 (7–145)	(4–24)	HNSCC, RT	Kaplan-Meier analysis revealed a significant difference in time from scan to OS between patients with positive FDG-PET/CT scans and those with negative ones. (20 mo vs 30.5 mo; Mantel-Cox P-value <0.0001). Positive PET/CT scan has an HR of 29.74 for OS (P-value<0.05)
Chan et al,[88] 2013	Taiwan	P	165	58 (7–98)	3	NPC (stages III and IVa–b), CRT (± induction)	The 3-y and 5-y OS rates of patients who showed a CMR on PET were higher than those without a CMR (94.8% vs 72.4% and 85.4% vs 64.6%, respectively). The 3-y and 5-y DFS rates of patients who showed a CMR on PET were also higher than those without a CMR (83.5% vs 51.7% and 80.5% vs 51.7%, respectively). The results of post-therapy PET were more predictive of DFS than TNM tumor stage.
Ito et al,[87] 2014	Japan	R	36	23.8 (4–47)	(2–3)	HNSCC, intra-arterial CRT	OS was significantly shorter in patients with higher SUVmax group (>6.1) than that in lower SUVmax group (<6.1) (12.1 mo, 95% CI, 6.3–18 vs 44.6 mo, 95% CI, 39.9–49.3; P-value <0.001). OS was significantly shorter in patients with positive PET/CT visual interpretation than in those with negative visual interpretation. (P-value <0.05) The SUVmax and visual interpretation of HNSCC on post-IACR FDG-PET/CT can provide prognostic survival estimates. OS was lower in the group with recurrence within 6-mo than in the group with recurrence after 6-mo (P<.01).

Studies compare survival in PET/CT detected vs clinically detected recurrence

Study	Country	Type	N		Interval	Cancer, treatment	Results
Sherriff et al,[89] 2012	UK	R	92 PET/CT group 209 non-PET/CT group	19 25	3 (2–8)	HNSCC, radical CRT	2-y LC rates were significantly lower in the PET/CT group than in the non-PET/CT group (68.75% vs 82.25%, P-value <0.02). 2-y OS rates were not significantly different between the PET/CT group and non-PET/CT groups (78.6% vs 78.97%; P-value 0.66).
Chan et al,[88] 2013	Taiwan	P	136 with PET 130 with CWU	58 (7–98)	3	NPC (stages III and IVa–b), CRT (± induction)	Overall, the result of post-therapy CWU were not a reliable predictor for OS (P-value 0.14) and DFS (P-value 0.10), whereas the result of post-therapy PET were significantly predict the OS and DFS (P-value <0.001 for both). Among patients with stage III, there is no significant difference in DFS rates in those with CMR on PET and those who showed CMR on the CWU (5-y DFS: 90.4% vs 88.5%). Among patients with stage IVa–b disease, there was a trend toward better 5-y DFS rates in patients with a CMR on PET than in those who showed a complete response in the Conventional wok up (5-y DFS: 70.7% vs 63.1%).
Ho et al,[74] 2013[b]	USA	R	175 77	36 (12–96)	3 and 12 3, 12, and 24	HNC, surgery, RT, or CRT	No difference in outcomes between PET/CT-detected and clinically detected recurrences, with similar 3-y DFS (41% vs 46%, P-value 0.91) and 3-y OS (60% vs 54%, P-value 0.70) rates.

Abbreviations: CMR, complete metabolic response; CWU, conventional work-up; mo, months; N, number; NPC, nasopharyngeal carcinoma; P, prospective; R, retrospective; RFS, relapse-free survival; RR, relative risk.
[a] The post-treatment PET/CT scans were performed at 2–4 months after treatment and then 6-month intervals thereafter.
[b] All included patients had negative 3-month PET/CT result and enrolled only if preceding interval scan were negative.
Data from Refs.[74–77,80,81,86–89]

the use of FDG-PET/CT improves the success of salvage treatment and OS in the whole group of patients.

SUMMARY

There is a growing body of evidence that point to the value of FDG-PET/CT in the management of HNC patients and predicting patient-related outcomes. FDG-PET/CT changes the baseline staging (compared with CT or MR imaging), guides appropriate therapy selection, separates the responders and non-responders for therapy assessment, adds value to clinical assessment in follow-up, and predicts patient survival outcomes. The high NPV of post-treatment FDG-PET/CT can be used to individualize follow-up regimens in patients who have been treated for HNC.

REFERENCES

1. Ferlay J, Shin HR, Bray F, et al. GLOBOCAN 2008 v1.2, Cancer Incidence and Mortality Worldwide: IARC CancerBase No.10 [Internet]. Lyon (France): International Agency for Research on Cancer; 2010. Available at: http://globocan.iarc.fr.
2. Siegel R, Ma J, Zou Z, et al. Cancer statistics, 2014. CA Cancer J Clin 2014;64:9–29.
3. Wissinger E, Griebsch I, Lungershausen J, et al. The economic burden of head and neck cancer: a systematic literature review. Pharmacoeconomics 2014;32(9):865–82.
4. Schoder H, Fury M, Lee N, et al. PET monitoring of therapy response in head and neck squamous cell carcinoma. J Nucl Med 2009;50(Suppl 1):74S–88S.
5. Brockstein B, Haraf DJ, Rademaker AW, et al. Patterns of failure, prognostic factors and survival in locoregionally advanced head and neck cancer treated with concomitant chemoradiotherapy: a 9-year, 337-patient, multi-institutional experience. Ann Oncol 2004;15: 1179–86.
6. Paidpally V, Chirindel A, Lam S, et al. FDG-PET/CT imaging biomarkers in head and neck squamous cell carcinoma. Imaging Med 2012;4:633–47.
7. Subramaniam RM, Truong M, Peller P, et al. Fluorodeoxyglucose-positron-emission tomography imaging of head and neck squamous cell cancer. AJNR Am J Neuroradiol 2010;31:598–604.
8. Lefebvre JL. Current clinical outcomes demand new treatment options for SCCHN. Ann Oncol 2005; 16(Suppl 6):vi7–12.
9. Isles MG, McConkey C, Mehanna HM. A systematic review and meta-analysis of the role of positron emission tomography in the follow up of head and neck squamous cell carcinoma following radiotherapy or chemoradiotherapy. Clin Otolaryngol 2008;33:210–22.
10. Dibble EH, Karantanis D, Mercier G, et al. PET/CT of cancer patients: part 1, pancreatic neoplasms. AJR Am J Roentgenol 2012;199:952–67.
11. Antoniou AJ, Marcus C, Tahari AK, et al. Follow-up or Surveillance 18F-FDG PET/CT and Survival Outcome in Lung Cancer Patients. J Nucl Med 2014;55:1062–8.
12. Davison J, Mercier G, Russo G, et al. PET-based primary tumor volumetric parameters and survival of patients with non-small cell lung carcinoma. AJR Am J Roentgenol 2013;200:635–40.
13. Agarwal A, Chirindel A, Shah BA, et al. Evolving role of FDG PET/CT in multiple myeloma imaging and management. AJR Am J Roentgenol 2013;200: 884–90.
14. Davison JM, Subramaniam RM, Surasi DS, et al. FDG PET/CT in patients with HIV. AJR Am J Roentgenol 2011;197:284–94.
15. Gupta T, Master Z, Kannan S, et al. Diagnostic performance of post-treatment FDG PET or FDG PET/CT imaging in head and neck cancer: a systematic review and meta-analysis. Eur J Nucl Med Mol Imaging 2011;38:2083–95.
16. Xie P, Li M, Zhao H, et al. 18F-FDG PET or PET-CT to evaluate prognosis for head and neck cancer: a meta-analysis. J Cancer Res Clin Oncol 2011;137: 1085–93.
17. Castaldi P, Leccisotti L, Bussu F, et al. Role of (18)F-FDG PET-CT in head and neck squamous cell carcinoma. Acta Otorhinolaryngol Ital 2013;33:1–8.
18. Jackson T, Chung MK, Mercier G, et al. FDG PET/CT interobserver agreement in head and neck cancer: FDG and CT measurements of the primary tumor site. Nucl Med Commun 2012;33:305–12.
19. Hadiprodjo D, Ryan T, Truong MT, et al. Parotid gland tumors: preliminary data for the value of FDG PET/CT diagnostic parameters. AJR Am J Roentgenol 2012;198:W185–90.
20. Tahari AK, Alluri KC, Quon H, et al. FDG PET/CT imaging of oropharyngeal squamous cell carcinoma: characteristics of human papillomavirus-positive and -negative tumors. Clin Nucl Med 2014;39:225–31.
21. Subramaniam RM, Alluri KC, Tahari AK, et al. PET/CT imaging and human papilloma virus-positive oropharyngeal squamous cell cancer: evolving clinical imaging paradigm. J Nucl Med 2014;55: 431–8.
22. Paidpally V, Chirindel A, Chung CH, et al. FDG volumetric parameters and survival outcomes after definitive chemoradiotherapy in patients with recurrent head and neck squamous cell carcinoma. AJR Am J Roentgenol 2014;203:W139–45.
23. Marcus C, Ciarallo A, Tahari AK, et al. Head and neck PET/CT: therapy response interpretation criteria (Hopkins Criteria)-interreader reliability, accuracy, and survival outcomes. J Nucl Med 2014; 55(9):1411–6.

24. Dibble EH, Alvarez AC, Truong MT, et al. 18F-FDG metabolic tumor volume and total glycolytic activity of oral cavity and oropharyngeal squamous cell cancer: adding value to clinical staging. J Nucl Med 2012;53:709–15.

25. Antoniou AJ, Marcus C, Subramaniam RM. Value of imaging in head and neck tumors. Surg Oncol Clin N Am 2014;23:685–707.

26. VanderWalde NA, Salloum RG, Liu TL, et al. Positron emission tomography and stage migration in head and neck cancer. JAMA Otolaryngol Head Neck Surg 2014;140(7):654–61.

27. Tantiwongkosi B, Yu F, Kanard A, et al. Role of (18) F-FDG PET/CT in pre and post treatment evaluation in head and neck carcinoma. World J Radiol 2014;6: 177–91.

28. Pfister DG, Ang KK, Brizel DM, et al. NCCN clinical practice guidelines in Oncology (NCCN): Head and neck cancers. Version 2.2013. National Comprehenesive Cancer Network, Inc, 2013.

29. Gold KA, Lee HY, Kim ES. Targeted therapies in squamous cell carcinoma of the head and neck. Cancer 2009;115:922–35.

30. Bonner JA, Harari PM, Giralt J, et al. Radiotherapy plus cetuximab for squamous-cell carcinoma of the head and neck. N Engl J Med 2006;354:567–78.

31. Pryor DI, Porceddu SV, Scuffham PA, et al. Economic analysis of FDG-PET-guided management of the neck after primary chemoradiotherapy for node-positive head and neck squamous cell carcinoma. Head Neck 2013;35:1287–94.

32. Wang D, Schultz CJ, Jursinic PA, et al. Initial experience of FDG-PET/CT guided IMRT of head-and-neck carcinoma. Int J Radiat Oncol Biol Phys 2006;65:143–51.

33. Deantonio L, Beldì D, Gambaro G, et al. FDG-PET/CT imaging for staging and radiotherapy treatment planning of head and neck carcinoma. Radiat Oncol 2008;3:29.

34. Abramyuk A, Appold S, Zophel K, et al. Modification of staging and treatment of head and neck cancer by FDG-PET/CT prior to radiotherapy. Strahlenther Onkol 2013;189:197–201.

35. Lonneux M, Hamoir M, Reychler H, et al. Positron emission tomography with [18F]fluorodeoxyglucose improves staging and patient management in patients with head and neck squamous cell carcinoma: a multicenter prospective study. J Clin Oncol 2010; 28:1190–5.

36. Ha PK, Hdeib A, Goldenberg D, et al. The role of positron emission tomography and computed tomography fusion in the management of early-stage and advanced-stage primary head and neck squamous cell carcinoma. Arch Otolaryngol Head Neck Surg 2006;132:12–6.

37. Rusthoven KE, Koshy M, Paulino AC. The role of fluorodeoxyglucose positron emission tomography in cervical lymph node metastases from an unknown primary tumor. Cancer 2004;101:2641–9.

38. Pavlidis N. Optimal therapeutic management of patients with distinct clinicopathological cancer of unknown primary subsets. Ann Oncol 2012;23(Suppl 10):x282–5.

39. Kwee TC, Kwee RM. Combined FDG-PET/CT for the detection of unknown primary tumors: systematic review and meta-analysis. Eur Radiol 2009;19: 731–44.

40. Xu GZ, Guan DJ, He ZY. (18)FDG-PET/CT for detecting distant metastases and second primary cancers in patients with head and neck cancer. A meta-analysis. Oral Oncol 2011;47:560–5.

41. Strobel K, Haerle SK, Stoeckli SJ, et al. Head and neck squamous cell carcinoma (HNSCC)–detection of synchronous primaries with (18)F-FDG-PET/CT. Eur J Nucl Med Mol Imaging 2009;36: 919–27.

42. Himeno S, Yasuda S, Shimada H, et al. Evaluation of esophageal cancer by positron emission tomography. Jpn J Clin Oncol 2002;32:340–6.

43. Hanamoto A, Takenaka Y, Shimosegawa E, et al. Limitation of 2-deoxy-2-[F-18]fluoro-D-glucose positron emission tomography (FDG-PET) to detect early synchronous primary cancers in patients with untreated head and neck squamous cell cancer. Ann Nucl Med 2013;27:880–5.

44. Yabuki K, Kubota A, Horiuchi C, et al. Limitations of PET and PET/CT in detecting upper gastrointestinal synchronous cancer in patients with head and neck carcinoma. Eur Arch Otorhinolaryngol 2013; 270:727–33.

45. Evangelista L, Cervino AR, Chondrogiannis S, et al. Comparison between anatomical cross-sectional imaging and 18F-FDG PET/CT in the staging, restaging, treatment response, and long-term surveillance of squamous cell head and neck cancer: a systematic literature overview. Nucl Med Commun 2014;35: 123–34.

46. Roh JL, Park JP, Kim JS, et al. 18F fluorodeoxyglucose PET/CT in head and neck squamous cell carcinoma with negative neck palpation findings: a prospective study. Radiology 2014;271:153–61.

47. Haerle SK, Strobel K, Ahmad N, et al. Contrast-enhanced (1)(8)F-FDG-PET/CT for the assessment of necrotic lymph node metastases. Head Neck 2010;33:324–9.

48. Lee HS, Kim JS, Roh JL, et al. Clinical values for abnormal F-FDG uptake in the head and neck region of patients with head and neck squamous cell carcinoma. Eur J Radiol 2014;83(8):1455–60.

49. Kanda T, Kitajima K, Suenaga Y, et al. Value of retrospective image fusion of (1)(8)F-FDG PET and MRI for preoperative staging of head and neck cancer: comparison with PET/CT and contrast-enhanced neck MRI. Eur J Radiol 2013;82:2005–10.

50. Suzuki H, Kato K, Fujimoto Y, et al. 18F-FDG-PET/CT predicts survival in hypopharyngeal squamous cell carcinoma. Ann Nucl Med 2013;27:297–302.

51. Suzuki H, Kato K, Fujimoto Y, et al. Prognostic value of (18)F-fluorodeoxyglucose uptake before treatment for pharyngeal cancer. Ann Nucl Med 2014; 28:356–62.

52. Pak K, Cheon GJ, Nam HY, et al. Prognostic value of metabolic tumor volume and total lesion glycolysis in head and neck cancer: a systematic review and meta-analysis. J Nucl Med 2014;55:884 90.

53. Koyasu S, Nakamoto Y, Kikuchi M, et al. Prognostic value of pretreatment 18F-FDG PET/CT parameters including visual evaluation in patients with head and neck squamous cell carcinoma. AJR Am J Roentgenol 2014;202:851–8.

54. Apostolova I, Steffen IG, Wedel F, et al. Asphericity of pretherapeutic tumour FDG uptake provides independent prognostic value in head-and-neck cancer. Eur Radiol 2014;24(9):2077–87.

55. Abd El-Hafez YG, Moustafa HM, Khalil HF, et al. Total lesion glycolysis: a possible new prognostic parameter in oral cavity squamous cell carcinoma. Oral Oncol 2013;49:261–8.

56. Ryan WR, Fee WE Jr, Le QT, et al. Positron-emission tomography for surveillance of head and neck cancer. Laryngoscope 2005;115:645–50.

57. Prestwich RJ, Subesinghe M, Gilbert A, et al. Delayed response assessment with FDG-PET-CT following (chemo) radiotherapy for locally advanced head and neck squamous cell carcinoma. Clin Radiol 2012;67:966–75.

58. Cheon GJ, Chung JK, So Y, et al. Diagnostic accuracy of F-18 FDG-PET in the assessment of posttherapeutic recurrence of head and neck cancer. Clin Positron Imaging 1999;2:197–204.

59. Ghanooni R, Delpierre I, Magremanne M, et al. (18) F-FDG PET/CT and MRI in the follow-up of head and neck squamous cell carcinoma. Contrast Media Mol Imaging 2011;6:260–6.

60. Mukundan H, Sarin A, Gill BS, et al. MRI and PET-CT: comparison in post-treatment evaluation of head and neck squamous cell carcinomas. Med J Armed Forces India 2014;70:111–5.

61. Kitagawa Y, Nishizawa S, Sano K, et al. Prospective comparison of 18F-FDG PET with conventional imaging modalities (MRI, CT, and 67Ga scintigraphy) in assessment of combined intraarterial chemotherapy and radiotherapy for head and neck carcinoma. J Nucl Med 2003;44:198–206.

62. Loeffelbein DJ, Souvatzoglou M, Wankerl V, et al. PET-MRI fusion in head-and-neck oncology: current status and implications for hybrid PET/MRI. J Oral Maxillofac Surg 2012;70:473–83.

63. Huang SH, Perez-Ordonez B, Weinreb I, et al. Natural course of distant metastases following radiotherapy or chemoradiotherapy in HPV-related oropharyngeal cancer. Oral Oncol 2013;49:79–85.

64. Yu J, Cooley T, Truong MT, et al. Head and neck squamous cell cancer (stages III and IV) induction chemotherapy assessment: value of FDG volumetric imaging parameters. J Med Imaging Radiat Oncol 2014;58:18–24.

65. Hentschel M, Appold S, Schreiber A, et al. Early FDG PET at 10 or 20 Gy under chemoradiotherapy is prognostic for locoregional control and overall survival in patients with head and neck cancer. Eur J Nucl Med Mol Imaging 2011;38:1203–11.

66. Yoon DH, Cho Y, Kim SY, et al. Usefulness of interim FDG-PET after induction chemotherapy in patients with locally advanced squamous cell carcinoma of the head and neck receiving sequential induction chemotherapy followed by concurrent chemoradiotherapy. Int J Radiat Oncol Biol Phys 2010;81:118–25.

67. Ceulemans G, Voordeckers M, Farrag A, et al. Can 18-FDG-PET during radiotherapy replace post-therapy scanning for detection/demonstration of tumor response in head-and-neck cancer? Int J Radiat Oncol Biol Phys 2010;81:938–42.

68. Beswick DM, Gooding WE, Johnson JT, et al. Temporal patterns of head and neck squamous cell carcinoma recurrence with positron-emission tomography/computed tomography monitoring. Laryngoscope 2012;122:1512–7.

69. Krabbe CA, Pruim J, Dijkstra PU, et al. 18F-FDG PET as a routine posttreatment surveillance tool in oral and oropharyngeal squamous cell carcinoma: a prospective study. J Nucl Med 2009;50:1940–7.

70. Abgral R, Querellou S, Potard G, et al. Does 18F-FDG PET/CT improve the detection of posttreatment recurrence of head and neck squamous cell carcinoma in patients negative for disease on clinical follow-up? J Nucl Med 2009;50:24–9.

71. Ng SH, Chan SC, Yen TC, et al. Comprehensive imaging of residual/recurrent nasopharyngeal carcinoma using whole-body MRI at 3 T compared with FDG-PET-CT. Eur Radiol 2010;20:2229–40.

72. Wierzbicka M, Popko M, Piskadlo K, et al. Comparison of positron emission tomography/computed tomography imaging and ultrasound in surveillance of head and neck cancer - the 3-year experience of the ENT Department in Poznan. Rep Pract Oncol Radiother 2011;16:184–8.

73. Zundel MT, Michel MA, Schultz CJ, et al. Comparison of physical examination and fluorodeoxyglucose positron emission tomography/computed tomography 4-6 months after radiotherapy to assess residual head-and-neck cancer. Int J Radiat Oncol Biol Phys 2011;81:e825–32.

74. Ho AS, Tsao GJ, Chen FW, et al. Impact of positron emission tomography/computed tomography surveillance at 12 and 24 months for detecting head

and neck cancer recurrence. Cancer 2013;119: 1349–56.

75. Paidpally V, Tahari AK, Lam S, et al. Addition of 18F-FDG PET/CT to clinical assessment predicts overall survival in HNSCC: a retrospective analysis with follow-up for 12 years. J Nucl Med 2013;54:2039–45.

76. Uzel EK, Ekmekcioglu O, Elicin O, et al. Is FDG -PET-CT a valuable tool in prediction of persistent disease in head and neck cancer. Asian Pac J Cancer Prev 2013;14:4847–51.

77. Kim JW, Roh JL, Kim JS, et al. (18)F-FDG PET/CT surveillance at 3-6 and 12 months for detection of recurrence and second primary cancer in patients with head and neck squamous cell carcinoma. Br J Cancer 2013;109:2973–9.

78. Robin P, Abgral R, Valette G, et al. Diagnostic performance of FDG PET/CT to detect subclinical HNSCC recurrence 6 months after the end of treatment. Eur J Nucl Med Mol Imaging 2014;42(1):72–8.

79. Lee JC, Kim JS, Lee JH, et al. F-18 FDG-PET as a routine surveillance tool for the detection of recurrent head and neck squamous cell carcinoma. Oral Oncol 2007;43:686–92.

80. Kunkel M, Forster GJ, Reichert TE, et al. Detection of recurrent oral squamous cell carcinoma by [18F]-2-fluorodeoxyglucose-positron emission tomography: implications for prognosis and patient management. Cancer 2003;98:2257–65.

81. Wong RJ, Lin DT, Schoder H, et al. Diagnostic and prognostic value of [(18)F]fluorodeoxyglucose positron emission tomography for recurrent head and neck squamous cell carcinoma. J Clin Oncol 2002; 20:4199–208.

82. Gao S, Li S, Yang X, et al. 18FDG PET-CT for distant metastases in patients with recurrent head and neck cancer after definitive treatment. A meta-analysis. Oral Oncol 2014;50:163–7.

83. Farber LA, Benard F, Machtay M, et al. Detection of recurrent head and neck squamous cell carcinomas after radiation therapy with 2-18F-fluoro-2-deoxy-D-glucose positron emission tomography. Laryngoscope 1999;109:970–5.

84. McDermott M, Hughes M, Rath T, et al. Negative predictive value of surveillance PET/CT in head and neck squamous cell cancer. AJNR Am J Neuroradiol 2013;34:1632–6.

85. Pignon JP, le Maitre A, Maillard E, et al. Meta-analysis of chemotherapy in head and neck cancer (MACH-NC): an update on 93 randomised trials and 17,346 patients. Radiother Oncol 2009;92:4–14.

86. Kim G, Kim YS, Han EJ, et al. FDG-PET/CT as prognostic factor and surveillance tool for postoperative radiation recurrence in locally advanced head and neck cancer. Radiat Oncol J 2012;29:243–51.

87. Ito K, Shimoji K, Miyata Y, et al. Prognostic value of post-treatment (18)F-FDG PET/CT for advanced head and neck cancer after combined intra-arterial chemotherapy and radiotherapy. Chin J Cancer Res 2014;26:30–7.

88. Chan SC, Kuo WH, Wang HM, et al. Prognostic implications of post-therapy (18)F-FDG PET in patients with locoregionally advanced nasopharyngeal carcinoma treated with chemoradiotherapy. Ann Nucl Med 2013;27:710–9.

89. Sherriff JM, Ogunremi B, Colley S, et al. The role of positron emission tomography/CT imaging in head and neck cancer patients after radical chemoradiotherapy. Br J Radiol 2012;85:e1120–6.

Lung Cancer

Tim Akhurst, MD, FRACP[a,b],*, Michael MacManus, MD, FRANZCR[b,c],
Rodney J. Hicks, MD, FRACP[a,b]

KEYWORDS

- Positron emission tomography • Lung cancer • Radiotherapy • Chemotherapy • CT scanning

KEY POINTS

- Undiagnosed ^{18}F-fluorodeoxyglucose–avid pulmonary nodules generally require further evaluation.
- PET-assisted staging of the mediastinum is much more accurate than computed tomography–based evaluation.
- PET imaging before planned surgery for apparently resectable lung cancer reduces the futile thoracotomy rate.
- Almost one-third of patients with apparent stage III non–small cell lung cancer will be found to have disease too advanced for curative radiation therapy after PET staging.
- PET-assisted radiation therapy planning greatly increases the accuracy of target volumes used in curative radiation therapy.

POSITRON EMISSION TOMOGRAPHY/COMPUTED TOMOGRAPHY IMAGING IN THE MANAGEMENT OF LUNG CANCER

Rational decision-making in oncology is dependent on high-quality data regarding the biological characteristics, location, and extent of malignancy. Although pathologic sampling of the presumed primary or suspected metastatic disease provides critical diagnostic information about tumor type and grade, economic and physical (morbidity) factors mandate noninvasive evaluation of the extent of disease. Medical imaging is pivotal in providing this information. Although computed tomography (CT) or MRI can provide detailed anatomic information, ^{18}F-fluorodeoxyglucose–positron emission tomography (FDG-PET) supplements this with metabolic data to generally improve both the sensitivity and specificity of staging. With the development of hybrid PET/CT and, more recently, PET/MRI, detailed anatomic and metabolic characterization of disease has become feasible in a single efficient and data-rich procedure.

It is important to recognize that imaging studies are not therapies in themselves and impact patient outcomes only insofar as they influence treatment choice and delivery. Patient survival and other oncological end-points are dependent on the efficacy of the therapy chosen, which relate to its delivery, the nature of the malignancy, and host factors. Traditionally, treatment choice has been based on disease stage, but increasingly molecular and genomic characterization of tumors is also guiding targeted approaches. Incorrect characterization of cancer, either of its biology or extent, can lead to errors of management that harm patients through the delivery of inappropriate therapy or incorrect amounts of an otherwise appropriate therapy. In this article, we consider the impact of PET imaging with FDG on the management of

The authors have nothing to disclose.
[a] Division of Radiation Oncology and Cancer Imaging, Centre for Molecular Imaging, Peter MacCallum Cancer Centre, East Melbourne, Victoria 3002, Australia; [b] The Sir Peter MacCallum Department of Oncology, The University of Melbourne, Melbourne, Victoria, Australia; [c] Division of Radiation Oncology and Cancer Imaging, Department of Radiation Oncology, Peter MacCallum Cancer Centre, East Melbourne, Victoria 3002, Australia
* Corresponding author. Centre for Molecular Imaging, Peter MacCallum Cancer Centre, St Andrew's Place, East Melbourne, Victoria 3002, Australia.
E-mail address: tim.akhurst@petermac.org

PET Clin 10 (2015) 147–158
http://dx.doi.org/10.1016/j.cpet.2014.12.002
1556-8598/15/$ – see front matter © 2015 Elsevier Inc. All rights reserved.

patients with non–small cell lung cancer (NSCLC). There is, perhaps, no other malignancy, that better epitomizes the value of FDG-PET/CT to patients for diagnosis, lesion characterization, staging, treatment selection, targeting of therapy, response assessment, and evaluation of relapse.

LUNG NODULE CHARACTERIZATION

As CT scans are increasingly performed for investigation of a range of diseases and, in some patients, as a screening procedure, the incidental detection of pulmonary nodules is becoming more common. FDG-PET can play a key role in characterizing many of these nodules. The Fleischner Society does not currently recommend FDG-PET/CT scanning of patients with nodules smaller than 8 mm.[1] These recommendations recognize that lesions smaller than twice the theoretic spatial resolution of the scanner (as defined by a parameter termed the full-width-at-half-maximum or FWHM) are subject to partial volume effect. Additionally, the effects of respiratory motion on lesion detectability are also exaggerated for small lesions. The net effect of partial volume averaging and lesion motion is an underestimation of the true activity in a lesion, thereby limiting the ability of PET to accurately exclude malignancy. Follow-up monitoring of these lesions for growth is advocated for this purpose.

As nodules increase in size, the risk of malignancy also increases and the hazards of an observational strategy are heightened by potentially allowing greater opportunity for metastatic spread. Accordingly, immediate characterization of such nodules is desirable. Although biopsy is the definitive method for this purpose, not all lesions are amenable to biopsy and, depending on the method used, can have significant associated morbidity and cost. Relatively early studies using stand-alone FDG-PET scanning of larger pulmonary nodules indicated the nodules without significant FDG-avidity can be safely observed with careful follow-up due to a relatively high negative predictive value.[2] The positive predictive value of FDG scans in indicating the presence of a lung cancer will depend on the relative pretest likelihoods of lung cancer or of another active pulmonary pathology being present. This reflects the fact that FDG is actively concentrated in both malignant and inflammatory cells. Factors that influence the a priori likelihood of malignancy as the etiology of an FDG-avid nodule include the patient's smoking history, ethnicity, and sex; the presence of a prior tumor; and the regional prevalence of tuberculosis or endemic granulomatous conditions, such as histoplasmosis.[3,4]

Although the intensity of FDG uptake as measured by the maximum standardized uptake value (SUVmax) has been suggested to be an indicator of tumor aggressiveness,[5] the relationship between this parameter and prognosis is not necessarily seen for all types of treatment.[6] Nevertheless, FDG uptake in the primary tumor mass does appear to influence the likelihood of nodal involvement.[7,8] The significance of a high SUV also may vary depending on histopathological subtype.[9] Despite its potential utility for characterization of disease biology, FDG uptake intensity does not currently determine the therapeutic approach to proven lung cancers in most centers. Nevertheless, in the exceptional cases in which biopsy is considered extremely risky to a patient with a high pretest probability of lung cancer, a pragmatic approach can be taken where FDG-avid lesions are treated as malignant, without an apparent adverse outcome.[10] Application of probabilistic models suggests that when the likelihood of malignancy is more than 85%, empiric treatment of lung nodules may be appropriate without recourse to biopsy in such patients.[11] PET also can help target biopsies to the most informative anatomic sites in patients found to have metastatic disease.

STAGING OF KNOWN NON–SMALL CELL LUNG CANCER

The most powerful adverse prognostic parameter in patients with NSCLC is the presence of metastatic disease (M status). Stage IV disease is defined by the presence of distant metastases (M1) and is independent of N-stage and T-stage because these cease to have independent prognostic significance in this setting. In the absence of distant metastases (M0), nodal (N) status (a surrogate for the later development of distant metastatic disease) becomes relevant to both treatment choices and prognosis. Finally, it is only in the absence of unresectable regional nodal disease (N2-3) that the resectability of the primary tumor itself (T status) becomes relevant. TNM staging reflects a surgical orientation to the management of lung cancer and in an era of multidisciplinary care of NSCLC, MNT-staging may be conceptually more appropriate. Although conventional imaging paradigms are focused on providing optimal assessment of T-stage, the major advantage of FDG-PET is its ability to more accurately define M-stage and N-stage. This information has the potential to significantly influence treatment choices and thereby influence patient outcomes. Accordingly, discussion of the advantages of FDG-PET/CT in staging NSCLC focuses on an MNT-staging paradigm.

M Status

In NSCLC, FDG-PET/CT is typically acquired from the base of the brain to the proximal thighs. This field-of-view is designed to acquire data over the expected red marrow distribution, thereby covering the dominant potential sites of osseous, as well as visceral and nodal metastasis. A meta-analysis of FDG-PET imaging in lung cancer published in 2001 found that the detection of metastatic disease altered therapy in 18% of 695 patients, with 12% of 581 patients having unsuspected extrathoracic metastases.[12] Technical developments in PET, including time-of-flight and improved reconstruction algorithms, plus the routine application of hybrid PET/CT, are likely to have further improved the sensitivity for detection of distant metastatic disease since that time. In an era in which more aggressive treatment of oligometastatic disease is being promoted, early detection of isolated systemic disease may have management implications. Of potential relevance to this scenario, it has been reported that potentially curable patients found to have more than one metastasis on PET have a significantly shorter survival than patients with a solitary PET-detected metastasis (5 months vs 12 months).[13] PET/CT is vastly more sensitive and specific in the detection of extracranial metastasis than a combination of CT and bone scanning, and upstaging by PET is frequent after conventional evaluation.[14] The likelihood that metastatic disease will be detected increases as locoregional disease extent increases. Our group reported that distant metastases, which were occult to conventional imaging, were found on FDG-PET scans in 7% of patients with pre-PET stage I, 18% of patients with pre-PET stage II, and 24% of patients pre-PET stage III disease.[15] These data are particularly pertinent to earlier studies regarding the accuracy and management impact of FDG-PET in lung cancer, which primarily focused on patients with early-stage disease for which pathologic validation was feasible as most patients came to surgery.

Nodal Status

It is now widely accepted that FDG-PET/CT has much higher diagnostic accuracy than CT in the characterization of mediastinal nodes in patients with NSCLC. The primary criterion for detection of nodal involvement on CT is nodal size. The threshold for categorization of malignant involvement of mediastinal nodes is generally a greatest short-axis diameter of more than 1 cm. A finite receiver-operating curve exists for all testing based on such linear data, such that improvements in sensitivity lead to falls in specificity and

vice versa. Evaluating intrathoracic nodal status, the 2001 meta-analysis discussed previously reported high sensitivity (88%), specificity (92%), and accuracy (91%) of FDG-PET in 1292 patients compared with 65%, 76%, and 73% in 1268 patients for CT. A separate meta-analysis by Gould and colleagues[16] recommended that enlarged nodes that are FDG negative need not be biopsied, as PET sensitivity in this group of patients is close to 100%. Where endemic infections are a common differential diagnosis, the specificity of FDG uptake will be reduced.[17] Many granulomatous infective processes affect both lungs so that inflammatory nodal uptake is often symmetric and low grade. Consequently, the recognition of this symmetric pattern allows specificity to be maintained. The addition of CT data to PET data allows classification of nodes with benign-appearing calcification as benign even in the presence of FDG uptake, thereby increasing specificity in patients who reside in areas in which tuberculosis is endemic.[18] Incorporating information with respect to nodal size and the relationship between uptake in nodes and the primary lesion can help to further define the likelihood of malignancy.[19] With the wider availability of endobronchial ultrasound, FDG-PET/CT can help to define metabolically active nodal stations that are most likely to influence management and thereby guide biopsy to confirm or exclude metastatic involvement (**Fig. 1**).[20]

T Status

The limited resolution of FDG-PET cameras and the effects of lesion motion restrict the ability of PET to determine invasion of structures unless gross invasion is present. Therefore, PET impacts T-stage less frequently than it does on either N-stage or M-stage. Nevertheless, in common clinical scenarios, such as when tumors are associated with atelectasis, PET can provide information crucial for treatment planning.[21] The contrast provided by PET compensates for the absence of contrast on CT between tissues of similar density, including collapsed lung, tumor, and other soft tissues. Where relevant to surgical planning, performing a dedicated contrast-enhanced diagnostic CT can provide complementary information that overcomes the limitations of stand-alone PET. Recent data suggest that the metabolic tumor volume assessed by FDG-PET/CT has prognostic value in NSCLC.[22]

As a result of changes in M-stage, N-stage, and T-stage, PET has been shown by many groups to have a significant impact on management in routine clinical practice and the validity of the

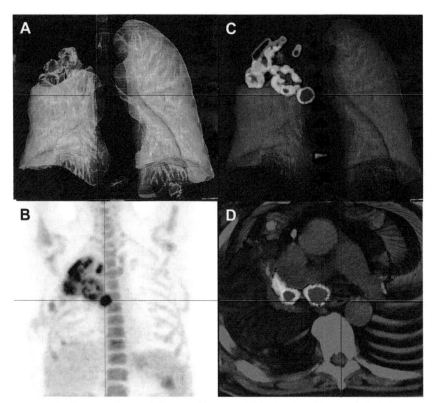

Fig. 1. The presence of collapse and consolidation of lung peripheral to an obstructing lesion limits the ability of CT to define the location and extent of the primary tumor (*A*) but the presence of infection within the collapsed lung also can potentially compromise assessment of draining nodes because the likelihood of reactive lymphadenopathy is increased (*B*). Fused images (*C*) allow identification of suspicious nodes and volume-rendered images (*D*) aid planning the optimal biopsy approach.

stage migration has been corroborated by associated improvement in prognostic stratification. A recent large series from a major comprehensive cancer center attests to the utility of FDG-PET/CT across a spectrum of disease stages.[23] Our own experience with FDG-PET/CT also indicates a high impact on management and prognostic stratification.[24] There is, however, some variation in the quantum and type of impact in patients who are surgical as opposed to radiotherapy candidates, as discussed in the next section.

IMPACT OF POSITRON EMISSION TOMOGRAPHY ON MANAGEMENT AND PROGNOSTIC STRATIFICATION IN SURGICAL CANDIDATES

In 2001, a study (using PET rather than PET-CT data) in a group of patients referred for surgical resection found that PET data predicted survival, whereas CT did not, but 10% of patients were overstaged with PET.[25] Accordingly, although this was less than the 32% overstaged by CT, the investigators recommended the need for

biopsy confirmation of suspected disease sites that would otherwise make the patient unsuitable for resection with curative intent. Invasive biopsy procedures can be intelligently planned using FDG-PET/CT data to target the most informative and accessible site of disease. Incorporating FDG-PET into the clinical workup of patients who would be considered surgically resectable after conventional imaging reduces the number of "futile" thoracotomies, with a randomized control study demonstrating a reduction from 41% to 21%.[26]

A recent pathologic reclassification of adenocarcinomas has added classifications of adenocarcinoma in situ (AIS) and minimally invasive (<5 mm invasive) adenocarcinoma (MIA) with the intention of describing a group of patients with close to 100% survival rates following surgical resection. The challenge in patients with AIS or MIA is in defining the minimum optimal treatment required to preserve quality of life, given their excellent prognosis. The recognition of these new pathologic entities has led to revised imaging guidelines.[27] FDG-PET/CT has little role in the management of these patients, as the pretest likelihood of nodal or metastatic disease is extremely low.

Importance of Contemporaneous Imaging and Definitive Therapy

Lung cancer can progress rapidly on serial PET scans. A study of a prospective series of 82 patients (61% stage III, 21% stage I, and 18% stage II) referred for radical (curative) radiotherapy reported in 2010 that a second FDG-PET/CT was acquired for radiotherapy-planning purposes in a subset of patients. Comparison of the 2 scans (staging and planning) revealed a median tumor-doubling time estimated at 55 days with a net result that 39% of the group was upstaged on TNM criteria, including 29% who were no longer suitable for a curative treatment approach and thus underwent palliative therapy.[28] Similarly, Geiger and colleagues[29] reported that radiation treatment planning with hybrid PET/CT scans repeated within 120 days of an initial staging PET/CT scan identified significant upstaging in more than half of patients. These publications suggest that near contemporaneous imaging before definitive therapy is essential. These data also suggest that time intervals between data collection points must be recorded in trials to ensure biases due to tumor progression before definitive therapy are avoided. In particular, surgical series evaluating the sensitivity of FDG-PET/CT for detection of nodal involvement should ideally exclude those cases with more than a few weeks between the staging scan and pathologic correlation.[30]

IMPACT OF POSITRON EMISSION TOMOGRAPHY ON MANAGEMENT AND PROGNOSTIC STRATIFICATION IN CANDIDATES FOR CURATIVE-INTENT RADIOTHERAPY

If resection of all known disease can be safely accomplished, radical surgery is generally the preferred treatment strategy for early-stage NSCLC, but in patients unfit for surgery or who refuse it, radiotherapy is a valid option. PET/CT is of particular value for such patients, as they will not have comprehensive evaluation of their mediastinal nodes at thoracotomy and hence will tend to be understaged by conventional imaging. PET/CT not only helps noninvasively to decide the need for irradiation of the mediastinum, but also detects distant metastasis in a significant proportion of cases.[31] Stereotactic body radiotherapy (SBRT) is a form of treatment that is becoming more frequently used in medically inoperable stage I NSCLC. Assessing outcomes of this

therapy compared with surgery is compromised by the severe comorbidities that prevent surgical resection,[32] as well as by the less rigorous staging that occurs in patients not undergoing surgery. Nevertheless, outcomes in radiotherapy and surgical patients with stage I lung cancer are different. A retrospective study comparing 462 patients who underwent surgical resection with 76 patients who received SBRT, revealed that overall survival at 3 years was better in the surgical group.[33] However, cancer-specific survival was not different ($P = .8$). There was a 7% (4/57) operative mortality in the highest-risk operative candidates in the study. Conventionally fractionated radiotherapy is rapidly being supplanted by SBRT on the basis of excellent phase II data showing rates of local control that are not dissimilar to surgery. As yet, no randomized data exist showing the superiority of SBRT to conventional radiotherapy, and an Australian randomized trial that will study this question is in progress.

Stage II to III lung cancer is a structurally diverse group. In stage II disease, surgery is still the preferred option in the absence of limiting comorbidities. Although some stage III patients may have "anatomically resectable" disease, radical chemoradiation is generally the preferred treatment approach. Such treatment requires that all known disease can be encompassed within a tolerable radiotherapy treatment volume. The likelihood of FDG-PET/CT finding distant metastatic disease in pre-PET stage III disease is greater than 20%.[15,34] It is therefore not surprising that when FDG-PET data are added to conventional imaging, combined structural and metabolic imaging reduces the likelihood of futile radical radiotherapy being prescribed.

Our group reported a prospective series of 153 patients referred for radical radiotherapy who underwent FDG-PET treatment planning scans.[31] Fully 30% of these patients were found to be unsuitable for chemoradiation with curative intent because of either the detection of metastatic disease or because of unexpectedly extensive intrathoracic nodal disease. In the group of patients who were treated radically, the stage of disease defined by FDG-PET was strongly associated with survival ($P = .0041$), whereas pre-PET, CT-based stage was not ($P = .19$). This strong association with survival suggests that, in this group of patients, PET staging data should have a powerful impact on decision-making.

Two separate groups have reported a similar reduction in futile radical radiotherapy rates. The first group, from Tubingen, reported in 2002 that 25 of 100 patients referred for radical radiotherapy were found to have occult distant metastases.[34] In a separate study from Warsaw, 25 of 100 patients referred for radical radiotherapy did not receive it after incorporation of FDG-PET/CT data into the management plan.[35] It appears that accepting a patient for radical radiotherapy based on CT alone will result in futile radiotherapy in approximately 25% to 30% of patients. They could be saved the morbidity of futile aggressive treatment if an FDG-PET/CT scan is added to their preradiotherapy workup.

Cohorts of patients with NSCLC who receive radiotherapy after PET-based selection will clearly have superior survival compared with conventionally staged cohorts, even if treatment is unchanged. Our group compared 2 cohorts of patients treated sequentially at the same center.[36] The first cohort was treated between 1989 and 1995 on a randomized study comparing 60 Gy conventionally fractionated radiotherapy with or without concurrent carboplatin. The second cohort included all radical radiotherapy candidates between 1996 and 1999 at our center who received radical radiotherapy after FDG-PET staging and fulfilled the same criteria for stage, Eastern Cooperative Oncology Group (ECOG) status, and weight loss. The median survival of patients in the first trial was 16 months and was nearly twice as long (31 months) in the patients accepted for therapy after FDG-PET. Although improvements in treatment will have accounted for some of this survival difference, it is likely that the use of PET-based patient selection was the major factor.

DEFINING THE TARGET FOR RADIOTHERAPY WITH CURATIVE INTENT

The radiotherapy lexicon includes a number of technical terms that describe the lesion to be targeted and its surrounds. The planning target volume (PTV) describes the volume within the patient that is to be irradiated. There is an element of clinical judgment as to how large the PTV needs to be to achieve optimal tumor control. Ideally, the PTV will include all of the tumor, its microscopic extensions, and a safety margin for factors such as variations in daily set-up on the treatment machine. If there is tumor outside the PTV, then treatment will usually fail. Data that assist in defining the PTV include knowledge of the visible gross tumor volume (GTV) seen on imaging. "Microscopic extension" of a tumor is a term used to describe the leading edge of malignant tumor infiltrating into surrounding tissues that appears normal on imaging. The term clinical target volume describes a volume that adds an empiric margin to the GTV that encompasses the estimated microscopic extension.[37] Two studies have suggested that the required

additional margin to account for microscopic extension of lung cancer is between 5 and 8 mm.[38,39] We believe that FDG-PET/CT is the imaging modality of choice for definition of GTV during the radiotherapy-planning process. Recent evidence suggests that its use will avoid geographic miss in more than a quarter of patients who would have had futile treatment if CT alone was used for treatment planning.[40] Use of PET/CT in this setting is associated with some of the best survival results ever reported in stage III NSCLC.

As noted previously, a common complication of centrally located primary NSCLC is intrinsic or extrinsic bronchial obstruction leading to distal collapse of the lung supplied by the involved bronchus. It can be very difficult to distinguish the tumor and the associated collapse on CT, as both appear dense/opaque. One of the roles of FDG-PET/CT is to help ensure that the radiotherapy plan will encompass the actual cancerous mass rather than its consequence, thereby limiting radiation damage to uninvolved lung (**Fig. 2**). The first task in radiotherapy planning, after acquisition of the imaging data used in the process, is to define the location of the tumor, its extensions, and all involved nodes in 3-dimensional (3D) space after the imaging study is imported into the radiotherapy-planning computer. Because of its proven accuracy, the PET/CT scan is the preferred 3D imaging modality for defining the target. The margins of the tumor lesions are defined by the radiation oncologist, ideally in consultation with the PET physician. This is generally performed using a visual (human) contouring approach,[41] in which the margin of the tumor is drawn, taking into account both PET and the CT information. Research is continuing into the use of automated computer-derived algorithms for defining tumor margins on PET scans, but none of these has yet been validated for routine use.[42]

A number of computationally intense algorithms have been designed to refine the delivery of radiotherapy to increase dose to the target and reduce normal tissue toxicity. These include 3D conformal radiotherapy and intensity-modulated radiation therapy. There has been an acknowledgment that lesions in patients with NSCLC can alter significantly in their position relative to other anatomic landmarks, leading to the increasing use of image-guided radiotherapy and, as an extension, gated radiotherapy.[43] Defining the target in radiotherapy can be inaccurate due to lesion motion. PET scans are acquired over multiple respiratory cycles. The FDG-avid GTV can be tracked in both space and time to give estimates of where the lesion is at any given point in the respiratory cycle. Lesions that can be categorized as

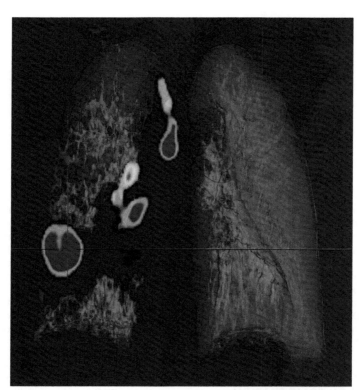

Fig. 2. Although primary tumors usually subtend the segment of lung collapse, hilar nodal disease also can cause secondary bronchial obstruction. In this case, a peripheral primary was masked by collapse caused by prominent central nodal involvement.

highly mobile may be suitable for the use of gated radiotherapy, in which treatment is delivered only at part of the respiratory cycle (**Fig. 3**). Gating or other forms of motion management, such as breath-holding techniques, can be used to minimize the target volumes and spare normal lung. Incorporating PET alters PTV in most series in which this has been studied.[44,45]

THE ROLES OF ^{18}F-FLUORODEOXYGLUCOSE–POSITRON EMISSION TOMOGRAPHY/COMPUTED TOMOGRAPHY IN THE POSTTREATMENT EVALUATION OF NON–SMALL CELL LUNG CANCER

The role of imaging after an attempt at cure in NSCLC remains controversial. Based on a lack of published evidence of benefit, most clinical guidelines do not recommend PET/CT, or even in some cases CT, for the routine follow-up of patients who have had therapy of lung cancer with curative intent.[46] The main justification for surveillance has been screening for complications of the previous therapy. In general terms, no test should be performed if the patient or the referring clinician is not prepared to act on the results.

There is a group of patients in whom the original attempt at cure leads to such a severe loss of physiologic reserve as to render them unsuitable for further salvage therapies, but there are some patients at risk of localized relapse in whom posttreatment surveillance could be beneficial by more sensitively detecting residual or recurrent disease and excluding distant metastases at recurrence.[47]

As with pretreatment staging, FDG-PET is able to detect lesions earlier than CT, leading to an improvement in the detection of curable recurrence. In a study of 100 patients treated with curative intent with chemoradiation, van Loon and colleagues[48] added an FDG-PET/CT scan 3 months after therapy. FDG-PET alone detected the 3 patients who were suitable for radical salvage therapy but CT did not. In 24 of 100 patients with progressive disease at 3 months, if the patient had symptoms (n = 16) or asymptomatic disease detectable by CT (n = 5), no curative therapy was possible. In a report from our own group, PET imaging at the time of suspected relapse was able to classify patients into groups with no disease, localized disease, or advanced disease, all with widely differing survival probabilities.[49]

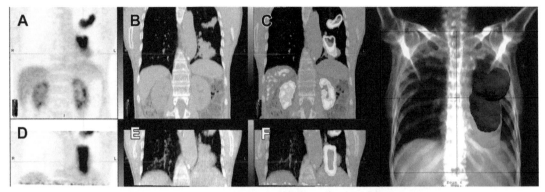

Fig. 3. Acquisition of FDG-PET during normal tidal volume breathing and CT at a random instant during the respiratory cycle with the subsequent fusion of these images as displayed in panels A to C, respectively, leads to respiratory blurring of the metabolic image, as indicated by the smudge of activity extending inferior to the primary tumor and the potential misregistration of the metabolic and anatomic information. Acquiring both the PET and CT studies gated to respiration and creating maximum intensity projection images of these same 3 datasets, as represented in panels D to F, respectively, demonstrates the high degree of respiratory movement in the inferiorly placed primary lesion. The far right panel represents radiation treatment volumes planned on the basis of both normal (3D) and gated (4D) acquisitions. The PTV, based on 3D PET-CT data is colored red with the added volume attributed to the 4D dataset seen in cyan. Concordant 3D and 4D PTVs are depicted as a color-wash of the 2 and are depicted as the puce-colored region. In this particular case, the PTV was enlarged to account for the 35-mm range of motion of the lesion in space.

THE ROLE OF ^{18}F-FLUORODEOXYGLUCOSE–POSITRON EMISSION TOMOGRAPHY/COMPUTED TOMOGRAPHY IN TREATMENT RESPONSE EVALUATION

Conventional response assessment of cancer after therapy using CT relies on unidimensional or bidimensional measures of tumor before and after treatment. This can be particularly problematic in lung cancer because of the presence of tumor-related atelectasis before treatment and the effects of treatment after its delivery. Posttherapy effects include radiation pneumonitis, infection, and postsurgical scarring, all of which can obscure tumor boundaries. Furthermore, because of the use of nodal size for assessing nodal response, a lymph node that responded only partially to treatment and reduced in size to smaller than 1 cm would wrongly be considered to have attained a complete response on CT.

When FDG-PET first became available for clinical use, there was a strong rationale for investigating its use for response assessment after potentially curative therapies. It was hoped that PET could overcome some of the limitations of CT listed previously. At that time, there were no established criteria for metabolic response assessment. Our group developed response assessment criteria that were based on visual rather than quantitative data and used them prospectively in cohorts of patients with lung cancer.[50,51] Patients were classified into 4 metabolic response category groups as follows:

1. Complete Metabolic Response: No abnormal tumor FDG uptake; activity in the tumor is absent or less than mediastinal blood pool.
2. Partial Metabolic Response: Absence of disease progression, any appreciable reduction in the intensity of tumor FDG uptake or tumor volume.
3. Stable Metabolic Disease: Absence of new sites of disease, and no appreciable change in intensity of tumor FDG uptake or volume.
4. Progressive Metabolic Disease: New sites of disease, and or an appreciable increase in intensity of tumor FDG uptake or volume of known sites of tumor.

In a group of 73 patients, we prospectively investigated disease status following chemoradiotherapy.[3] PET visual assessment of response at a median of 70 days posttreatment predicted survival better than CT performed at the same time. In only 40% of cases, FDG and CT assessments of response were identical. There were more complete responders on FDG criteria (n = 34) compared with CT (n = 10), whereas fewer patients were classed as nonresponders (12 vs 20) or non-evaluable (0 vs 6) by PET than CT. PET criteria were able to stratify those patients with assessable disease on CT, better than CT, even after adjusting for known prognostic factors, such as pretreatment stage, ECOG stats, and weight loss. Despite the superiority of PET for response assessment, there have been no large prospective studies that define how this information can be used to adapt further treatment or surveillance strategies. Whether qualitative or semiquantitative parameters should be used also remains controversial. A recent investigation of various semiquantitative measures suggests that posttreatment SUV may be a useful predictor of survival after definitive chemoradiation.[52] In anecdotal cases, residual PET-detected disease has been resected curatively after chemoradiation when the mediastinum has been cleared.

In contrast to the situation of assessing response to already completed treatment, the role of FDG-PET/CT in assessing response to neoadjuvant therapy before definitive resection has been the subject of more intense scrutiny. In 1993, Pisters and colleagues[53] described excellent postoperative outcomes (54% alive at 5 years) in a group of 21 of 73 patients treated with preoperative chemotherapy who were found to have a pathologic complete response (pCR) at a subsequent thoracotomy. The 5-year survival rate was only 15% in those patients without a pCR. It was recognized at the time that although objective responses were seen in all of the 21 with a pCR, only 43% of these patients had a complete response on CT imaging. The lack of predictive power of CT led Vansteenkiste and colleagues[54] to design a study of the utility of metabolic response based on prechemotherapy and postchemotherapy FDG-PET scanning in patients with surgically staged stage IIIa (N2) disease who subsequently had induction therapy before definitive surgical resection. CT was assessed with bidimensional measurements of nodes, and PET used an assessment of visual response by comparing lesion uptake with mediastinal blood pool. Of 15 patients who satisfied study entry criteria, 3 of 9 with persistent N2 nodes on CT criteria were alive at the time of report, whereas 2 of 6 who had mediastinal downstaging subsequently died. On PET criteria, all 7 who had persistent nodal uptake died within the study period, whereas only 1 of 8 patients who had a PET complete response died. The poor predictive value of CT response resulted in no difference in survival based on CT criteria ($P = .73$), whereas survival was strongly predicted by PET response ($P = .0142$). These data suggested that PET could be used to inform decisions concerning surgery after induction therapy. In a further study of 30 patients, Dooms and colleagues[55] subsequently reported that persistent major residual FDG uptake in mediastinal nodes after induction therapy was associated with a dismal prognosis, suggesting that surgery would be inappropriate for such patients. Recent data suggest that semiquantitative measures may provide prognostic stratification in the setting of induction chemotherapy.[56] An area of recent interest has been whether metabolic response early in radiotherapy may also predict eventual response and allow adaptation of treatment.[57,58]

With increasing understanding of the genomic drivers of lung cancer, subgroups of patients with specific mutations are amenable to treatment with biologically targeted therapies. Mutations in the epidermal growth factor receptor constitute one such target. There is accumulating evidence that FDG-PET/CT can provide significantly earlier identification of patients likely to benefit from such therapy than can CT.[59-62]

SUMMARY

The role of PET is continually evolving in lung cancer, but it is already firmly established as the primary noninvasive imaging modality for the staging of patients with lung cancer who are candidates for curative therapies. In the developed world, it is now routine to have an FDG-PET/CT scan before surgery is contemplated for apparently localized NSCLC. The impact of PET in patients with more advanced disease, especially for those being considered for definitive chemoradiation, is even greater. FDG-PET/CT is the imaging modality of choice for targeting tumors during the radiotherapy-planning process. It is also clear that PET is extremely useful in the posttreatment setting. It has a role in decision-making after induction therapy, for assessment of the overall effect of a course of treatment, and for the diagnosis of relapsed disease. At each of these points, it gives prognostic information that is superior to CT. However, there is a dearth of well-conducted prospective trials investigating the best way to use this information and further research is needed to clarify its role in these vital areas.

REFERENCES

1. MacMahon H, Austin JH, Gamsu G, et al. Guidelines for management of small pulmonary nodules detected on CT scans: a statement from the Fleischner Society. Radiology 2005;237(2):395–400.
2. Abou-Zied M, Zubeldia J, Nabi H. Follow-up of patients with single pulmonary nodules and negative 18F-fluorodeoxyglucose positron emission tomography scans. Clin Positron Imaging 2000;3(4):184.
3. Croft DR, Trapp J, Kernstine K, et al. FDG-PET imaging and the diagnosis of non-small cell lung cancer in a region of high histoplasmosis prevalence. Lung Cancer 2002;36(3):297–301.
4. Deppen SA, Blume JD, Kensinger CD, et al. Accuracy of FDG-PET to diagnose lung cancer in areas

with infectious lung disease: a meta-analysis. JAMA 2014;312(12):1227–36.

5. Vansteenkiste JF, Stroobants SG, Dupont PJ, et al. Prognostic importance of the standardized uptake value on (18)F-fluoro-2-deoxy-glucose-positron emission tomography scan in non-small-cell lung cancer: an analysis of 125 cases. Leuven Lung Cancer Group. J Clin Oncol 1999;17(10):3201–6.

6. Lin MY, Wu M, Brennan S, et al. Absence of a relationship between tumor (1)(8)F-fluorodeoxyglucose standardized uptake value and survival in patients treated with definitive radiotherapy for non-small-cell lung cancer. J Thorac Oncol 2014;9(3):377–82.

7. Downey RJ, Akhurst T, Gonen M, et al. Preoperative F-18 fluorodeoxyglucose-positron emission tomography maximal standardized uptake value predicts survival after lung cancer resection. J Clin Oncol 2004;22(16):3255–60.

8. Higashi K, Ito K, Hiramatsu Y, et al. 18F-FDG uptake by primary tumor as a predictor of intratumoral lymphatic vessel invasion and lymph node involvement in non-small cell lung cancer: analysis of a multicenter study. J Nucl Med 2005;46(2):267–73.

9. Schuurbiers OC, Meijer TW, Kaanders JH, et al. Glucose metabolism in NSCLC is histology-specific and diverges the prognostic potential of 18FDG-PET for adenocarcinoma and squamous cell carcinoma. J Thorac Oncol 2014;9:1485–93.

10. Haidar YM, Rahn DA 3rd, Nath S, et al. Comparison of outcomes following stereotactic body radiotherapy for non-small cell lung cancer in patients with and without pathological confirmation. Ther Adv Respir Dis 2014;8(1):3–12.

11. Louie AV, Senan S, Patel P, et al. When is a biopsy-proven diagnosis necessary before stereotactic ablative radiotherapy for lung cancer? A decision analysis. Chest 2014;146(4):1021–8.

12. Hellwig D, Ukena D, Paulsen F, et al, Onko-PET der Deutschen Gesellschaft fur Nuklearmedizin. Meta-analysis of the efficacy of positron emission tomography with F-18-fluorodeoxyglucose in lung tumors. Basis for discussion of the German Consensus Conference on PET in Oncology 2000. Pneumologie 2001;55(8):367–77 [in German].

13. MacManus MR, Hicks R, Fisher R, et al. FDG-PET-detected extracranial metastasis in patients with non-small cell lung cancer undergoing staging for surgery or radical radiotherapy–survival correlates with metastatic disease burden. Acta Oncol 2003; 42(1):48–54.

14. Kalff V, Hicks RJ, MacManus MP, et al. Clinical impact of (18)F fluorodeoxyglucose positron emission tomography in patients with non-small-cell lung cancer: a prospective study. J Clin Oncol 2001;19(1):111–8.

15. MacManus MP, Hicks RJ, Matthews JP, et al. High rate of detection of unsuspected distant metastases

by PET in apparent stage III non-small-cell lung cancer: implications for radical radiation therapy. Int J Radiat Oncol Biol Phys 2001;50(2):287–93.

16. Gould MK, Kuschner WG, Rydzak CE, et al. Test performance of positron emission tomography and computed tomography for mediastinal staging in patients with non-small-cell lung cancer: a meta-analysis. Ann Intern Med 2003;139(11):879–92.

17. Sebro R, Aparici CM, Hernandez-Pampaloni M. FDG PET/CT evaluation of pathologically proven pulmonary lesions in an area of high endemic granulomatous disease. Ann Nucl Med 2013;27(4):400–5.

18. Kim YK, Lee KS, Kim BT, et al. Mediastinal nodal staging of nonsmall cell lung cancer using integrated 18F-FDG PET/CT in a tuberculosis-endemic country: diagnostic efficacy in 674 patients. Cancer 2007;109(6):1068–77.

19. Moloney F, Ryan D, McCarthy L, et al. Increasing the accuracy of 18F-FDG PET/CT interpretation of "mildly positive" mediastinal nodes in the staging of non-small cell lung cancer. Eur J Radiol 2014;83(5):843–7.

20. Kalade AV, Eddie Lau WF, Conron M, et al. Endoscopic ultrasound-guided fine-needle aspiration when combined with positron emission tomography improves specificity and overall diagnostic accuracy in unexplained mediastinal lymphadenopathy and staging of non-small-cell lung cancer. Intern Med J 2008;38(11):837–44.

21. Nestle U, Walter K, Schmidt S, et al. 18F-deoxyglucose positron emission tomography (FDG-PET) for the planning of radiotherapy in lung cancer: high impact in patients with atelectasis. Int J Radiat Oncol Biol Phys 1999;44(3):593–7.

22. Im HJ, Pak K, Cheon GJ, et al. Prognostic value of volumetric parameters of F-FDG PET in non-small-cell lung cancer: a meta-analysis. Eur J Nucl Med Mol Imaging 2014. http://dx.doi.org/10.1007/s00259-014-2903-7. [Epub ahead of print].

23. Takeuchi S, Khiewvan B, Fox PS, et al. Impact of initial PET/CT staging in terms of clinical stage, management plan, and prognosis in 592 patients with non-small-cell lung cancer. Eur J Nucl Med Mol Imaging 2014;41(5):906–14.

24. Gregory DL, Hicks RJ, Hogg A, et al. Effect of PET/CT on management of patients with non-small cell lung cancer: results of a prospective study with 5-year survival data. J Nucl Med 2012;53(7):1007–15.

25. Dunagan D, Chin R Jr, McCain T, et al. Staging by positron emission tomography predicts survival in patients with non-small cell lung cancer. Chest 2001;119(2):333–9.

26. van Tinteren H, Hoekstra OS, Smit EF, et al. Effectiveness of positron emission tomography in the preoperative assessment of patients with suspected non-small-cell lung cancer: the PLUS multicentre randomised trial. Lancet 2002;359(9315): 1388–93.

27. Naidich DP, Bankier AA, MacMahon H, et al. Recommendations for the management of subsolid pulmonary nodules detected at CT: a statement from the Fleischner Society. Radiology 2013;266(1):304–17.

28. Everitt S, Herschtal A, Callahan J, et al. High rates of tumor growth and disease progression detected on serial pretreatment fluorodeoxyglucose-positron emission tomography/computed tomography scans in radical radiotherapy candidates with nonsmall cell lung cancer. Cancer 2010;116(21):5030–7.

29. Geiger GA, Kim MB, Xanthopoulos EP, et al. Stage migration in planning PET/CT scans in patients due to receive radiotherapy for non-small-cell lung cancer. Clin Lung Cancer 2014;15(1):79–85.

30. Booth K, Hanna GG, McGonigle N, et al. The mediastinal staging accuracy of 18F-fluorodeoxyglycose positron emission tomography/computed tomography in non-small cell lung cancer with variable time intervals to surgery. Ulster Med J 2013;82(2):75–81.

31. Mac Manus MP, Hicks RJ, Ball DL, et al. F-18 fluorodeoxyglucose positron emission tomography staging in radical radiotherapy candidates with nonsmall cell lung carcinoma: powerful correlation with survival and high impact on treatment. Cancer 2001;92(4):886–95.

32. Siva S, Shaw M, Chesson B, et al. Analysis of the impact of chest wall constraints on eligibility for a randomized trial of stereotactic body radiotherapy of peripheral stage I non-small cell lung cancer. J Med Imaging Radiat Oncol 2012;56(6):654–60.

33. Crabtree TD, Denlinger CE, Meyers BF, et al. Stereotactic body radiation therapy versus surgical resection for stage I non-small cell lung cancer. J Thorac Cardiovasc Surg 2010;140(2):377–86.

34. Eschmann SM, Friedel G, Paulsen F, et al. FDG PET for staging of advanced non-small cell lung cancer prior to neoadjuvant radio-chemotherapy. Eur J Nucl Med Mol Imaging 2002;29(6):804–8.

35. Kolodziejczyk M, Kepka L, Dziuk M, et al. Impact of [18F]fluorodeoxyglucose PET-CT staging on treatment planning in radiotherapy incorporating elective nodal irradiation for non-small-cell lung cancer: a prospective study. Int J Radiat Oncol Biol Phys 2011;80(4):1008–14.

36. Mac Manus MP, Wong K, Hicks RJ, et al. Early mortality after radical radiotherapy for non-small-cell lung cancer: comparison of PET-staged and conventionally staged cohorts treated at a large tertiary referral center. Int J Radiat Oncol Biol Phys 2002;52(2):351–61.

37. Denham JW, Dobbs HJ, Hamilton CS. ICRU 50: a commentary. Australas Radiol 1994;38(3):204–7.

38. Giraud P, Antoine M, Larrouy A, et al. Evaluation of microscopic tumor extension in non-small-cell lung cancer for three-dimensional conformal radiotherapy planning. Int J Radiat Oncol Biol Phys 2000;48(4):1015–24.

39. Li WL, Yu JM, Liu GH, et al. A comparative study on radiology and pathology target volume in non-small-cell lung cancer. Zhonghua Zhong Liu Za Zhi 2003; 25(6):566–8 [in Chinese].

40. Mac Manus MP, Everitt S, Bayne M, et al. The use of fused PET/CT images for patient selection and radical radiotherapy target volume definition in patients with non-small cell lung cancer: results of a prospective study with mature survival data. Radiother Oncol 2013;106(3):292–8.

41. Bayne M, Hicks RJ, Everitt S, et al. Reproducibility of "intelligent" contouring of gross tumor volume in non-small-cell lung cancer on PET/CT images using a standardized visual method. Int J Radiat Oncol Biol Phys 2010;77(4):1151–7.

42. Macmanus MP, Hicks RJ. Where do we draw the line? Contouring tumors on positron emission tomography/computed tomography. Int J Radiat Oncol Biol Phys 2008;71(1):2–4.

43. Kubo HD, Len PM, Minohara S, et al. Breathing-synchronized radiotherapy program at the University of California Davis Cancer Center. Med Phys 2000; 27(2):346–53.

44. Vanuytsel LJ, Vansteenkiste JF, Stroobants SG, et al. The impact of (18)F-fluoro-2-deoxy-D-glucose positron emission tomography (FDG-PET) lymph node staging on the radiation treatment volumes in patients with non-small cell lung cancer. Radiother Oncol 2000;55(3):317–24.

45. Erdi YE, Rosenzweig K, Erdi AK, et al. Radiotherapy treatment planning for patients with non-small cell lung cancer using positron emission tomography (PET). Radiother Oncol 2002;62(1):51–60.

46. Colt HG, Murgu SD, Korst RJ, et al. Follow-up and surveillance of the patient with lung cancer after curative-intent therapy: diagnosis and management of lung cancer, 3rd ed: American College of Chest Physicians evidence-based clinical practice guidelines. Chest 2013;143(5 Suppl):e437S–54S.

47. Dane B, Grechushkin V, Plank A, et al. PET/CT vs. non-contrast CT alone for surveillance 1-year post lobectomy for stage I non-small-cell lung cancer. Am J Nucl Med Mol Imaging 2013;3(5):408–16.

48. van Loon J, Grutters J, Wanders R, et al. Follow-up with 18FDG-PET-CT after radical radiotherapy with or without chemotherapy allows the detection of potentially curable progressive disease in non-small cell lung cancer patients: a prospective study. Eur J Cancer 2009;45(4):588–95.

49. Hicks RJ, Kalff V, MacManus MP, et al. The utility of (18)F-FDG PET for suspected recurrent non-small cell lung cancer after potentially curative therapy: impact on management and prognostic stratification. J Nucl Med 2001;42(11):1605–13.

50. Mac Manus MP, Hicks RJ, Matthews JP, et al. Positron emission tomography is superior to computed tomography scanning for response-assessment

after radical radiotherapy or chemoradiotherapy in patients with non-small-cell lung cancer. J Clin Oncol 2003;21(7):1285–92.

51. Mac Manus MP, Hicks RJ, Matthews JP, et al. Metabolic (FDG-PET) response after radical radiotherapy/chemoradiotherapy for non-small cell lung cancer correlates with patterns of failure. Lung Cancer 2005;49(1):95–108.

52. Machtay M, Duan F, Siegel BA, et al. Prediction of survival by [18F]fluorodeoxyglucose positron emission tomography in patients with locally advanced non-small-cell lung cancer undergoing definitive chemoradiation therapy: results of the ACRIN 6668/RTOG 0235 trial. J Clin Oncol 2013;31(30):3823–30.

53. Pisters KM, Kris MG, Gralla RJ, et al. Pathologic complete response in advanced non-small-cell lung cancer following preoperative chemotherapy: implications for the design of future non-small-cell lung cancer combined modality trials. J Clin Oncol 1993;11(9):1757–62.

54. Vansteenkiste JF, De Leyn PR, Deneffe GJ, et al. Vindesine-ifosfamide-platinum (VIP) induction chemotherapy in surgically staged IIIA-N2 non-small-cell lung cancer: a prospective study. Leuven Lung Cancer Group. Ann Oncol 1998;9(3):261–7.

55. Dooms C, Verbeken E, Stroobants S, et al. Prognostic stratification of stage IIIA-N2 non-small-cell lung cancer after induction chemotherapy: a model based on the combination of morphometric-pathologic response in mediastinal nodes and primary tumor response on serial 18-fluoro-2-deoxy-glucose positron emission tomography. J Clin Oncol 2008;26(7):1128–34.

56. Bahce I, Vos CG, Dickhoff C, et al. Metabolic activity measured by FDG PET predicts pathological response in locally advanced superior sulcus NSCLC. Lung Cancer 2014;85(2):205–12.

57. Kong FM, Frey KA, Quint LE, et al. A pilot study of [18F]fluorodeoxyglucose positron emission tomography scans during and after radiation-based therapy in patients with non small-cell lung cancer. J Clin Oncol 2007;25(21):3116–23.

58. Usmanij EA, de Geus-Oei LF, Troost EG, et al. 18F-FDG PET early response evaluation of locally advanced non-small cell lung cancer treated with concomitant chemoradiotherapy. J Nucl Med 2013;54(9):1528–34.

59. Mileshkin L, Hicks RJ, Hughes BG, et al. Changes in 18F-fluorodeoxyglucose and 18F-fluorodeoxythymidine positron emission tomography imaging in patients with non-small cell lung cancer treated with erlotinib. Clin Cancer Res 2011;17(10):3304–15.

60. Dingemans AM, de Langen AJ, van den Boogaart V, et al. First-line erlotinib and bevacizumab in patients with locally advanced and/or metastatic non-small-cell lung cancer: a phase II study including molecular imaging. Ann Oncol 2011;22(3):559–66.

61. Bengtsson T, Hicks RJ, Peterson A, et al. 18F-FDG PET as a surrogate biomarker in non-small cell lung cancer treated with erlotinib: newly identified lesions are more informative than standardized uptake value. J Nucl Med 2012;53(4):530–7.

62. van Gool MH, Aukema TS, Schaake EE, et al. (18)F-fluorodeoxyglucose positron emission tomography versus computed tomography in predicting histopathological response to epidermal growth factor receptor-tyrosine kinase inhibitor treatment in resectable non-small cell lung cancer. Ann Surg Oncol 2014;21(9):2831–7.

PET Imaging of Breast Cancer
Role in Patient Management

Lizza Lebron, MD, Daniel Greenspan, MD, Neeta Pandit-Taskar, MD*

KEYWORDS

- Breast cancer imaging • FDG PET • Metabolic imaging • Prognosis • Fluoroestradiol imaging • FES

KEY POINTS

- Metabolic imaging plays an important role in management of breast cancer.
- Fluorodeoxyglucose (FDG) PET imaging is currently the PET imaging tracer approved by the US Food and Drug Administration.
- FDG PET is not routinely indicated in early stage breast cancer but is recommended (National Comprehensive Cancer Network 2B) for advanced disease patients.
- FDG PET affects management by affecting change in the staging, early assessment of response and provides prognostic and predictive information.
- F16α-[^{18}F]fluoro-17β-estradiol imaging allows assessment of estrogen receptor status of primary and metastatic lesions and may play a role in management of antiestrogen targeted therapy.

INTRODUCTION

Breast cancer is the most common type of cancer in women and the second most fatal cancer. Approximately 12.3% of women will be diagnosed with breast cancer at some point during their lifetime, based on 2008 through 2010 Surveillance, Epidemiology, and End Results Program (SEER) data.[1] Despite the increasing incidence of breast cancer in recent decades, mortality rates are decreasing because of earlier diagnosis and new treatment strategies that incorporate the molecular impact of breast cancer. Initial cancer staging and prediction of prognosis are important aspects in the development of a treatment plan and for deciding personal treatment strategies.

The American Society of Clinical Oncology recommends routine physical examination and periodic mammography for surveillance purposes.[2]

MR imaging may play a role in the evaluation of equivocal lesions seen on mammography, and in identifying disease in those at high risk and with dense breasts.[3,4] Once breast cancer is diagnosed, imaging plays a critical role in the staging of breast cancer (see the American Joint Committee on Cancer [AJCC] guidelines at https://cancerstaging.org/references-tools/quick references/Documents/BreastLarge.pdf). Most conventional imaging methods reflect mainly morphologic change in tumor site and are often inconclusive, particularly after treatment. Molecular imaging studies using PET tracers have the ability to image cellular function and physiology rather than anatomic features, which may play an important role in detecting recurrent disease when posttreatment alteration of anatomy is present.

The authors have nothing to disclose.
Molecular Imaging and Therapy Service, Department of Radiology, Memorial Sloan Kettering Cancer Center, 1275 York Avenue, New York, NY 10065, USA
* Corresponding author.
E-mail address: Pandit-n@mskcc.org

PET Clin 10 (2015) 159–195
http://dx.doi.org/10.1016/j.cpet.2014.12.004

The National Comprehensive Cancer Network (NCCN) guidelines recommend selective use of imaging (**Table 1**). Bone scans are recommended for patients with symptoms or elevated alkaline phosphatase levels. For stage IIIA or higher invasive cancers, bone scan and fluorodeoxyglucose (FDG) PET/Computed tomography (CT) are categorized as 2B, and FDG PET/CT imaging is recommended as optional for evaluation of patients with stage IIIA and higher disease.[5]

MODALITIES FOR MOLECULAR IMAGING WITH RADIOPHARMACEUTICALS IN BREAST CANCER
PET/Computed Tomography Scanners

This modality is based on coincidence imaging of the gamma rays that generate from annihilation of the positron in the tissue, after injection of the positron-emitting tracer. PET/CT is the most commonly clinically used scanning method. FDG is a

Table 1
National Comprehensive Cancer Network guidelines: recommended imaging modalities for workup

Type	Recommendation (US/Mammography)	MR Imaging
Ductal carcinoma in situ/stage 0	Diagnostic mammogram Postoperative mammogram q 12 mo	MR imaging optional (Use of MR imaging has not shown to increase likelihood of negative margins or decrease conversion to mastectomy) FDG PET and bone scan (99m Tc MDP or NaF) not recommended
Stage I, IIa, IIB	Diagnostic mammogram US as needed	MR imaging optional, special consideration for mammography occult tumors For stage I–IIb: additional studies if signs and symptoms Bone scan indicated if bone pain or elevated alkaline phosphatase. Abdominal and/or pelvic CT/MR imaging in case of elevated alkaline phosphatase, abnormal liver function, or abnormal physical examination of abdomen or pelvis Chest CT if pulmonary symptoms are seen
Stage IIIa	Diagnostic mammogram US as needed	MR imaging optional, special consideration for mammography occult tumors Consider: Abdominal and/or pelvic CT/MR imaging, chest CT, bone scan (99m Tc MDP or NaF) - category 2B, and FDG PET scan - category 2B
Stage IIIB	Diagnostic mammogram US as needed	MR imaging optional, special consideration for mammography occult tumors Consider: Abdominal and/or pelvic CT/MR imaging, chest CT, FDG PET scan - category 2B, and bone scan (99m Tc MDP or NaF) - category 2B (not needed if FDG clearly shows bone metastasis)
Stage IV or recurrent disease	Diagnostic mammogram US as needed	Chest CT Abdominal and/or pelvic CT/MR imaging Brain MR imaging for suspected CNS symptoms FDG PET scan - category 2B Bone scan (99m Tc MDP or NaF) - category 2B (not needed if FDG clearly shows bone metastasis) X-rays of asymptomatic bones and long, weight-bearing bones abnormal on bone scan.

Abbreviations: 99m Tc MDP, technetium medronic acid; CNS, central nervous system; FDG, fluorodeoxyglucose; NaF, ^{18}F-sodium fluoride; US, ultrasonography.

glucose analog labeled to the positron-emitting radioisotope fluoride-18 ($t_{1/2} = 110$ min). After intravenous injection of the 18 FDG, images are acquired on a PET/CT scanner that allows for overlay of PET and CT images, which can be evaluated in multiple projections (axial, coronal, and sagittal) for assessment of lesions. The imaging protocol is detailed in **Box 1**.

Positron Emission Mammography

Positron emission mammography is a dedicated PET system for breast imaging. There are several systems that primarily differ from each other in detector geometry and the detector mobility. The positron emission mammography system has 2 flat detectors used for imaging the breast in a manner similar to mammography. The breast is placed and mildly compressed between the 2 detectors and imaged to match the mammography. Limited tomographic reconstruction allows generating images to match mammography. The first commercially available, approved system approved by the US Food and Drug Administration (FDA) was the Flex Solo II PEM (Naviscan, Inc). The system's in-plane resolution is about 2.4 mm, which is one-half of the general PET body scanners.[6] Another commercially available system is the Mammography with Molecular Imaging (MAMMI; Oncovision, Valencia, Spain). This system is based on monolithic LYSO crystals coupled to position-sensitive photomultiplier tubes, has a full ring of detectors, uses full tomographic imaging, and has spatial resolution of 1.6 mm.[7] A meta-analysis that evaluated 8 studies comprising 873 breast lesions showed a pooled

sensitivity of 85% (95% CI, 83%–88%) and a specificity of 79% (95% CI, 74%–83%) on a lesion basis, using FDG imaging with positron emission mammography in women with suspected breast malignancy (**Fig. 1**).[8] Using MAMMI, a feasibility study in 35 women showed greater heterogeneity in tumor uptake compared with the standard PET/CT.[9]

PET MR Imaging

Technical advances in recent years have led to the development of the PET MR scanner, which combines information from dual functional modalities. In a pilot study, simultaneous FDG PET MR whole body imaging was performed in 36 patients with invasive ductal carcinoma. Although more lesions were seen on MR imaging than PET, combined information from both led to improved diagnostic accuracy and confidence. Change in management was noted in 33% of patients.[10] Currently, PET MR imaging is not available in many centers and not used universally in the imaging of breast cancer. The advantages of combined PET MR imaging in the routine evaluation of breast cancer is yet to be explored and delineated, although it is possible that it will improve assessment of equivocal lesions, posttreatment changes, and evaluation of bone or marrow-related disease. Currently, it is used mainly as a research tool.

RADIOPHARMACEUTICALS IN MOLECULAR IMAGING OF BREAST CANCER

A number of PET tracers have been used for targeted imaging of breast cancer (**Table 2**), which are based on a unique mechanism of uptake and reflect a different metabolic function. Of these, FDG PET is FDA-approved for clinical use in breast cancer imaging.

18 Fluorodeoxyglucose PET

As a molecular imaging agent, FDG PET has changed the management of patients in a number of cancers, and is playing an increasing role in the active assessment of breast cancer, enabling confirmation of disease in equivocal lesions, and in early detection of metastatic disease. The uptake of FDG may be related to tumor vascularity, number of tumor cells or disease burden, and the mitotic activity index. FDG uptake in breast tumors is variable in different tumor types and sites[11–13] and is influenced by the phenotype, higher grade, or Ki-67 proliferation index.[14]

FDG has variable sensitivity in detecting disease, depending on the histologic tumor type. Several studies have correlated FDG PET

Box 1
Procedure guidelines for FDG PET imaging

Fasting for 4–6 hours before scan

Screen for diabetes, insulin injection

Finger stick and fasting glucose level check before injection (should be < 200 mg/dL)

Inject tracer IV (10–20 mCi) – generally 10–12 mCi[a]

Image at 45–60 minutes after injection

Void bladder before imaging

Image from skull base to mid thigh

CT (either low dose or diagnostic) done first

Emission scan 5–6 fields, 3 min per field of view

[a]Adult dose.

SNM guidelines. Available at: www.snm.org/guidelines. Accessed date October 20, 2014.

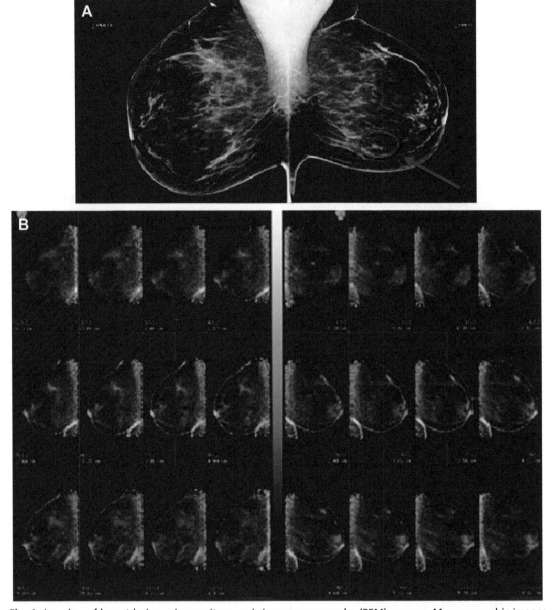

Fig. 1. Imaging of breast lesion using positron emission mammography (PEM) scanner. Mammographic images (*A, B*) show an area of density (*arrow*). PEM (*C, D*) shows no significant uptake favoring a benign etiology. Biopsy confirmed a benign lesion (fibroadenoma). (*Courtesy of* Dr Gustavo Mercier, Boston, MA.)

maximum standardized uptake value (SUV$_{max}$) values with histologic grade, tumor size, or hormonal receptor expression status, all of which are known to be important prognostic indicators for long-term survival of breast cancer patients.[15,16] The standardized uptake values (SUVs) are generally lower in invasive lobular carcinomas (**Fig. 2**).[11,17,18] This is probably owing to the lower density of tumor cells in lobular carcinomas, lower expression of GLUT1, lower proliferation rates, and diffuse infiltrative tumor growth patterns to surrounding tissue, that may lead to false-negative scans.[19] In contrast, greater SUV$_{max}$ values have been found in patients with ductal carcinoma than in other pathologic subtypes of carcinoma (**Fig. 3**).[20] Intratumoral necrosis, usually seen in malignant and rapidly growing tumors, reflects more

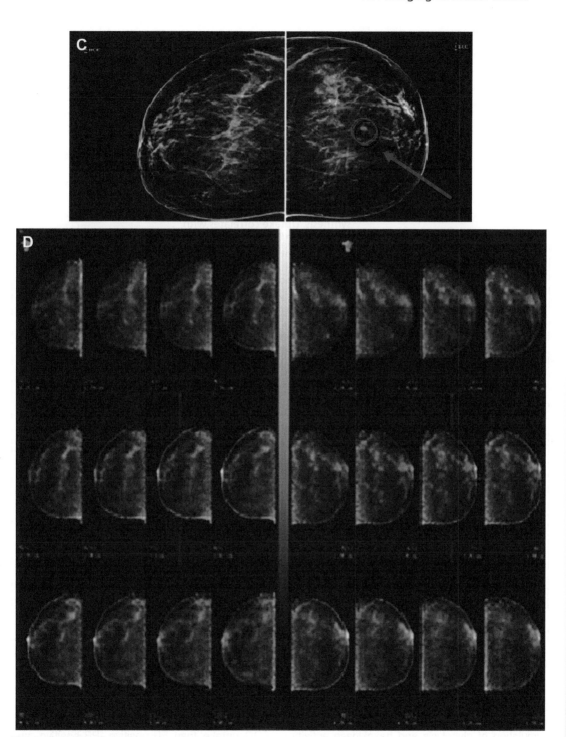

Fig. 1. (*continued*)

aggressive behavior and is associated with high FDG uptake.[17] Poorly differentiated tumors are more aggressive tumors and are more FDG avid (**Fig. 4**).

Variability of FDG uptake is also noted to be related to the receptor expression. Those with high estrogen receptor (ER) expression generally have lower uptake[21,22] than those with negative

Table 2
PET tracers in imaging of breast cancer

PET Tracers	Class	Biochemical Mechanism	Clinical Application
F18-FDG	Glucose metabolism	Uptake based on increased glycolysis and glucose transporters of tumor cells	Staging in advanced disease, detection of recurrent disease, Prognostic value, and assessment of therapeutic response
F18-FLT	Cell proliferation	Substrates for cytosolic thymidine kinase-1 (TK1) which catalyzes the initial metabolic step of thymidine triphosphate synthesis. Uptake correlates with proliferation index ki-67	Staging, monitoring, and prediction of response to treatment
F18-FES	Estrogen receptor	Estrogen receptor analog. Uptake correlates with estrogen receptor concentration.	Molecular information of ER expression in both primary tumor and metastasis. Prediction of response to antiestrogen therapy.
F18-FFNP	Progesterone receptor	Progesterone analogue, uptake based on presence of progesterone receptor.	Molecular information of PR status in primary and metastatic disease.
64Cu or 68Ga-trastuzumab or 89Zr-trastuzumab)	HER2 receptor	Targets HER2 receptor	Assessing human epidermal growth factor receptor 2 (HER2) expression status in tumors. Potential for prognostic information and prediction of response to Her2 targeted therapy.
11C-choline or 18F-choline	Membrane Lipid Synthesis	Intracellular phosphorylation by choline kinase to phosphoryl choline. Associated with phospholipids of cell membrane and tumor growth.	Assessment of tumor progression and Monitoring response to therapy
11C-methionine	Amino Acid Transport	Uptake related to amino acid transport in tumor cells	Assessment of disease, response to therapy and distinguishing responders from nonresponders
18F-fluoride-PET	Skeletal imaging	Bone seeking. Uptake related to increased local blood flow, osteoblastic activity, and bone mineralization	Staging; and evaluation of metastatic disease in advanced tumors and recurrent disease.

Abbreviations: F18-FDG, 2-[18F]-fluoro-2-deoxy-D-glucose; F18-FES, 16α-[18F]-fluoro-17β-estradiol; F18-FFNP, 18F-fluoro furanyl norprogesterone; F18-FLT, 3′-deoxy-3′[18F]fluorothymidine.

ER expression.[20,23,24] Tumors with influence of estradiol may show greater uptake through the stimulation of glycolysis and hexokinase activity via membrane-initiated E(2) action that activates the PI3K-Akt pathway.[22] Those with triple-negative disease (ER-, progesterone receptor [PR]-, HER2/neu-) disease have poor prognosis and more aggressive disease. Koolen and colleagues[25] showed that FDG imaging is more useful in those with triple-negative disease, which tend to show higher FDG uptake (**Fig. 5**). Similar findings have been reported by others with triple-negative breast tumors being associated with higher FDG uptake than ER-positive, PR-positive, and HER2-negative tumors.[26,27] A study by Koo and colleagues[18] showed a 1.67-fold higher SUV_{max} value in triple-negative tumors compared with luminal A tumors ($P<.001$) after adjustment for invasive tumor size, lymph node involvement status, and histologic grade in the multivariate regression analysis, which is similar to results for SUV_{max} from other studies. HER2-positive breast cancers

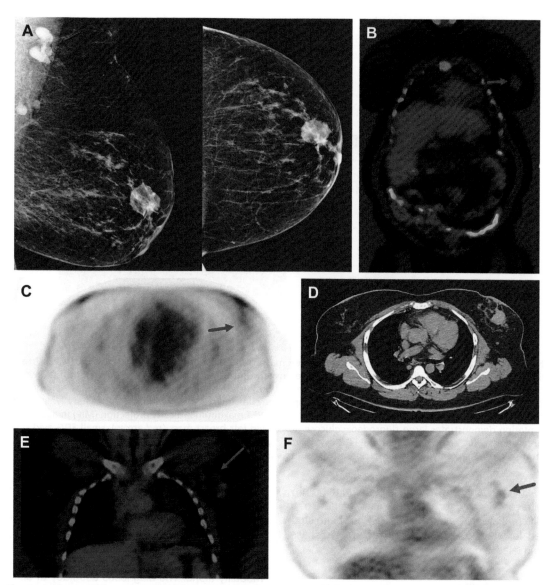

Fig. 2. A 54-year-old woman with left invasive lobular cancer and lobular carcinoma in situ metastatic to lymph nodes. Left mammogram craniocaudal and mediolateral oblique projections demonstrating a dense spiculated mass (*A, pink arrow*) with irregular margins in the upper outer quadrant, anterior third depth, suspicious for malignancy. Prominent round axillary lymph nodes are also visualized (*A, purple arrow*). Coronal fused PET/CT image (*B*) and axial PET image (*C*) showing the spiculated mass in the left breast with minimal fluorodeoxyglucose avidity (*B, purple arrow; C, red arrow*; standardized uptake value [SUV] of 2.1) corresponding to the mass on axial CT image (*D*). Coronal PET/CT fused (*E*) and PET images (*F*) show mild uptake in the enlarged left axillary lymph nodes (*red arrows*; SUV of 1.6–2.2).

are characterized by a high expression of HER2 gene, which promotes tumor growth and progression and therefore tends to be more aggressive and FDG avid. They are less responsive to hormone treatment. Clinically, the HER2-positive subtype is associated with a higher rate of recurrence and mortality, although anti-HER2 treatment has improved survival outcomes in the last decade. False-positive scans may be seen in patients with benign conditions like granulomatous

lymphadenitis or sarcoidosis, which are especially common in mediastinal nodes (**Fig. 6**).[28,29] Fat necrosis may also show increased FDG uptake and mimic disease.[30] Additionally, acute and chronic inflammation, physiologic lactation (**Fig. 7**), and benign breast masses, including silicone granuloma, fibroadenoma, and postoperative changes, may show increased FDG uptake on PET/CT.[31] A good correlation with clinical history and physical condition of the patient and correlation with other

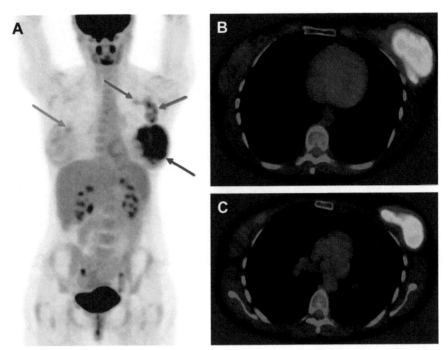

Fig. 3. A 62-year-old woman with a small, spiculated mass in the right breast and large mass in the left breast. Biopsies revealed poorly differentiated, high-grade, invasive ductal adenocarcinoma on the right and invasive ductal adenocarcinoma with lobular features on the left, both triple negative. Axillary lymph nodes were positive bilaterally. The patient was treated with right lumpectomy, left mastectomy, and bilateral axillary lymph node dissection, with adjuvant chemoradiation. (*A*) Whole body PET maximum intensity projection (MIP) image at presentation demonstrates large fluorodeoxyglucose (FDG) avid left breast mass (*red arrow*), small FDG avid right breast mass (*blue arrow*), and bilateral FDG avid axillary lymph nodes (*green arrows*). Axial fused images demonstrate a large markedly FDG avid left breast mass and small FDG avid right breast mass (*B, C*).

imaging (including findings on mammography, ultrasonography, or MR imaging) can help to differentiate malignancy. FDG PET has been studied for staging, evaluation of recurrent disease, and assessment of tumor response.

Role in Staging

Several studies have suggested that FDG PET/CT has a higher detection rate of metastases compared with conventional imaging procedures, based on histologic confirmation of additional lesions or imaging follow-up. FDG PET has limited role in early stage cancers; however, it can detect local and distant metastatic sites in advanced cancers and high-risk cancer.[32–36] In early stage disease, the yield of FDG imaging is low, although the specificity is high.[37] For those with early disease and small tumors, when standard conventional imaging is negative for axillary nodal disease, the value of FDG PET is limited and not recommended for routine evaluation.[38]

In combination with ultrasonography, it improves the accuracy of axillary node detection. Using the criteria of positivity as an axillary lymph node with focal uptake (with an SUV of ≥ 2 and a length-to-width ratio of ≤ 1.5, cortical thickening of ≥ 3 mm, or compression of the hilum on ultrasonography in the ipsilateral axilla on FDG PET), it was found that the combined sensitivity of ultrasonography and FDG was greater than for either modality alone. The diagnostic accuracy of ultrasonography was 78.8%, for FDG PET it was 76.4%, and for combined ultrasonography and FDG PET is was 91.6%.[39] Inflammatory breast cancer, an uncommon and aggressive malignant form, may benefit from FDG PET imaging (**Fig. 8**). In 59 patients with inflammatory breast cancer, FDG PET detected ipsilateral axillary nodes in 90% and extra-axillary areas in 56% of patients. About 31% of cases showed distant disease by FDG. Compared with clinical examination, the axillary lymph node status by FDG PET upstaged disease in 35 and downstaged in 5 patients. Pathologically, 86% were true positives by FDG PET.[40] FDG PET has incremental value over contrast-enhanced CT in locoregional and distant metastasis in inflammatory cancers.[41] FDG PET in advanced breast cancer is helpful in local staging and particularly helpful in evaluation of internal

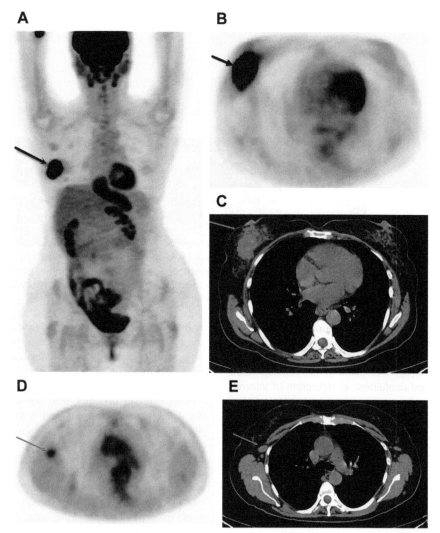

Fig. 4. A 62-year-old female with large right breast mass. Pathology revealed poorly differentiated ductal adeno-carcinoma, HER2$^+$, with biopsy-proven axillary lymph node metastases. (*A*) Whole body PET MIP image at presentation demonstrates intensely FDG avid right breast mass (SUV 10.3, *black arrow*) Axial PET image (*B, black arrow*) with correlating noncontrast CT image (*C*) demonstrates FDG avid right breast mass (*blue arrow*). Axial PET image (*D*) and corresponding axial non-contrast CT image (*E*) at the level of the axilla demonstrates enlarged, FDG avid right axillary lymphadenopathy (*blue arrows*, SUV 2.4).

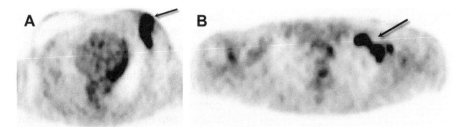

Fig. 5. A 67-year-old woman with history of lobular carcinoma of the right breast, status post total mastectomy 10 years prior, presented with discomfort of the left breast. Further investigation revealed a triple-negative adenocarcinoma with squamous differentiation. (*A*) Axial PET image demonstrates a large CRT left breast mass (*arrow*). (*B*) Axial PET image demonstrating FDG avid left subpectoral lymphadenopathy (*arrow*). The patient was treated with left mastectomy and chemoradiotherapy.

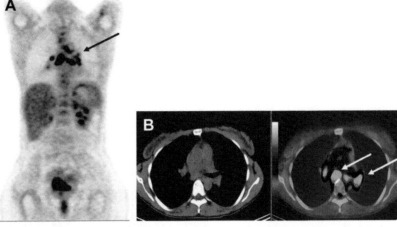

Fig. 6. Patient for follow-up of recurrent disease was imaged with fluorodeoxyglucose (FDG) PET. Coronal PET image (*A*) and axial CT and fused PET/CT images (*B*) show multiple nodes in the mediastinum, including subcarinal, bilateral hilar, and paratracheal adenopathy (*black and white arrows*). Patient had history of sarcoidosis, which was the likely cause of uptake. Patient did not have any other sites of disease.

mammary nodes and distant nodal metastasis. In many cases, distant nodes that are otherwise not suspicious owing to small size can be detected (**Figs. 9** and **10**). An initial small retrospective study reported usefulness in detection of internal

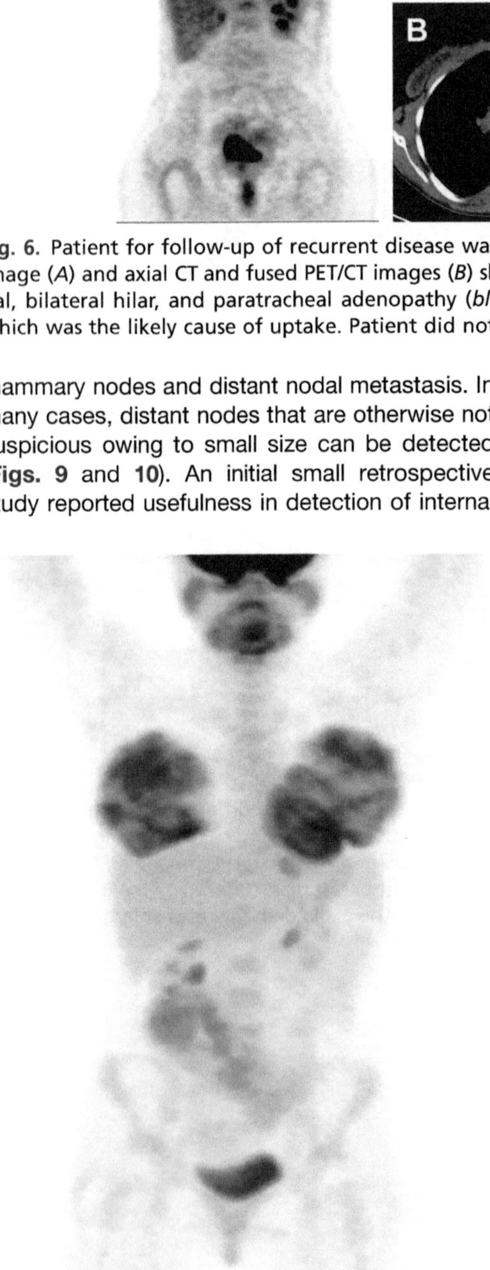

Fig. 7. Fluorodeoxyglucose (FDG) accumulation in the breasts of a lactating patient.

mammary nodes in locally advanced cancer.[42] The study was limited by lack of pathologic correlation and clinical follow-up was used to determine usefulness of FDG uptake in internal mammary nodes.

Most data in patients with stage I and early stage II breast cancer suggest a low diagnostic yield for FDG PET/CT[43,44]; a basis for NCCN consensus guidelines that systemic staging, including FDG PET/CT, is not indicated for early stage breast cancer in the absence of signs or symptoms suggesting metastasis.[5] Owing to the low FDG avidity of lobular carcinoma or low-grade malignancy that inherently are not FDG avid, the benefit of routine use is limited (**Fig. 11**). In addition, the low avidity leads to greater false-negative results in these patients. Small lesions may also be missed, particularly nodes or small lung nodules. The incremental value of FDG PET has mainly been the ability to help evaluate the equivocal findings on standard imaging. It is recommended in advanced and aggressive tumors with greater risk for metastatic disease.[5] In some cases, unknown sites of distant metastasis can be detected even though the standard imaging is negative for lesions (see **Figs. 4** and **5**).

Limited data exist for the use of combined PET MR for routine staging. A recent small retrospective analysis in 36 patients with histologically confirmed invasive ductal carcinoma, which were imaged with PET MR for primary staging, showed best diagnostic confidence score with PET MR imaging compared with each modality alone. PET MR was able to detect unsuspected contralateral disease in 2 of 36 patients (5.5%). About 23 of 47 satellite lesions that were detected on DCE

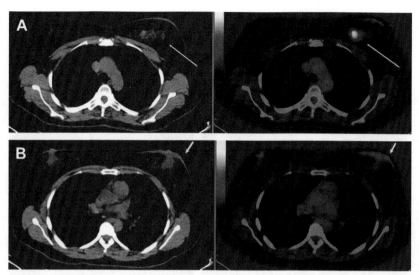

Fig. 8. Fluorodeoxyglucose (FDG) PET in inflammatory carcinoma. (*A, B*) Uptake is seen in primary tumor (*arrow*) and associated skin thickening (*short arrows*).

MR imaging were FDG avid, and 21 patients showed multifocality and multicentricity of disease. The performance of MR imaging was slightly better and distant disease was found in 22% of patients, with significantly more sites seen on MR imaging compared with FDG (105 vs 91 metastatic lesions, respectively). Overall, PET MR imaging led to a change in management for 12 patients (33.3%).[10] More studies and larger datasets are needed to confirm these findings.

Role in Assessment of Response to Neoadjuvant Therapy

The ability of FDG PET to show metabolic changes to treatment allows for early detection of response and prediction of the efficacy of treatment (**Fig. 12**). Those who are unlikely to respond generally show an increase in uptake or sites of disease. Significant data exist in support of FDG PET in the clinical management of patients. Most of the prospective response evaluation studies are done with 18F-FDG as a tracer. The evaluation has been performed predominantly in the neoadjuvant setting with reference to subsequent pathologic response at definitive surgery. The changes in FDG uptake have been found to be the strongest indicator for the evaluation of response to treatment.[45] In this context, changes in FDG uptake, quantified using SUVs, are evaluable serially and as early as after the first cycles of chemotherapy, and can differentiate between responding and nonresponding tumors.[46,47] Serial imaging is generally needed and comparison with baseline imaging is done to evaluate for lesion uptake and number of sites seen (**Fig. 13**). Prospective data in the

metastatic setting are more limited but indicate that in mixed skeletal and visceral disease the change in lesion SUV_{max} on sequential 18F-FDG PET/CT similarly differentiates between responders and nonresponders after a single cycle of chemotherapy.[48] Most data evaluated are from patients with advanced disease. The reported sensitivity and specificity are as high as 83.3% and 78.9%, respectively,[49] for differentiation of responders from nonresponders; however, the specificity is lower. FDG improves patient management by avoiding unnecessary chemotherapy[50] and detecting increased metabolic activity, uptake of FDG, and new sites of disease (**Fig. 14**).

In patients receiving docetaxel neoadjuvant chemotherapy, an SUV_{max} reduction rate of less than 18% was associated with a lack of significant responses and may be an indicator of nonresponse to docetaxel.[51] However, there are no uniform data of a similar threshold of SUV change that can predict response in neoadjuvant therapy. FDG uptake in locoregional disease measured as SUV_{max} is associated with prognostic factors, such as tumor size, grade, and histology, and is predictive of response.[52] FDG uptake and change after 1 course of chemotherapy in luminal HER2-negative breast tumors have shown to be early surrogate markers of patient survival, and those with persistent hypermetabolic activity reflecting poor response in tumors were correlated with poor prognosis at 5 years and can be identified early.[53]

A meta-analysis of FDG PET in early assessment of response to treatment, from 15 studies and a total of 745 patients, showed an overall sensitivity of 80% (95% CI, 74%–83%) and specificity of 79% (95% CI, 74.1%–83%).[54] The

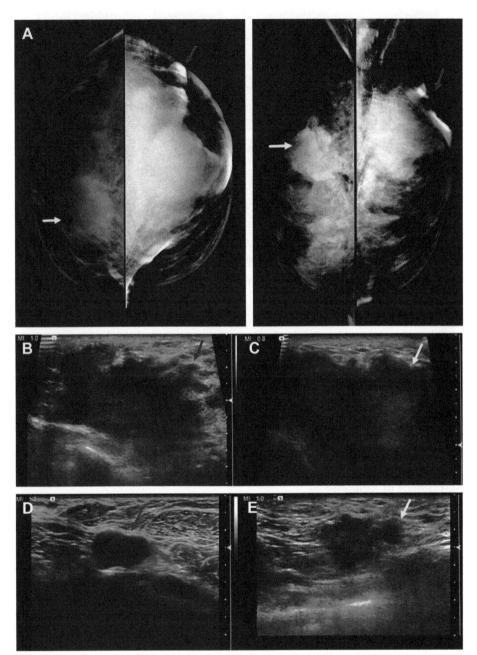

Fig. 9. A 47-year-old woman with bilateral palpable breast masses, biopsy-proven estrogen receptor/progesterone receptor–positive invasive ductal carcinomas bilaterally. (*A*) Bilateral mammogram (craniocaudal and mediolateral oblique views) demonstrates an extremely dense breast parenchymal pattern and mass in the right upper inner quadrant, with microcalcifications (*yellow arrow*). A large, ulcerated mass is present in the superior left breast occupying the medial and lateral quadrants from anterior to posterior depth, extending from the chest wall to the skin (*pink arrow*). Ultrasonography (*B*) and (*C*) shows hypoechoic, irregular masses with posterior acoustic shadowing, in the right breast at 2:00 axis (*B, pink arrow*) and superior left breast (*C, yellow arrow*), corresponding to the mammographic findings and abnormal right and left axillary lymph nodes (*D, pink arrow; E, pink arrow*). PET maximum intensity projection image (*F*) and fused image (*G*) demonstrating intense fluorodeoxyglucose (FDG) uptake in bilateral breast cancers (*F* and *G, pink arrows*; standard uptake volume of 6.2, 7.8 - right and left breast, respectively), and masses on axial CT image (*H*). Additionally, FDG avid suspicious metastatic disease sites were seen in lymph nodes (*F, purple arrows*), sternum (*F, yellow arrow*), and liver (*F* and *I, turquoise arrow*).

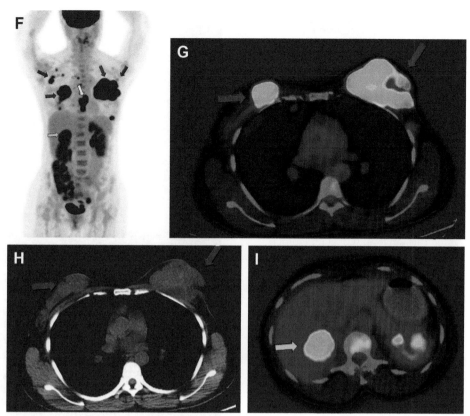

Fig. 9. (*continued*)

evaluation in the preoperative setting is, however, less sensitivity with FDG compared with MR imaging in microscopic or minimal residual disease setting.[55] FDG imaging can also be used to evaluate response to receptor-targeted therapy with aromatase inhibitors and trastuzumab therapy and has prognostic value.[56] A meta-analysis of 73 studies showed that FDG PET is not sensitive enough to detect small primary and metastatic tumors. A complete biochemical response identified

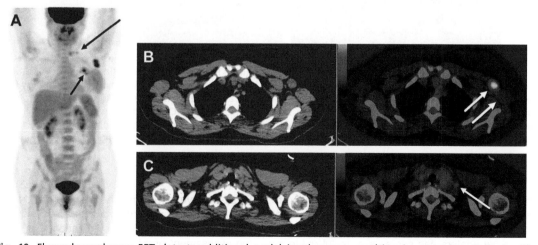

Fig. 10. Fluorodeoxyglucose PET detects additional nodal involvement, resulting in upstaging. Patient with breast carcinoma. Uptake is seen in primary tumor on maximum intensity projection (MIP) images (*A, arrows*). In addition, left axillary node and small left supraclavicular nodes are also seen (fused images; *B, C arrows*, and *long arrow* on MIP [*A*]) that were positive for metastatic disease on pathology.

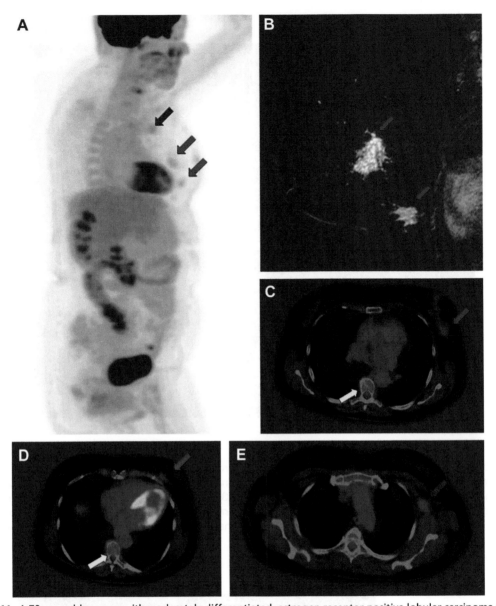

Fig. 11. A 70-year-old woman with moderately differentiated, estrogen receptor-positive lobular carcinoma with signet ring cell features. (*A*) Maximum intensity projection (MIP) PET image demonstrating minimal fluorodeoxyglucose (FDG) avidity (less than mediastinal blood pool) in left breast masses and left axillary adenopathy (*purple arrow*). Contrast-enhanced breast MR image (*B*), showing 2 left breast masses measuring up to 3.2 cm (*pink arrows*), correlating to the 2 masses seen on PET/CT. Fused PET/CT images (*C, D, E*) demonstrating minimally FDG avid left breast masses and left axillary adenopathy (*purple arrow*). Additional lesions were seen in spine on CT; however, they were non–FDG avid, as expected given the low FDG avidity of primary tumor (*C, D, yellow arrow*).

by FDG PET should not be relied on to mean an absence of disease because the technique cannot detect residual microscopic elements.[57] FDG imaging parameters can serve as a useful guide in stratifying patients for therapy.[58] Those with greater uptake are likely more aggressive and hence may need prompt and intense treatment.

False-positive results may be seen owing to post-treatment inflammatory processes, or may be masked by physiologic accumulation that limits the assessment of minimal disease, for example, in the liver. In certain cases, for example, if pleural effusion has been treated by pleurodesis, changes may lead to FDG uptake that may mimic tumor

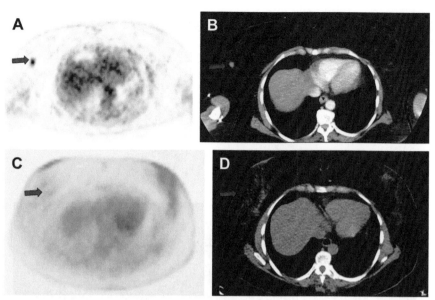

Fig. 12. A 52-year-old woman with right breast estrogen/progesterone receptor–positive HER2/neu equivocal, invasive ductal carcinoma. PET/CT was performed to evaluate treatment response. (*A*) Axial PET image shows fluorodeoxyglucose (FDG) avid focus (*pink arrow*) corresponding with a 6-mm right breast lesion seen on axial CT image (*B, pink arrow*). Postchemotherapy PET/CT scan (*C*) shows resolution of FDG avidity in the right breast (*pink arrow*) along the lesion that has near completely resolved on CT (*D, pink arrow*).

uptake. Distinction of pleurodesis-related uptake versus tumor may be difficult and CT may help in delineating chronic changes of pleurodesis (**Fig. 15**). It is limited in its use for assessment of those with low FDG avidity and small lesions that cannot be detected by PET. Limited preliminary data suggest improved detection and prediction of response to treatment with combined

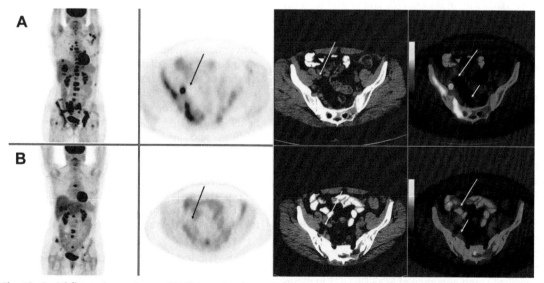

Fig. 13. Serial fluorodeoxyglucose (FDG) imaging for evaluation of treatment response. After the worsening (see **Fig. 14**), the patient's treatment was changed to a new chemotherapeutic agent. Maximum intensity projection (MIP) image (*A*) shows multiple foci of uptake seen to localize in the skeleton. In addition, focal uptake is seen in right pelvic external iliac node (*arrow*) and liver (*long arrow*). Follow-up imaging at 6 months (MIP; *B*) after systemic treatment shows significant decrease in number and uptake of FDG-avid sites in skeleton (*short white arrow*), lesions in liver (*A, B, short arrow*), and resolution of the iliac node (transaxials, *long white arrow*).

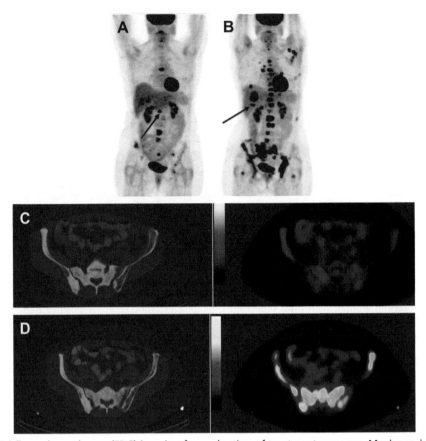

Fig. 14. Serial fluorodeoxyglucose (FDG) imaging for evaluation of treatment response. Maximum intensity projection (MIP) image (*A*) shows multiple foci of uptake in the skeleton (*C*) at multiple sites, and also in the liver (*arrow*). Follow-up imaging 4 months later (MIP; *B*) after systemic treatment shows significant increase in number of FDG-avid sites in skeleton (*D*) and in liver (*B, arrow*).

FDG and F16α-[^{18}F]fluoro-17β-estradiol (FES) imaging.[59]

Role in Evaluation of Recurrent Disease

FDG PET has an average sensitivity and specificity of 96% and 77%, respectively, in the detection of recurrent breast cancer. It has greater sensitivity than conventional imaging, although specificity is lower for tumor detection, especially of certain histology and small size tumors (**Fig. 16**).[60]

The predominant advantage of FDG PET is in detecting distant metastatic sites, disease in normal-sized nodes (**Figs. 17** and **18**), confirming disease in equivocal disease, and detection of more sites as compared with CT.[61] The sensitivity, specificity, and accuracy of FDG PET/CT in recurrent disease is reported as high as 97%, 92%, and 95%, respectively. In 32 of 56 patients (57%), PET/CT localized more tumor sites. Distant metastases and additional sites of disease were detected in significantly more patients compared with conventional imaging (45%), and changed management in 48% of them. In 36% of patients, extensive surgery was prevented and treatment was changed to palliative treatment.[62] FDG imaging can, therefore, change management in patients (**Fig. 19**).[63,64] Assessment of small lung nodules and liver disease may be limited. A meta-analysis of 73 studies showed that FDG PET is not sensitive enough to detect small metastatic tumors and small volume recurrent disease. A complete response or lack of disease identified by FDG PET is not reliable because the sensitivity for residual microscopic disease is low.[57]

Prognostic Value and Impact on Management of Fluorodeoxyglucose PET Imaging

The prognosis of breast cancer patients has significantly improved over the last decade, reaching an overall 5-year relative survival of 79%. The 5-year relative survival decreases to 55% and 18% in cases of locally advanced tumors and metastatic

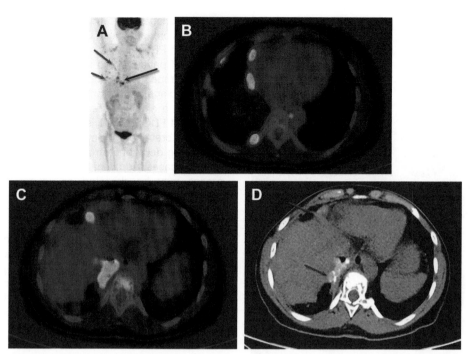

Fig. 15. A 54-year-old female with high-grade invasive ductal adenocarcinoma, ER/PR+, HER-, of the right breast, status post-lumpectomy and lymph node dissection. Later, patient presented with shortness of breath and was found to have malignant large right pleural effusion and had pleurodesis. Two years later, patient underwent PET scan for evaluation of recurrent disease. (*A*) MIP whole body PET image demonstrates multiple foci of increased FDG activity (*red and black arrows*), which localized to pleural nodularity (axial fused images *B* and *C*), corresponding to the nodular pleural calcifications seen on noncontrast axial CT (*D*) images (*red arrows*). The uptake mostly corresponds to the dense calcified regions, and may be secondary to post-plerodesis changes; however, associated malignant tissue can also cause this. Therefore, in these cases, distinction of tumor versus post-pleurodesis change is difficult to differentiate on PET. Associated CT findings and follow-up studies generally help distinguish.

disease, respectively.[1] Thus, a precise knowledge of the extent of disease is essential for adequate management and prognostic stratification in newly diagnosed breast cancer.

FDG PET/CT provides more accurate staging information to stratify prognostic risk, more in advanced cancers, compared with conventional imaging alone. High uptake reflects aggressive tumors and has poor prognosis (see **Fig. 2**). Additionally, tumor burden as detected by FDG and its correlation with histology is predictive of outcomes and impacts management of disease. FDG uptake correlates with tumor aggressiveness and prognostic factors, such as histologic type, grade, proliferation index, and receptor status; therefore, those with greater uptake on FDG carry a poorer prognosis than those with low FDG uptake (**Fig. 20**).[65] In comparison with the MR diffusion-weighted imaging, both FDG SUV and apparent diffusion coefficient were helpful parameters in

differentiating benign from malignant breast tumors and showing an inverse relationship. Although an high preoperative SUV has been associated with poor prognosis, the prognostic value of the apparent diffusion coefficient was small.[65] FDG PET impacts management by upstaging or downstaging the disease (**Fig. 21**). In a study of 79 patients with stage II to IV disease, 21% were upstaged by PET/CT, of which 8% had either stage II or III disease and were upstaged to stage IV disease. In addition, 16% of patients were downstaged; 3% went from stage IV to stage II or III. PET/CT changed management planning in 13% of patients. Although the staging with conventional imaging was associated significantly with progression-free survival (PFS), FDG staging provided stronger prognostic stratification and was associated with PFS.[66] The extent of disease and disease burden seen in FDG PET scan is prognostic in a recurrent disease setting (see **Fig. 19**).

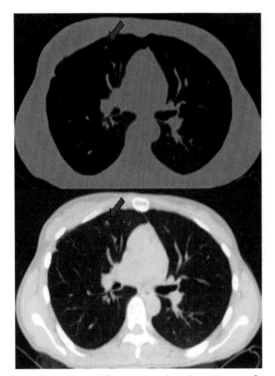

Fig. 16. Patient with invasive ductal carcinoma for evaluation of recurrent disease. A small, subcentimeter nodule in the right lung is not avid (*arrow*). This was metastatic disease. Assessment in general is limited for small-sized lung nodules and the histology.

In a retrospective analysis of FDG scans in more than 400 operative breast cancer patients, recurrence was correlated with TNM staging. FDG uptake in axillary nodes, pathologic T stage, pathologic nodal disease, ER, PR, stage grouping, and neoadjuvant chemotherapy history were prognostic for early recurrence, although primary tumor SUV$_{max}$, age, and ER or PR status were not significant on logistic regression. On multivariate analysis, only the stage and neoadjuvant chemotherapy identified patients at an increased risk for recurrence within 2 years.[67] In a large review of 3561 PET/CT scans performed on 1906 postoperative breast cancer patients, the estimated 3-year PFS rate was 48.6%. The SUV$_{max}$ cutoff of 2.7 and size of 1.4 cm were the best discriminative values for predicting clinical outcome. The SUV$_{max}$ and size of extra-axillary nodal recurrences were correlated significantly with PFS on both univariate and multivariate analyses.[68] The presence of extranodal sites and involvement of systemic organs has poor prognosis. FDG-avid sites may also be useful to guide biopsies (see **Figs. 18** and **19**).

FDG provides complementary information to conventional imaging and plays an important role in the management and treatment planning of advanced breast cancer. Cochet and colleagues[66] found that PET/CT provides high-stage migration in 37% of patients, and has a significant impact on the therapeutic management in 13% of patients. These findings are not only relevant clinically, but can have a significant economic impact. Avril[58] found that FDG PET/CT is useful as a prognostic factor for breast carcinoma risk classification and for making decisions on adjuvant chemotherapy. In many cases, additional sites involving multiple organs may be detected or unusual sites of involvement may be found that are the only sites of recurrent disease. In aggressive cancers, metastasis to the brain, peritoneum, skin, soft tissue, or colon may be seen (**Figs. 22–24**). In inflammatory breast cancer, using FDG imaging, a univariate analysis of the first enrolled patients (n = 42) showed that, among 28 patients who showed intense tumoral uptake (standard uptake value [max] of >5), the 11 patients with distant lesions had a worse prognosis than the 17 patients without distant lesions (*P* = .04).[40]

Male Breast Carcinomas

Male breast carcinomas comprise 0.6% of all breast carcinomas and constitute 1% of all cancers in men.[69] Although men have been known to have poorer prognosis than women with breast carcinoma, recent studies have shown similar prognoses in women and men. T stage, axillary lymph node metastasis, and age greater than 65 years are prognostic factors that affect survival rates.

Given the low incidence, the data of role of FDG in the male population are limited. In a retrospective analysis of male patients, with 30 FDG studies performed in 15 men, the findings of FDG PET/CT were compared with that of conventional imaging and the impact on management was evaluated. Most tumors were ER positive and 1 had HER2 overexpression. PET/CT sensitivity, specificity, positive predictive value, negative predictive value, and accuracy to detect distant metastases were 100%, 67%, 86%, 100%, and 89%, respectively. PET/CT was more sensitive than conventional imaging in 40% of studies and led to modification in the planned treatment in 13 of 30 cases (43%). Findings supported the use of FDG PET for staging, restaging, and treatment response assessment in male patients.[70]

Breast Cancer Bone Metastasis

Conventional skeletal staging options in high-risk, early breast cancer or at suspicion of bone relapse include the 99mTc-diphosphonate bone scan (eg, 99mTc-methylene diphosphonate [MDP]) or

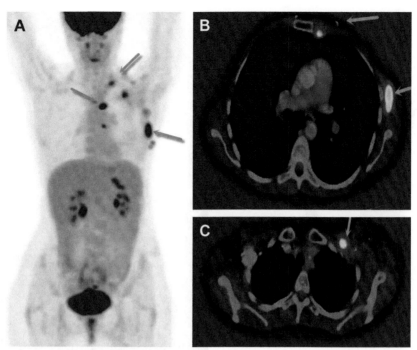

Fig. 17. Patient with triple-negative breast cancer presented for evaluation of recurrent disease. Whole body maximum intensity projection (MIP) PET image (*A*) and axial fused images (*B, C*) demonstrate fluorodeoxyglucose (FDG) avid left axillary and internal mammary lymph nodes (*arrows*), consistent with recurrence.

cross-sectional imaging with CT using bone windows, MR imaging, or plain radiographs. ^{99m}Tc-MDP bone scintigraphy images the osteoblastic changes that occur secondary to bone destruction by tumor cells. The advantage includes high sensitivity and ability to assess the entire skeleton, unlike cross-sectional imaging. However, it is also a nonspecific imaging technique and false-positive results are seen in a number of benign conditions, including fracture or degenerative change. The sensitivity is low for lytic disease, which is commonly seen in breast cancer. Also, assessment of bone lesions that are responding to treatment is difficult; bone scan remains positive owing to uptake related to osteoblastic process and CT scan may be interpreted as persistent disease or worsening owing to increased sclerosis seen in lesions (**Figs. 25** and **26**). FDG PET is superior for evaluation of lytic bone disease and comparable with bone scan for blastic disease; it may be more specific in the assessment of treatment response in bone lesions.[60,71–74] The PET tracer ^{18}F-sodium fluoride (NaF) is used for imaging bone metastasis. The mechanism of uptake is similar to MDP and is, therefore, nonspecific. The combined PET/CT imaging allows for distinction of the uptake in benign versus malignant lesions by simultaneous evaluation of CT images. There are limited data of use in breast cancer, although

some reports have observed greater detection and possible evaluation of marrow disease.[60,72] In patients with marrow rebound phenomenon, focal activity of FDG may be confusing and NaF imaging may be useful to distinguish.[75]

Imaging Breast Cancer with Receptor-Targeting Agents

Approximately two-thirds of breast cancers depend on estrogen or progesterone, or both, for their growth. The stimulatory effect of estrogen and progesterone is mediated through nuclear ERs and PRs (PgRs). To control the growth of hormone-dependent breast cancer, these receptors have been targeted by endocrine agents. The most widely used endocrine therapies include aromatase inhibitors, which deplete estrogen levels in vivo and within the tumor by disrupting estrogen synthesis selective ER modulators, such as tamoxifen, and selective ER downregulators, such as fulvestrant. The presence of ER and PgR in the tumor also is known to be an important prognostic factor for breast cancer; their presence typically indicates that the tumor is less aggressive and more indolent than ER-negative (ER−) or PgR-negative (PgR−) tumors. Currently, the ER status of a breast tumor is assessed through an immunohistochemistry assay performed on thin sections

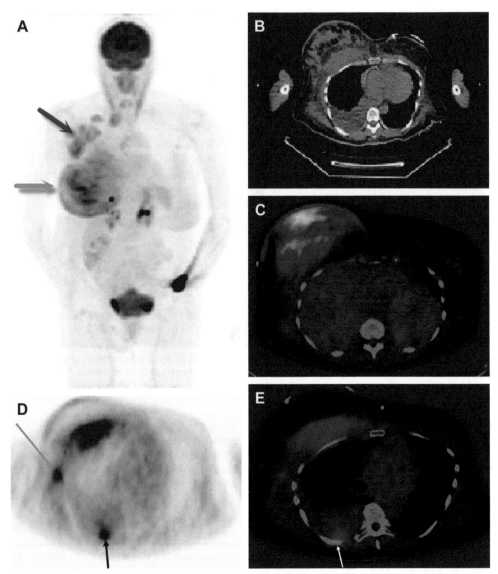

Fig. 18. A 60-year-old woman with a prior history of biopsy-proven right invasive ductal adenocarcinoma, estrogen/progesterone receptor–negative, HER2-, treated with lumpectomy and adjuvant chemoradiation therapy. The patient presented for evaluation of recurrent disease. (*A*) Maximum intensity projection PET image demonstrates a large fluorodeoxyglucose (FDG)-avid breast mass (*blue arrow*) and right axillary adenopathy (*red arrow*). Axial CT (*B*) and fused images (*C*) demonstrate markedly FDG-avid right breast mass, with chest wall involvement (*D, blue arrow*). Axial PET image (*D*) demonstrates focus of FDG activity posteriorly that corresponds to the posterior pleura (*black arrow*) as seen on fused image (*E, arrow*). Also, the pleural effusion is mildly avid (*E*). Thoracentesis and pleural biopsy of the FDG-avid site were positive for metastases.

of tumor tissue.[76] However, this method has high and consistent rates of intralaboratory and interlaboratory variability, which in turn makes it difficult to determine the true rates of ER positivity. Also, there is intrinsic heterogeneity of receptor content within the same lesion, as well as variations in receptor status among the primary and metastatic sites.[77,78]

The presence of the ER receptor (ER+) in a tumor is not predictive of a functional ER. This is evident in that not all patients with ER+ breast cancers respond to endocrine therapy. This assay provides limited information about the functional status of the receptors and the sensitivity of a given tumor to endocrine therapy; only 55% to 60% of patients with ER+ and fewer than 10%

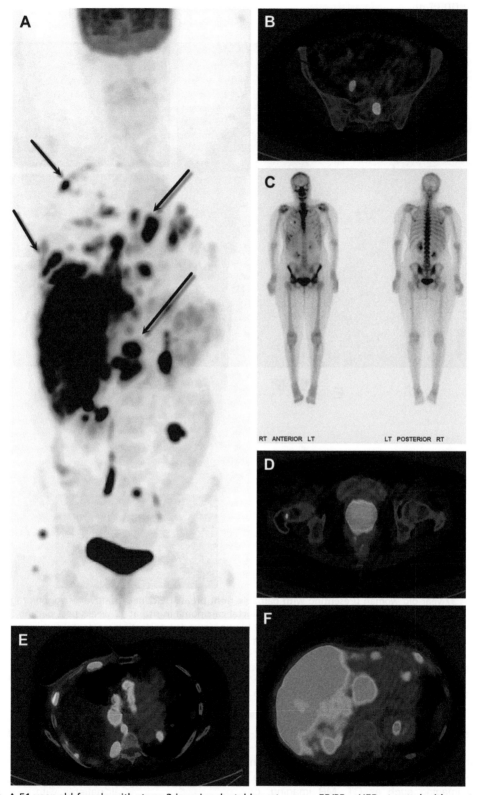

Fig. 19. A 51-year-old female with stage 2 invasive ductal breast cancer, ER/PR+, HER-, treated with mastectomy and adjuvant chemoradiation. Patient was imaged for evaluation of recurrent disease. (*A*) FDG PET MIP showed extensive metastatic disease involving the bone (*black arrows*). Fused image (*B*) shows uptake in sacrum and node (*arrow*). Bone scan (*C*) shows no suspicious foci; costochondral uptake in right third rib was considered benign. Fused image (*D*) shows uptake in right femur and FDG also showed extensive disease in liver and nodal metastasis (Images *E* and *F*).

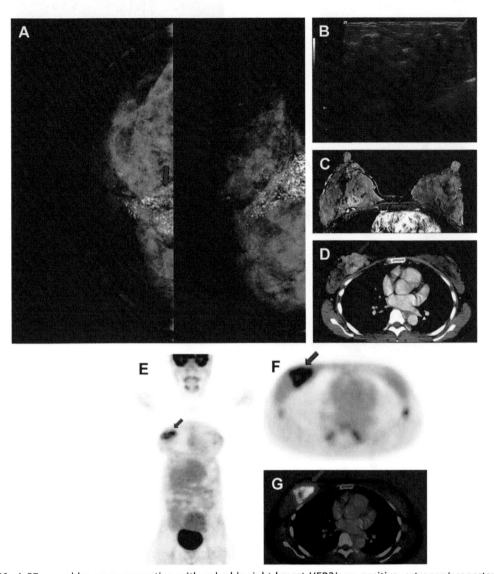

Fig. 20. A 37-year-old woman presenting with palpable right breast HER2/neu–positive, estrogen/progesterone receptora–negative, invasive ductal carcinoma and ductal carcinoma in situ at 12 weeks post partum. (*A*) Right breast mammogram craniocaudal and mediolateral oblique views demonstrating segmental suspicious calcifications at the 12:00 axis, mid and posterior third depths (*purple arrows*). (*B*) Right breast ultrasound demonstrating an irregular, hypoechoic mass with posterior acoustic shadowing at the 12:00 axis (*pink arrow*), corresponding to mammographic abnormality, the heterogeneously enhancing mass seen on contrast-enhanced MR imaging (*C, purple arrow*) and on axial CT image (*D, purple arrow*). Fluorodeoxyglucose PET scan shows moderately FDG-avid right breast mass (*E–G, purple arrows*); there was no evidence of distant metastatic disease.

of ER- disease respond to hormonal therapy.[79] There is heterogeneity of ER expression in tumors.[80] Currently, follow-up of patients on hormone therapy is a challenge. No single test can indicate accurately and reliably tumor response. Routine imaging such as CT, MR imaging, or bone scans may take weeks or months to show a change. Lack of early information on response may lead the treating physician to abandon the less toxic hormone treatment in favor of more toxic chemotherapy. The role of FDG in the assessment of the effects of hormone therapy is not well established, although preliminary studies have shown possible use.[56]

PET-Targeted Imaging of Estrogen Receptor Imaging

FES PET shows promise as a noninvasive test that can simultaneously measure the in vivo delivery and binding of estrogens, and thus ER expression. FES is metabolized by the liver and excreted

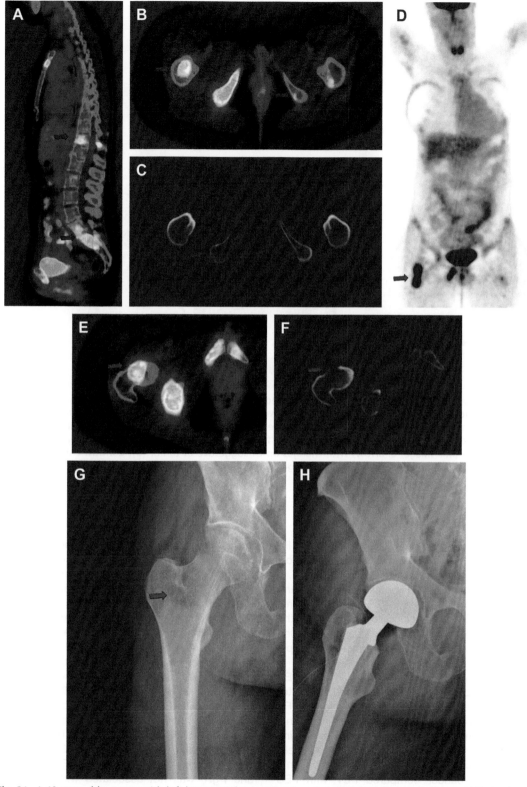

Fig. 21. A 40-year-old woman with left breast triple-negative invasive ductal carcinoma status post bilateral mastectomies (prophylactic on the right) for evaluation of extent of disease. PET/CT imaging showed fluorodeoxyglucoseavid lytic osseous metastases in right proximal femur, right ischium, and right intertrochanteric femur (*A, B,* and *C, purple arrows; D, E,* and *F, pink arrows*) that were otherwise not known. These corresponded with lytic lesions on CT (*C, purple arrow; F, pink arrow*). Axial CT image (*F*) demonstrates lytic metastasis to right intertrochanteric region with cortical thinning, occupying more than 50% of bone width, at risk for pathologic fracture. Frontal radiograph of the right femur (*G*) was done to confirm cortical thinning (*pink arrow*). The patient underwent prophylactic right hip hemiarthroplasty (*H*).

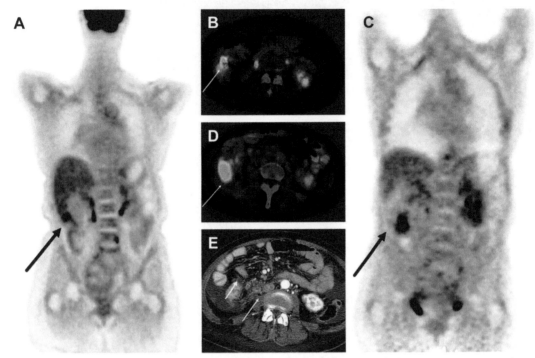

Fig. 22. Fluorodeoxyglucose (FDG) detects unsuspected disease. Patient with breast carcinoma was evaluated with FDG PET for recurrent disease. No abnormal sites were seen in breast, bone, or liver (maximum intensity projection [MIP] image; *A*). Focal increased uptake was seen in the right upper quadrant along hepatic flexure (*arrow*). No CT correlate (*B*) was seen. Patient received follow-up scanning, which showed increased uptake in hepatic flexure (MIP image; *C, arrow*) with changes on CT suggestive of tumor (*D*). Contrast-enhanced CT also showed stranding and mesenteric infiltration, suggestive of peritoneal carcinomatosis (*E, arrow*).

primarily through the hepatobiliary system and intestines; therefore, FES activity within these organs is not related to tumor estrogen binding. It localizes in primary and metastatic cancer, and uptake is generally seen in ER-positive patients (**Fig. 27**). FES PET imaging allows imaging of the whole body and, therefore, as a single imaging test can detect ER expressing tumors at multiple sites.

FES imaging correlates with in vivo ER testing[81] and therefore may help to identify tumors with heterogeneous ER expression.[82] FES imaging has been used as a marker of functional ER status and to assess response to endocrine therapy.[23,80,83–87] Preliminary studies by Dehdashti and colleagues[23] in a subset of patients with breast cancer compared PET with FES and FDG, and correlated PET uptake with in vitro receptor assay results. Correlation of ER positivity and FES was found in 88% of cases, whereas no correlation was noted between tumor FDG uptake and ER status, or between tumor FDG and FES uptake. FES was

superior in predicting ER expression and FDG uptake in ER+ and ER- breast cancers was not different. Other authors have also found superiority of FES over FDG in determining estrogen expression of tumors.[88] FES PET is therefore thought to be a more sensitive and discriminatory test than FDG in patients with ER+ breast cancer. In a larger study involving FES imaging in preoperative patients, FES identified 5 ER + patients with axillary nodal uptake (median SUV, 3.0; range, 1.7–6.9; **Fig. 28**). FES SUV was associated with immunohistochemistry ER expression and tumor size. The sensitivity and specificity of the FES PET for the breast lesion were 0.85 and 0.75, respectively. Estrogen and progesterone gene expression (ESR1, ESR2, and PgR) was not associated with FES SUV. FES uptake did not correlate with ductal histology, grade, HER2/neu overexpression, PgR, estradiol, body mass index, or lean body mass index (logistic regression). ER expression (*P*<.001) and tumor size (*P*<.0001) were significant on multivariate regression analysis.[89]

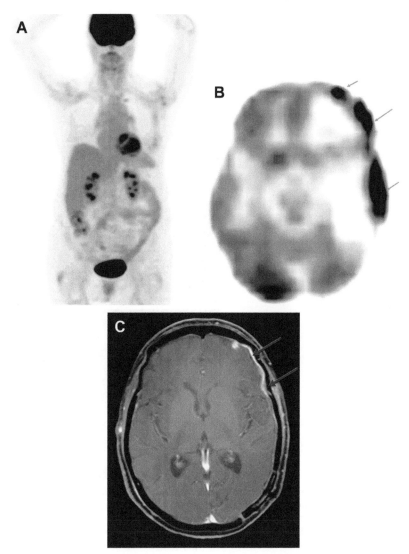

Fig. 23. Patient with triple-negative breast cancer. Fluorodeoxyglucose (FDG) PET was performed to evaluate for recurrent disease. Maximum intensity projection (MIP) image (*A*) shows no systemic foci of abnormal uptake in the body. Brain axial PET image (*B*) revealed FDG activity overlying the left frontal–parietal lobes (*blue arrows*), which corresponded with enhancing dural-based lesions seen on gadolinium-enhanced axial MR imaging of the brain (*C*) along the left frontal lobe (*pink arrows*), consistent with dural metastasis.

Some false positives have been noted in benign conditions owing to inflammation.[90] It is possible to detect unknown, distant sites of disease with FES (**Fig. 29**).

FES scanning has been evaluated in assessing and predicting response to endocrine therapy.[91,92] Those with positive FES uptake are more likely to benefit and respond to antiestrogen therapy than those who do not show uptake on FES scan.[93,94] The FES positivity, as measured by SUV, predicts response to endocrine therapy with selective ER

modulators or aromatase inhibitors in first-line therapy or salvage settings.[83,95] Typically, a significantly greater tumor SUV is noted in responders compared with nonresponders. However, patients with tumors that bind and concentrate estrogen do not uniformly respond or benefit from treatment— this may be linked to the heterogenous distribution and ER expression.[96] FES demonstrates intrapatient and interpatient variability of uptake and ER expression[80] and can be of prognostic value. Aromatase inhibitors, which affect the ligand, do not

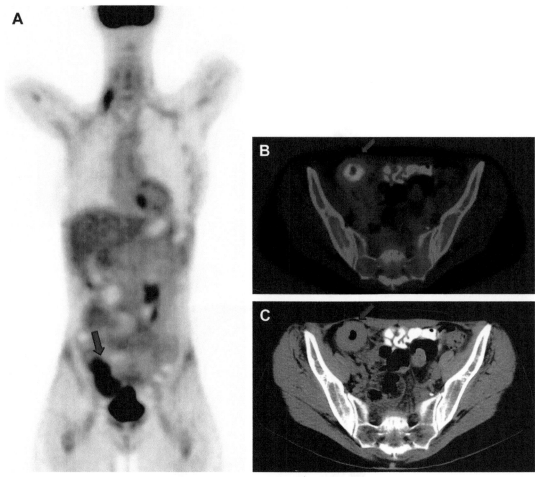

Fig. 24. A 63-year-old woman with estrogen receptor–positive, multifocal invasive lobular and tubular carcinoma of the right breast status post mastectomy, chemotherapy, and radiation. The patient was evaluated for recurrent disease. Coronal PET (*A*) image demonstrates fluorodeoxyglucose uptake in the right lower quadrant (*pink arrow*) that on (*B*) fused axial PET/CT image corresponds with the circumferential thickening of the colon seen on (*C*) axial CT image. Pathology was consistent with biopsy-proven metastatic breast cancer (*pink arrow*).

affect FES uptake, but blocking therapies such as tamoxifen (a selective ER modulator) or fulvestrant (a selective ER downregulator) result in a marked decline in FES uptake.[83] These observations could be exploited in drug development of novel therapeutics aimed to block or degrade ER to determine whether the target ER is affected by the potential therapeutic agent. Although the current data support significance of FES, further evaluation in a larger patient population in multi-institutional studies is needed to establish its role.

Imaging the Progesterone Receptors

Approximately two-thirds of breast cancers are ER+ and approximately one-half of these patients also express PgR, an estrogen-regulated gene whose expression is considered to indicate a functioning ER pathway. There may be a better correlation between PgR status than ER status and responsiveness to endocrine therapy. ER+/PgR+ tumors are more likely to benefit from endocrine therapy, whereas ER+/PgR− tumors are less likely to respond to endocrine therapy.[97] PgR status is therefore a routine assessment in patients.

A radioligand for assessment of PgR, 18F-fluoro furanyl norprogesterone (FFNP) has high affinity and selectivity for PgR.[98–100] There are limited clinical data of utility of this tracer in imaging breast cancer. PgR level increases after treatment with tamoxifen in hormone-sensitive

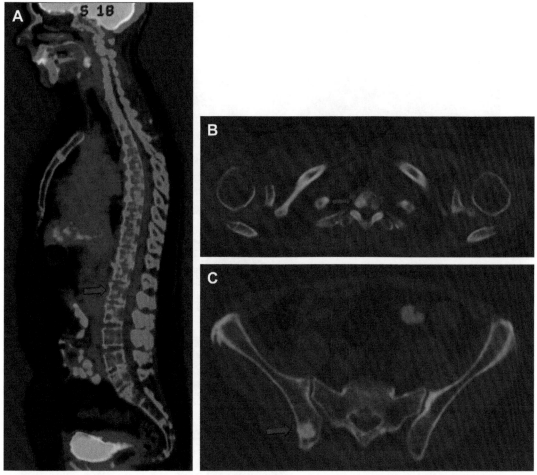

Fig. 25. A 56-year-old woman with biopsy-proven, estrogen receptor–positive breast cancer metastatic to the bones, status post breast conservation therapy. (*A*) Fused sagittal PET/CT images demonstrating non–fluorodeoxyglucose-avid blastic osseous metastases to the spine (*purple arrow*). (*B*) Axial CT image at the level of the cervical spine demonstrating a sclerotic lesion in T1 vertebral body and at the level of the pelvis (*C*) showing a sclerotic lesion in the right iliac bone (*purple arrows on B and C*).

breast cancer,[98] and thus may be a good target for imaging and predicting response to hormones, especially in those with low ER expression where ER binding agents may be less sensitive. Currently, imaging data in patients are limited and future studies are needed to assess the value of FFNP-PET in predicting the response to endocrine therapy, either by change in FFNP uptake after a brief antiestrogen therapy or estradiol challenge.

HER2 Receptor Imaging

HER2/neu is a member of the family of tyrosine kinase receptors that has an important role in cell growth and survival. Overexpression of the HER2

receptor occurs in approximately 20% to 30% of primary breast cancers and has been associated with relatively poor prognosis. In addition, it has been shown that tumors with HER2 overexpression differ from tumors without HER2 overexpression in their response to systemic therapy.

HER2-targeted therapies have been shown to improve survival and reduce the development of distant metastatic disease in HER2-positive breast cancer. HER2 expression is routinely assessed using immunohistochemistry and fluorescence in situ hybridization and plays a role in selection of therapy. Similar to ER, there is intratumoral and intertumoral heterogeneity in HER2 expression, and targeted imaging could play an important for prognosis and assessment of response to therapy.

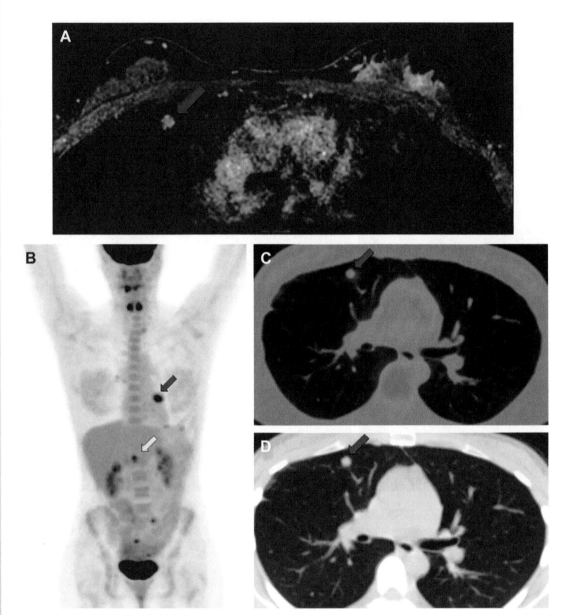

Fig. 26. A 33-year-old woman with poorly differentiated estrogen/progesterone receptor–positive invasive ductal carcinoma and ductal carcinoma in situ of the right breast, status post lumpectomy and chemotherapy, was referred for evaluation of recurrent disease. (*A*) Axial breast MR imaging was negative for local recurrence. Incidentally, a right lung nodule was noted (*A, pink arrow*) that required further evaluation. Bilateral lung nodules and osseous metastases were found on PET/CT. Maximum intensity projection image shows a left lower lobe fluorodeoxyglucose (FDG)-avid nodule (*B, pink arrow*) and osseous lesion in the lumbar spine (*yellow arrow; B*); fused image shows minimal uptake in the right lung nodule originally detected on breast MR imaging (*C, pink arrow*); corresponding to the nodule seen on CT axial image (*D, pink arrow*). L2 vertebra metastasis on sagittal MR imaging (*E, pink arrow*) correlating to FDG-avid lytic lesion on PET/CT (*F, pink arrow*) and lytic osseous metastasis on CT (*H, pink arrow*). New systemic therapy was initiated. Posttherapy scan for evaluation of response showed resolved uptake in L2 metastasis (*G, pink arrow*), increased sclerosis of the lesion on CT (*I, pink arrow*).

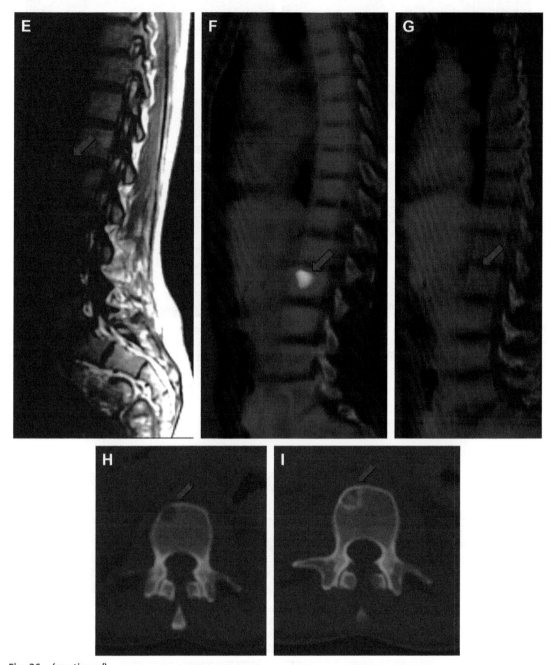

Fig. 26. (continued)

Several imaging agents labeled with single photon radionuclides (such as indium-111–labeled trastuzumab and 99mTc-ICR12) and positron-emitting radionuclides (such as 64Cu-trastuzumab, 64Cu-DOTA-ZHER2:477, 68Ga-trastuzumab F[ab']2 fragments, 68Ga-ABY-002, and 89Zr-trastuzumab) for noninvasive in vivo evaluation of HER2 expression have been

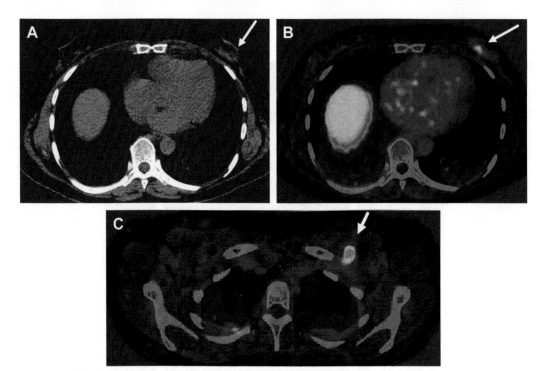

Fig. 27. F16α-[¹⁸F]fluoro-17β-estradiol (FES) imaging in breast cancer. Woman with biopsy-proven left breast cancer. A 2.1×1.6-cm mass in left breast is seen on axial CT image (*A*) with increased uptake on FES scan fused image (*B*); standardized uptake value (SUV) of 2.8. Intense uptake was also seen in a level II axillary lymph node (image *C, small arrow*); SUV of 6.8.

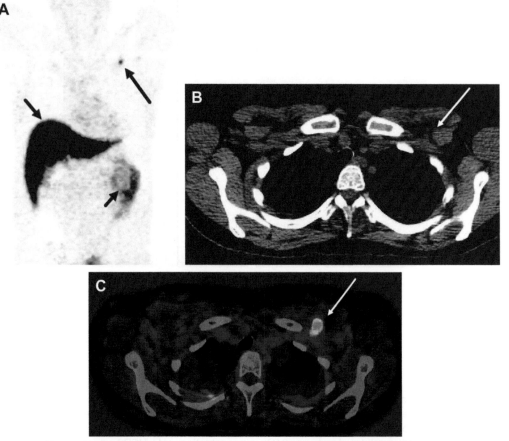

Fig. 28. F16α-[¹⁸F]fluoro-17β-estradiol (FES) imaging in patient with left breast cancer. Maximum intensity projection image (*A*) shows physiologic uptake in liver and gastrointestinal tract (*short arrows*). CT (*B*) fused images of the chest show increased uptake of FES seen in left level II axillary lymph node (*C, long arrow*).

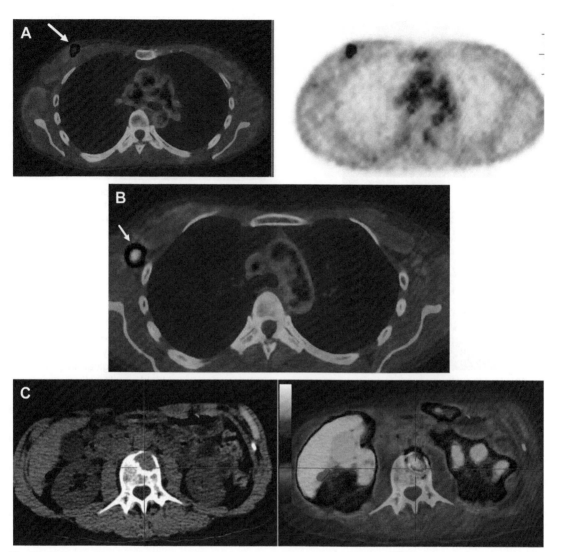

Fig. 29. Patient with recently diagnosed breast cancer was evaluated with F16α-[¹⁸F]fluoro-17β-estradiol (FES) imaging before surgery. Uptake was seen in the primary tumor (*A, arrow*) and in a right axillary lymph node (*B, short arrow*). In addition, FES imaging detected vertebral metastases that were otherwise not known (*C, D, cross bar*). Management was changed and the patient did not undergo surgery.

developed (**Figs. 30** and **31**).[101–109] Currently, there are limited clinical data in the utilization of these tracers in breast cancer. A recent study with ⁶⁴Cu-DOTA-trastuzumab PET in 8 patients showed feasibility and safety of the tracer. Tumor targeting of metastatic disease was seen.[106] Using ⁸⁹Zr-trastuzumab PET, HER2 expression in breast cancers has been studied.[108,109] In small patient studies, ⁸⁹Zr-trastuzumab showed good uptake in lesions.[108] Additional clinical studies are needed to evaluate further the role of these tracers in breast cancer management.

Other Tracers

Increased cell proliferation is the hallmark of cancer phenotype and is among the important key features of tumor behavior. Cell proliferation is commonly measured by immunohistochemistry using the Ki-67 antibody MIB-1. The radiotracer [(18)F]fluoro-3'-deoxy-3'-L-fluorothymidine (FLT)] images cell proliferation. The tracer is phosphorylated by thymidine kinase-1 and because of its structure (fluorination at the 3' position) is not incorporated into the DNA synthesis and is

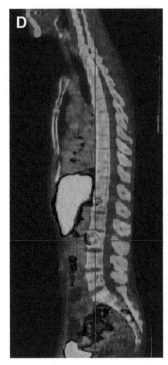

Fig. 29. (*continued*)

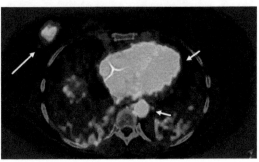

Fig. 31. Patient with HER2/neu-positive breast carcinoma for evaluation of disease with 64Cu-trastuzumab imaging. Focus of uptake is seen in right breast at the primary tumor site (*long arrow*). Physiologic biodistribution in the blood pool (heart and aorta; *short arrows*).

trapped within the proliferating cells using the salvage pathway for DNA synthesis. A meta-analysis shows that FLT uptake correlates with Ki-67 expression.[110] FLT uptake is heterogenous; however, it can help to assess treatment effectiveness.[111–113] One advantage of FLT is its lack of accumulation in inflammation, a process typically associated with cancer therapy that can result in false-positive results. Physiological uptake of FLT in bone marrow, a highly proliferative organ, and high accumulation in the liver owing to metabolism may limit its use in evaluating these organs. More studies are needed to establish the role of FLT in breast cancer. Currently, it is an investigational tracer and not part of routine evaluation or follow-up. Other investigational tracers include radiolabeled choline compounds, ^{11}C-choline, or ^{18}F-choline, whose uptake is related to cell membrane synthesis. There are limited data of its use in breast cancer, although it seems to target breast

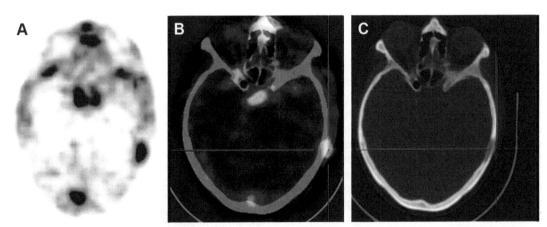

Fig. 30. Patient with HER2/neu-positive breast carcinoma for evaluation of disease with 68Ga-trastuzumab imaging. Images show uptake in the region the skull (*A, B*) corresponding to a lytic lesion seen on axial CT image (*C, crossbar*).

cancer well.[114,115] Physiologic uptake of radiolabeled choline in the liver, kidneys, pancreas, and bowel may limit its use in evaluating these organs.

REFERENCES

1. DeSantis C, Ma J, Bryan L, et al. Breast cancer statistics, 2013. CA Cancer J Clin 2014;64:52–62.
2. Khatcheressian JL, Hurley P, Bantug E, et al. Breast cancer follow-up and management after primary treatment: American Society of Clinical Oncology clinical practice guideline update. J Clin Oncol 2013;31:961–5.
3. Gilbert FJ, van den Bosch HC, Petrillo A, et al. Comparison of gadobenate dimeglumine-enhanced breast MRI and gadopentetate dimeglumine-enhanced breast MRI with mammography and ultrasound for the detection of breast cancer. J Magn Reson Imaging 2014;39:1272–86.
4. Gareth ED, Nisha K, Yit L, et al. MRI breast screening in high-risk women: cancer detection and survival analysis. Breast Cancer Res Treat 2014;145:663–72.
5. NCCN guidelines. 2014. Available at: http://www.nccnorg/professionals/physician_gls. Accessed date October, 2014.
6. MacDonald L, Edwards J, Lewellen T, et al. Clinical imaging characteristics of the positron emission mammography camera: PEM Flex Solo II. J Nucl Med 2009;50:1666–75.
7. Moliner L, Gonzalez AJ, Soriano A, et al. Design and evaluation of the MAMMI dedicated breast PET. Med Phys 2012;39:5393–404.
8. Caldarella C, Treglia G, Giordano A. Diagnostic performance of dedicated positron emission mammography using fluorine-18-fluorodeoxyglucose in women with suspicious breast lesions: a meta-analysis. Clin Breast Cancer 2014;14:241–8 [Systematic review or meta-analysis].
9. Koolen BB, Vidal-Sicart S, Benlloch Baviera JM, et al. Evaluating heterogeneity of primary tumor (18)F-FDG uptake in breast cancer with a dedicated breast PET (MAMMI): a feasibility study based on correlation with PET/CT. Nucl Med Commun 2014;35:446–52.
10. Taneja S, Jena A, Goel R, et al. Simultaneous whole-body F-FDG PET-MRI in primary staging of breast cancer: a pilot study. Eur J Radiol 2014;83(12):2231–9.
11. Garcia Vicente AM, Soriano Castrejon A, Leon Martin A, et al. Molecular subtypes of breast cancer: metabolic correlation with (1)(8)F-FDG PET/CT. Eur J Nucl Med Mol Imaging 2013;40:1304–11.
12. Ong LC, Jin Y, Song IC, et al. 2-[18F]-2-deoxy-D-glucose (FDG) uptake in human tumor cells is related to the expression of GLUT-1 and hexokinase II. Acta Radiol 2008;49:1145–53.
13. Koga H, Matsuo Y, Sasaki M, et al. Differential FDG accumulation associated with GLUT-1 expression in a patient with lymphoma. Ann Nucl Med 2003; 17:327–31.
14. Tchou J, Sonnad SS, Bergey MR, et al. Degree of tumor FDG uptake correlates with proliferation index in triple negative breast cancer. Mol Imaging Biol 2010;12:657–62.
15. Groheux D, Giacchetti S, Moretti JL, et al. Correlation of high 18F-FDG uptake to clinical, pathological and biological prognostic factors in breast cancer. Eur J Nucl Med Mol Imaging 2011;38: 426–35.
16. Avril N, Menzel M, Dose J, et al. Glucose metabolism of breast cancer assessed by 18F-FDG PET: histologic and immunohistochemical tissue analysis. J Nucl Med 2001;42:9–16.
17. Bos R, van Der Hoeven JJ, van Der Wall E, et al. Biologic correlates of (18)fluorodeoxyglucose uptake in human breast cancer measured by positron emission tomography. J Clin Oncol 2002;20: 379–87.
18. Koo HR, Park JS, Kang KW, et al. 18F-FDG uptake in breast cancer correlates with immunohistochemically defined subtypes. Eur Radiol 2014;24: 610–8.
19. Maffione AM, Lisato LC, Rasi A, et al. Lobular breast carcinoma: a case of rare possible 18F-FDG PET/CT and bone scan false negative. Clin Nucl Med 2014;40:e134–6.
20. Song BI, Hong CM, Lee HJ, et al. Prognostic value of primary tumor uptake on F-18 FDG PET/CT in patients with invasive ductal breast cancer. Nucl Med Mol Imaging 2011;45:117–24.
21. Brown RS, Leung JY, Fisher SJ, et al. Intratumoral distribution of tritiated-FDG in breast carcinoma: correlation between Glut-1 expression and FDG uptake. J Nucl Med 1996;37:1042–7.
22. Ko BH, Paik JY, Jung KH, et al. 17beta-estradiol augments 18F-FDG uptake and glycolysis of T47D breast cancer cells via membrane-initiated rapid PI3K-Akt activation. J Nucl Med 2010;51: 1740–7.
23. Dehdashti F, Mortimer JE, Siegel BA, et al. Positron tomographic assessment of estrogen receptors in breast cancer: comparison with FDG-PET and in vitro receptor assays. J Nucl Med 1995;36: 1766–74.
24. Yoon HJ, Kang KW, Chun IK, et al. Correlation of breast cancer subtypes, based on estrogen receptor, progesterone receptor, and HER2, with functional imaging parameters from (6)(8)Ga-RGD PET/CT and (1)(8)F-FDG PET/CT. Eur J Nucl Med Mol Imaging 2014;41:1534–43.
25. Koolen BB, Pengel KE, Wesseling J, et al. FDG PET/CT during neoadjuvant chemotherapy may predict response in ER-positive/HER2-negative

and triple negative, but not in HER2-positive breast cancer. Breast 2013;22:691–7.

26. Basu S, Chen W, Tchou J, et al. Comparison of triple-negative and estrogen receptor-positive/progesterone receptor-positive/HER2-negative breast carcinoma using quantitative fluorine-18 fluorodeoxyglucose/positron emission tomography imaging parameters: a potentially useful method for disease characterization. Cancer 2008;112:995–1000.

27. Kim BS, Sung SH. Usefulness of 18F-FDG uptake with clinicopathologic and immunohistochemical prognostic factors in breast cancer. Ann Nucl Med 2012;26:175–83.

28. Ugurluer G, Kibar M, Yavuz S, et al. False positive 18F-FDG uptake in mediastinal lymph nodes detected with positron emission tomography in breast cancer: a case report. Case Rep Med 2013;2013:459753.

29. Ataergin S, Arslan N, Ozet A, et al. Abnormal 18F-FDG uptake detected with positron emission tomography in a patient with breast cancer: a case of sarcoidosis and review of the literature. Case Rep Med 2009;2009:785047.

30. Akkas BE, Ucmak Vural G. Fat necrosis may mimic local recurrence of breast cancer in FDG PET/CT. Rev Esp Med Nucl Imagen Mol 2013;32:105–6.

31. Adejolu M, Huo L, Rohren E, et al. False-positive lesions mimicking breast cancer on FDG PET and PET/CT. Am J Roentgenol 2012;198:W304–14.

32. Manohar K, Mittal BR, Bhoil A, et al. Role of 18F-FDG PET/CT in identifying distant metastatic disease missed by conventional imaging in patients with locally advanced breast cancer. Nucl Med Commun 2013;34:557–61.

33. Koolen BB, Valdes Olmos RA, Vogel WV, et al. Pre-chemotherapy 18F-FDG PET/CT upstages nodal stage in stage II-III breast cancer patients treated with neoadjuvant chemotherapy. Breast Cancer Res Treat 2013;141:249–54.

34. Hama Y, Nakagawa K. Early distant relapse in early stage triple-negative breast cancer: usefulness of FDG-PET for diagnosis of distant metastases. Breast Cancer 2013;20:191–3.

35. Groheux D, Giacchetti S, Delord M, et al. 18F-FDG PET/CT in staging patients with locally advanced or inflammatory breast cancer: comparison to conventional staging. J Nucl Med 2013;54:5–11.

36. Groheux D, Espie M, Giacchetti S, et al. Performance of FDG PET/CT in the clinical management of breast cancer. Radiology 2013;266:388–405.

37. Koolen BB, van der Leij F, Vogel WV, et al. Accuracy of 18F-FDG PET/CT for primary tumor visualization and staging in T1 breast cancer. Acta Oncol 2014;53:50–7.

38. Jeong YJ, Kang DY, Yoon HJ, et al. Additional value of F-18 FDG PET/CT for initial staging in breast cancer with clinically negative axillary nodes. Breast Cancer Res Treat 2014;145:137–42.

39. Ahn JH, Son EJ, Kim JA, et al. The role of ultrasonography and FDG-PET in axillary lymph node staging of breast cancer. Acta Radiol 2010;51:859–65.

40. Alberini JL, Lerebours F, Wartski M, et al. 18F-fluorodeoxyglucose positron emission tomography/computed tomography (FDG-PET/CT) imaging in the staging and prognosis of inflammatory breast cancer. Cancer 2009;115:5038–47.

41. Champion L, Lerebours F, Cherel P, et al. (1)(8)F-FDG PET/CT imaging versus dynamic contrast-enhanced CT for staging and prognosis of inflammatory breast cancer. Eur J Nucl Med Mol Imaging 2013;40:1206–13.

42. Bellon JR, Livingston RB, Eubank WB, et al. Evaluation of the internal mammary lymph nodes by FDG-PET in locally advanced breast cancer (LABC). Am J Clin Oncol 2004;27:407–10.

43. Pritchard KI, Julian JA, Holloway CM, et al. Prospective study of 2-[(1)(8)F]fluorodeoxyglucose positron emission tomography in the assessment of regional nodal spread of disease in patients with breast cancer: an Ontario clinical oncology group study. J Clin Oncol 2012;30:1274–9.

44. Peare R, Staff RT, Heys SD. The use of FDG-PET in assessing axillary lymph node status in breast cancer: a systematic review and meta-analysis of the literature. Breast Cancer Res Treat 2010;123:281–90 [Systematic review or meta-analysis].

45. Dalus K, Rendl G, Rettenbacher L, et al. FDG PET/CT for monitoring response to neoadjuvant chemotherapy in breast cancer patients. Eur J Nucl Med Mol Imaging 2010;37:1992–3.

46. Rousseau C, Devillers A, Campone M, et al. FDG PET evaluation of early axillary lymph node response to neoadjuvant chemotherapy in stage II and III breast cancer patients. Eur J Nucl Med Mol Imaging 2011;38:1029–36.

47. Couturier O, Jerusalem G, N'Guyen JM, et al. Sequential positron emission tomography using [18F]fluorodeoxyglucose for monitoring response to chemotherapy in metastatic breast cancer. Clin Cancer Res 2006;12:6437–43.

48. Kolesnikov-Gauthier H, Vanlemmens L, Baranzelli MC, et al. Predictive value of neoadjuvant chemotherapy failure in breast cancer using FDG-PET after the first course. Breast Cancer Res Treat 2012;131:517–25.

49. Cheng X, Li Y, Liu B, et al. 18F-FDG PET/CT and PET for evaluation of pathological response to neoadjuvant chemotherapy in breast cancer: a meta-analysis. Acta Radiol 2012;53:615–27.

50. Ogino K, Nakajima M, Kakuta M, et al. Utility of FDG-PET/CT in the evaluation of the response of

locally advanced breast cancer to neoadjuvant chemotherapy. Int Surg 2014;99:309–18.

51. Hirakata T, Yanagita Y, Fujisawa T, et al. Early predictive value of non-response to docetaxel in neoadjuvant chemotherapy in breast cancer using 18F-FDG-PET. Anticancer Res 2014;34: 221–6.

52. Garcia Garcia-Esquinas M, Garcia-Saenz JA, Arrazola Garcia J, et al. 18F-FDG PET-CT imaging in the neoadjuvant setting for stages II-III breast cancer: association of locoregional SUVmax with classical prognostic factors. Q J Nucl Med Mol Imaging 2014;58:66–73.

53. Humbert O, Berriolo-Riedinger A, Cochet A, et al. Prognostic relevance at 5 years of the early monitoring of neoadjuvant chemotherapy using (18)F-FDG PET in luminal HER2-negative breast cancer. Eur J Nucl Med Mol Imaging 2014;41:416–27.

54. Mghanga FP, Lan X, Bakari KH, et al. Fluorine-18 fluorodeoxyglucose positron emission tomography-computed tomography in monitoring the response of breast cancer to neoadjuvant chemotherapy: a meta-analysis. Clin Breast Cancer 2013;13:271–9 [Systematic review or meta-analysis].

55. Dose-Schwarz J, Tiling R, Avril-Sassen S, et al. Assessment of residual tumour by FDG-PET: conventional imaging and clinical examination following primary chemotherapy of large and locally advanced breast cancer. Br J Cancer 2010;102:35–41.

56. Kurland BF, Gadi VK, Specht JM, et al. Feasibility study of FDG PET as an indicator of early response to aromatase inhibitors and trastuzumab in a heterogeneous group of breast cancer patients. EJNMMI Res 2012;2:34.

57. Escalona S, Blasco JA, Reza MM, et al. A systematic review of FDG-PET in breast cancer. Med Oncol 2010;27:114–29 [Systematic review or meta-analysis].

58. Avril N. Metabolic FDG-PET imaging in breast cancer: implications for treatment stratification. Nat Clin Pract Oncol 2007;4:336–7.

59. Yang ZY, Sun YF, Xue J, et al. Can positron emission tomography/computed tomography with the dual tracers fluorine-18 fluoroestradiol and fluorodeoxyglucose predict neoadjuvant chemotherapy response of breast cancer? A pilot study. PLoS One 2013;8:e78192.

60. Gaeta CM, Vercher-Conejero JL, Sher AC, et al. Recurrent and metastatic breast cancer PET, PET/CT, PET/MRI: FDG and new biomarkers. Q J Nucl Med Mol Imaging 2013;57:352–66.

61. Eubank WB. Diagnosis of recurrent and metastatic disease using F-18 fluorodeoxyglucose-positron emission tomography in breast cancer. Radiol Clin North Am 2007;45:659–67, vi.

62. Aukema TS, Rutgers EJ, Vogel WV, et al. The role of FDG PET/CT in patients with locoregional breast cancer recurrence: a comparison to conventional imaging techniques. Eur J Surg Oncol 2010;36: 387–92.

63. Wolfort RM, Li BD, Johnson LW, et al. The role of whole-body fluorine-18-FDG positron emission tomography in the detection of recurrence in symptomatic patients with stages II and III breast cancer. World J Surg 2006;30:1422–7.

64. Kim TS, Moon WK, Lee DS, et al. Fluorodeoxyglucose positron emission tomography for detection of recurrent or metastatic breast cancer. World J Surg 2001;25:829–34.

65. Baba S, Isoda T, Maruoka Y, et al. Diagnostic and prognostic value of pretreatment SUV in 18F-FDG/PET in breast cancer: comparison with apparent diffusion coefficient from diffusion-weighted MR imaging. J Nucl Med 2014;55:736–42.

66. Cochet A, Dygai-Cochet I, Riedinger JM, et al. (1)(8)F-FDG PET/CT provides powerful prognostic stratification in the primary staging of large breast cancer when compared with conventional explorations. Eur J Nucl Med Mol Imaging 2014;41:428–37.

67. O JH, Choi WH, Han EJ, et al. The prognostic value of (18)F-FDG PET/CT for early recurrence in operable breast cancer: comparison with TNM stage. Nucl Med Mol Imaging 2013;47:263–7.

68. Oh JK, Chung YA, Kim YS, et al. Value of F-18 FDG PET/CT in detection and prognostication of isolated extra-axillary lymph node recurrences in postoperative breast cancer. Biomed Mater Eng 2014;24: 1173–84.

69. DeSantis CE, Lin CC, Mariotto AB, et al. Cancer treatment and survivorship statistics, 2014. CA Cancer J Clin 2014;64:252–71 [Systematic review or meta-analysis].

70. Groheux D, Hindie E, Marty M, et al. (18)F-FDG-PET/CT in staging, restaging, and treatment response assessment of male breast cancer. Eur J Radiol 2014;83:1925–33 [Systematic review or meta-analysis].

71. Mandegaran R, Debard A, Alvarez M, et al. Disseminated osteomyelitis or bone metastases of breast cancer: (18)F-FDG-PET/CT helps unravel an unusual presentation. Ann Nucl Med 2014;28: 167–71.

72. Harisankar CN, Agrawal K, Bhattacharya A, et al. F-18 fluoro-deoxy-glucose and F-18 sodium fluoride cocktail PET/CT scan in patients with breast cancer having equivocal bone SPECT/CT. Indian J Nucl Med 2014;29:81–6.

73. D'Amico A, Kowalska T. Paradoxal metabolic flare detected by 18F-fluorodeoxyglucose positron emission tomography in a patient with metastatic breast cancer treated with aromatase inhibitor

and biphosphonate. Indian J Nucl Med 2014;29: 34–7.

74. Lin CY, Chen YW, Chang CC, et al. Bone metastasis versus bone marrow metastasis? Integration of diagnosis by (18)F-fluorodeoxyglucose positron emission/computed tomography in advanced malignancy with super bone scan: two case reports and literature review. Kaohsiung J Med Sci 2013; 29:229–33.

75. Avery R, Kuo PH. 18F sodium fluoride PET/CT detects osseous metastases from breast cancer missed on FDG PET/CT with marrow rebound. Clin Nucl Med 2013;38:746–8.

76. Fisher ER, Anderson S, Dean S, et al. Solving the dilemma of the immunohistochemical and other methods used for scoring estrogen receptor and progesterone receptor in patients with invasive breast carcinoma. Cancer 2005;103:164–73.

77. Castagnetta L, Traina A, Di Carlo A, et al. Do multiple oestrogen receptor assays give significant additional information for the management of breast cancer? Br J Cancer 1989;59:636–8.

78. van Netten JP, Armstrong JB, Carlyle SJ, et al. Cellular distribution patterns of estrogen receptor in human breast cancer. Eur J Cancer Clin Oncol 1988;24:1899–901.

79. Vollenweider-Zerargui L, Barrelet L, Wong Y, et al. The predictive value of estrogen and progesterone receptors' concentrations on the clinical behavior of breast cancer in women: clinical correlation on 547 patients. Cancer 1986;57:1171–80.

80. Kurland BF, Peterson LM, Lee JH, et al. Between-patient and within-patient (site-to-site) variability in estrogen receptor binding, measured in vivo by 18F-fluoroestradiol PET. J Nucl Med 2011;52: 1541–9.

81. Peterson LM, Mankoff DA, Lawton T, et al. Quantitative imaging of estrogen receptor expression in breast cancer with PET and F-18-fluoroestradiol. J Nucl Med 2008;49:367–74.

82. Mankoff DA, Tewson TJ, Peterson LM, et al. The heterogeneity of estrogen receptor (ER) expression in metastatic breast cancer is measured by [F-18]-fluoroestradiol (FES) PET. J Nucl Med 2000;41:28.

83. Linden HM, Kurland BF, Peterson LM, et al. Fluoroestradiol positron emission tomography reveals differences in pharmacodynamics of aromatase inhibitors, tamoxifen, and fulvestrant in patients with metastatic breast cancer. Clin Cancer Res 2011; 17:4799–805.

84. McGuire AH, Dehdashti F, Siegel BA, et al. Positron tomographic assessment of 16 alpha-[18F] fluoro-17 beta-estradiol uptake in metastatic breast carcinoma. J Nucl Med 1991;32:1526–31.

85. Mintun MA, Welch MJ, Siegel BA, et al. Breast cancer: PET imaging of estrogen receptors. Radiology 1988;169:45–8.

86. Mortimer JE, Dehdashti F, Siegel BA, et al. Positron emission tomography with 2-[18F]Fluoro-2-deoxy-D-glucose and 16alpha-[18F]fluoro-17beta-estradiol in breast cancer: correlation with estrogen receptor status and response to systemic therapy. Clin Cancer Res 1996;2:933–9.

87. Peterson LM, Kurland BF, Link JM, et al. Factors influencing the uptake of 18F-fluoroestradiol in patients with estrogen receptor positive breast cancer. Nucl Med Biol 2011;38:969–78.

88. Kumar P, Mercer J, Doerkson C, et al. Clinical production, stability studies and PET imaging with 16-alpha-[18F]fluoroestradiol ([18F]FES) in ER positive breast cancer patients. J Pharm Pharm Sci 2007;10:256s–65s.

89. Gemignani ML, Patil S, Seshan VE, et al. Feasibility and predictability of perioperative PET and estrogen receptor ligand in patients with invasive breast cancer. J Nucl Med 2013;54:1697–702.

90. Yang ZY, Sun YF, Yao ZF, et al. Increased F-18-fluoroestradiol uptake in radiation pneumonia. Ann Nucl Med 2013;27:931–4.

91. Mankoff DA, Peterson LM, Stekhova S, et al. Uptake of [F-18]-fluoroestradiol (FES) predicts response of recurrent or metastatic breast cancer to hormonal therapy. J Nucl Med 2003;44:126.

92. Linden HM, Stekhova SA, Link JM, et al. Quantitative fluoroestradiol positron emission tomography imaging predicts response to endocrine treatment in breast cancer. J Clin Oncol 2006; 24:2793–9.

93. Linden HM, Link JM, Stekhova S, et al. Changes in estrogen binding to ER during endocrine therapy measured by serial [F-18]-fluoroestradiol positron emission tomography (FES PET). Breast Cancer Res Treat 2005;94:S237.

94. Gennari A, Amadori D, Brain E, et al. Early prediction of efficacy of endocrine therapy in breast cancer (BC): pilot study and validation with 18F fluoroestradiol (18F-FES) PET/CT. J Clin Oncol 2013;31(15): TPS649.

95. Mankoff DA, Linden HM, Link J, et al. NCI-sponsored phase II study of [(18)f]fluoroestradiol (FES) as a marker of hormone sensitivity of metastatic breast cancer: initial results. J Clin Oncol 2011;29.

96. Yang ZY, Sun YF, Zhang YP, et al. Can fluorine-18 fluoroestradiol positron emission tomography-computed tomography demonstrate the heterogeneity of breast cancer in vivo? Clin Breast Cancer 2013;13:359–63.

97. Burstein HJ, Temin S, Anderson H, et al. Adjuvant endocrine therapy for women with hormone receptor-positive breast cancer: American Society of Clinical Oncology clinical practice guideline focused update. J Clin Oncol 2014;32:2255–69 [Systematic review or meta-analysis].

98. Zhou D, Sharp TL, Fettig NM, et al. Evaluation of a bromine-76-labeled progestin 16 alpha,17 alpha-dioxolane for breast tumor imaging and radiotherapy: in vivo biodistribution and metabolic stability studies. Nucl Med Biol 2008;35:655–63.

99. Fowler AM, Chan SR, Sharp TL, et al. Small-animal PET of steroid hormone receptors predicts tumor response to endocrine therapy using a preclinical model of breast cancer. J Nucl Med 2012;53:1119–26.

100. Dence CS, Fowler A, Zhou D, et al. Metabolism of [F-18]fluoro furanyl norprogesterone (FFNP) in mice used in clinical evaluation of therapies involving the progesterone receptor (PR) in breast tumors. J Labelled Compd Rad 2011;54:S403.

101. Price EW, Zeglis BM, Lewis JS, et al. H6phospa-trastuzumab: bifunctional methylenephosphonate-based chelator with 89Zr, 111In and 177Lu. Dalton Trans 2014;43:119–31.

102. Holloway CM, Scollard DA, Caldwell CB, et al. Phase I trial of intraoperative detection of tumor margins in patients with HER2-positive carcinoma of the breast following administration of 111In-DTPA-trastuzumab Fab fragments. Nucl Med Biol 2013;40:630–7.

103. Chan C, Cai Z, Reilly RM. Trastuzumab labeled to high specific activity with (1)(1)(1)In by conjugation to G4 PAMAM dendrimers derivatized with multiple DTPA chelators exhibits increased cytotoxic potency on HER2-positive breast cancer cells. Pharm Res 2013;30:1999–2009.

104. Boyle AJ, Liu P, Lu Y, et al. The effect of metal-chelating polymers (MCPs) for 111In complexed via the streptavidin-biotin system to trastuzumab Fab fragments on tumor and normal tissue distribution in mice. Pharm Res 2013;30:104–16.

105. The MICAD Research Team. (68)Ga-Trastuzumab F(ab') fragment. 2007 May 18 [updated 2007 Jun 25]. Molecular Imaging and Contrast Agent Database (MICAD) [Internet]. Bethesda (MD): National Center for Biotechnology Information (US); 2004–2013. Available from http://www.ncbi.nlm.nih.gov/books/NBK23296/. PubMed PMID: 20641498.

106. Mortimer JE, Bading JR, Colcher DM, et al. Functional imaging of human epidermal growth factor receptor 2-positive metastatic breast cancer using (64)Cu-DOTA-trastuzumab PET. J Nucl Med 2014;55:23–9.

107. Gaykema SB, Brouwers AH, Hovenga S. et al. Zirconium-89-trastuzumab positron emission tomography as a tool to solve a clinical dilemma in a patient with breast cancer. J Clin Oncol 2012;30:e74–5.

108. Dijkers EC, Oude Munnink TH, Kosterink JG, et al. Biodistribution of 89Zr-trastuzumab and PET imaging of HER2-positive lesions in patients with metastatic breast cancer. Clin Pharmacol Ther 2010;87:586–92.

109. Oude Munnink TH, Korte MA, Nagengast WB, et al. (89)Zr-trastuzumab PET visualises HER2 downregulation by the HSP90 inhibitor NVP-AUY922 in a human tumour xenograft. Eur J Cancer 2010;46:678–84.

110. Chalkidou A, Landau DB, Odell EW, et al. Correlation between Ki-67 immunohistochemistry and 18F-fluorothymidine uptake in patients with cancer: a systematic review and meta-analysis. Eur J Cancer 2012;48:3499–513 [Systematic review or meta-analysis].

111. Contractor K, Aboagye EO, Jacob J, et al. Monitoring early response to taxane therapy in advanced breast cancer with circulating tumor cells and [(18)F] 3 -deoxy-3 -fluorothymidine PET: a pilot study. Biomark Med 2012;6:231–3.

112. Contractor KB, Kenny LM, Stebbing J, et al. [18F]-3'Deoxy-3'-fluorothymidine positron emission tomography and breast cancer response to docetaxel. Clin Cancer Res 2011;17:7664–72.

113. Kenny L, Coombes RC, Vigushin DM, et al. Imaging early changes in proliferation at 1 week post chemotherapy: a pilot study in breast cancer patients with 3'-deoxy-3'-[18F]fluorothymidine positron emission tomography. Eur J Nucl Med Mol Imaging 2007;34:1339–47.

114. Kenny LM, Contractor KB, Hinz R, et al. Reproducibility of [11C]choline-positron emission tomography and effect of trastuzumab. Clin Cancer Res 2010;16:4236–45.

115. Contractor KB, Kenny LM, Stebbing J, et al. [11C]choline positron emission tomography in estrogen receptor-positive breast cancer. Clin Cancer Res 2009;15:5503–10.

PET with Fluorodeoxyglucose F 18/Computed Tomography in the Clinical Management and Patient Outcomes of Esophageal Cancer

Robert M. Kwee, MD, PhD[a], Charles Marcus, MD[b],
Sara Sheikhbahaei, MD, MPH[b], Rathan M. Subramaniam, MD, PhD, MPH[b,c,d],*

KEYWORDS

- ^{18}F-Fluorodeoxyglucose • Positron emission tomography • Computed tomography
- Esophageal cancer • Management

KEY POINTS

- FDG PET/CT is valuable in staging of distant metastasis and thus selecting appropriate therapy for patients.
- Baseline FDG PET/CT SUVmax and metabolic tumor volume are prognostic markers of patient survival.
- FDG PET/CT may be valuable in neoadjuvant chemoradiation therapy assessment and may impact on subsequent management.
- FDG PET/CT is valuable in detecting recurrence in patients with clinical suspicion.

INTRODUCTION

Esophageal cancer is a disease with dismal prognosis and high mortality. The incidence of esophageal cancers has increased sharply over the past few decades. The American Cancer Society has estimated a total of 18,170 new cases and 15,450 deaths from esophageal cancer in 2014.[1–3] Esophageal cancer is more common in men and is associated with obesity and heavy alcohol and tobacco use. The risk increases with age, with a median age of 67 years at diagnosis.[2,4]

More than 90% of esophageal cancers are either squamous cell carcinoma or adenocarcinoma by histology.[4] The incidence of esophageal adenocarcinomas has been increasing rapidly in the last few decades.[5] Chemoradiotherapy followed by surgery is now considered the standard

Author Disclosure: Dr. Subramaniam received an honorarium from Philips Health Care for attending the Molecular Imaging Advisory Board meeting, and from Oakstone Publications for being the Administrative Editor for Nuclear Medicine Review. Dr. Kwee, Dr. Marcus, and Dr. Sheikhbahaei have nothing to disclose.

[a] Department of Radiology, Maastricht University Medical Center, PO Box 5800, Maastricht 6202 AZ, The Netherlands; [b] Russell H Morgan Department of Radiology and Radiologic Sciences, Johns Hopkins University, JHOC 3230, 601 N Caroline Street, Baltimore, MD 21287, USA; [c] Sidney Kimmel Comprehensive Cancer Center, Johns Hopkins School of Medicine, 601 North Caroline Street, Baltimore, MD, USA; [d] Department of Health Policy and Management, Johns Hopkins Bloomberg School of Public Health, Johns Hopkins University, 624 North Broadway, Baltimore, MD 21205, USA
* Corresponding author. Russell H Morgan Department of Radiology, Johns Hopkins Medical Institutions, JHOC 3230, Baltimore, MD 21287.
E-mail address: rsubram4@jhmi.edu

PET Clin 10 (2015) 197–205
http://dx.doi.org/10.1016/j.cpet.2014.12.003
1556-8598/15/$ – see front matter © 2015 Elsevier Inc. All rights reserved.

of care in patients with potentially curable esophageal or esophagogastric junction cancer.[6,7] The 5-year survival rates in esophageal cancer vary widely from 39.6% in localized esophageal cancer to less than 4% in patients with distant metastasis. This underscores the importance of early and accurate selection of patients who might benefit from curatively intended therapy.[5]

PET with fluorodeoxyglucose F 18/computed tomography (^{18}F-FDG PET/CT) has evolved into an indispensable imaging technique in the management of patients with solid tumors.[8–14] In this article, the current clinical value of ^{18}F-FDG PET/CT in primary staging, assessment of prognosis, treatment planning, monitoring of treatment response, and restaging in patients with esophageal cancer are outlined.

PRIMARY STAGING

After a diagnosis of esophageal cancer has been made by endoscopic biopsy, the disease is commonly staged according to the TNM classification[15–17] to ascertain the treatment plan, determine prognosis, and distinguish patients with potentially curable disease from incurable advanced local or metastatic disease. Tumors confined to the esophageal wall or with less extensive extension into the periesophageal adventitia are considered potentially resectable with or without neoadjuvant chemoradiotherapy (T1–T3).[18] Patients with unresectable disease (T4b, M1) may undergo primary chemoradiotherapy, brachytherapy, stent placement, or other less invasive palliative forms of treatment. Because of the considerable morbidity and mortality associated with chemoradiotherapy and esophagectomy, appropriate patient selection is critical.[7]

In clinical practice, patients usually undergo endoscopic ultrasonography (EUS), which has excellent sensitivity and specificity in accurately determining T stage and locoregional node involvement in esophageal cancer and is superior to ^{18}F-FDG PET/CT in this context.[19] However, PET/CT may be complementary to EUS for assessment of T4b disease.[18] Increased ^{18}F-FDG uptake can be appreciated in 68% to 100% of primary tumors, whereas those showing minimal or no ^{18}F-FDG uptake are usually T1 and T2 tumors, which could be attributed to the lower degree of cellular proliferation in smaller tumors.[20] Sensitivity of ^{18}F-FDG PET/CT in detecting locoregional lymph node metastases is poor (55%; 95% confidence interval [CI], 34%–74%), whereas specificity is moderate (76%; 95% CI, 66%–83%).[21] It should be noted, however, that locoregional lymph node assessment may be clinically less significant, because these nodes are likely to be resected with

the primary tumor and may also be included in the radiation field.[22] The more important advantage of ^{18}F-FDG PET/CT is its ability to detect remote nodal involvement and systemic metastatic disease. To our knowledge, published formal studies investigating the diagnostic accuracy of integrated ^{18}F-FDG PET/CT in the M staging of esophageal cancer are limited. It has been shown that ^{18}F-FDG PET/CT provides incremental staging information and changes management in about one-third of patients, compared with EUS and CT.[22] In addition, a 2011 study by Schreurs and colleagues[23] of 216 patients with esophageal cancer has shown that EUS had limited impact beyond ^{18}F-FDG PET/CT in staging esophageal tumors, in terms of curative resectability.

Synchronous neoplasm is detected by ^{18}F-FDG PET/CT in a considerable number of patients with esophageal cancer who undergo staging, resulting in a significant impact on treatment (**Fig. 1**). A study by Malik and colleagues[24] evaluated 591 patients with biopsy-proved esophageal cancer who underwent a staging ^{18}F-FDG PET/CT. Suspicion of a synchronous neoplasm was raised in 9.3% of the patients. The most common sites suspected were the colon and head and neck regions. Malignancy was confirmed in 18.6% of the patients who underwent further investigations, resulting in a change in management in all these patients.

ASSESSMENT OF PROGNOSIS

Tumor stage is currently the most important clinical prognostic factor for survival of esophageal cancer.[16,17] A combination of other factors including male gender, African American race, obesity, tobacco and alcohol use, and presence of Barrett mucosa are additional negative prognostic factors.[5]

Recent studies suggest that FDG PET/CT imaging parameters can provide valuable prognostic information in patients with esophageal cancers (**Fig. 2**).[22,25–27] A meta-analysis of 11 studies depicted that high pretreatment standardized uptake value (SUV) was a significant predictor of poor overall survival (hazard ratio [HR], 1.86; 95% CI, 1.53–2.27) and disease-free survival (HR, 2.52; 95% CI, 1.98–3.21).[26] However, another review article that synthesized the results of 15 individual studies showed that pretreatment SUV of the primary tumor was not an unequivocal predictor of survival. Although 12 of the 15 studies showed that pretreatment SUV was a predictor of survival by univariate analysis, only two studies showed SUV to be a predictor of survival by multivariate analysis.[27] This could partly be explained by the partial-volume effect and the dependence of

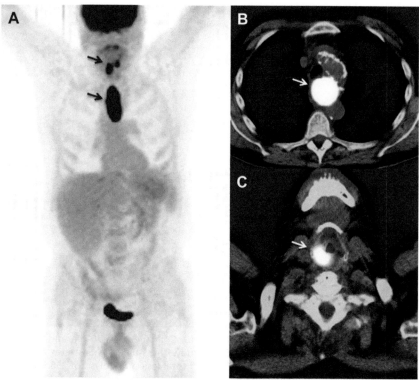

Fig. 1. Synchronous second primary. Anterior Maximum Intensity Projection (MIP) (*A*) and axial fused PET/CT (*B, C*) images of a 67-year-old man with a new diagnosis of esophageal squamous cell carcinoma, who underwent a staging FDG PET/CT study. The study demonstrates an intensely FDG-avid esophageal mass (*arrows* in *A, B*), consistent with the patient's known malignancy. The PET/CT study also demonstrated a second hypermetabolic lesion in the right pyriform sinus (*arrow* in *C*), consistent with a synchronous, second primary malignancy, which was later confirmed to be a squamous cell carcinoma of the right pyriform sinus by histopathology.

the maximum SUV (SUVmax) on tumor size.[28] In this respect, it is crucial to apply appropriate partial-volume correction methods while evaluating these tumors.[29] Other studies highlighted that assessing SUV reduction ratio before and after neoadjuvant therapy could predict the metabolic response to neoadjuvant treatment and long-term survival, independent of the previously mentioned limitation.[30]

Pretreatment metabolic tumor volume is another parameter that could be a better predictor for overall survival than SUVmax, as has been demonstrated in a retrospective study by Hyun and colleagues[28] of 151 patients. The study evaluated the prognostic significance of metabolic tumor volume, SUVmax, and other clinicopathologic variables. In the multivariate analysis, metabolic tumor volume (HR, 1.013; P = .021) was significantly associated with overall survival, whereas SUVmax (HR, 0.97; P = .061) was not. This finding needs confirmation by larger prospective studies.

Novel ¹⁸F-FDG PET/CT–defined tumor variables have been evaluated for their prognostic significance in patients with esophageal cancer. A study

by Foley and colleagues[31] of 103 patients with esophageal cancer has demonstrated an independent statistical association between pretreatment ¹⁸F-FDG PET/CT parameters including total lesion glycolysis (HR, 1.002; P = .018); metastatic length of disease, which is the total length of disease within nonregional lymph node metastasis and distant metastasis (HR, 1.035; P = .011); total local nodal metastatic count, which is the total count of involved local lymph node metastases on PET/CT (HR, 0.048; P = .015); and survival.[31]

An important issue that should be dealt with before incorporating any ¹⁸F-FDG PET–derived parameter other than TNM staging in a clinical prognostic model is the standardization of methods of acquisition and image analysis.[31,32]

RADIATION THERAPY PLANNING

Accurate delineation and subsequent irradiation of the gross tumor volume is a prerequisite for successful radiation therapy.[20] The addition of PET to CT-based radiation treatment planning has improved target volume definition through more

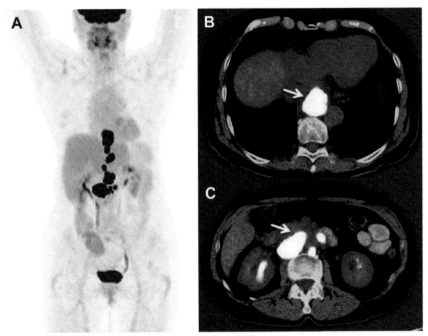

Fig. 2. Prognosis. Anterior MIP (*A*) and axial fused PET/CT (*B, C*) images of a 70-year-old man with esophageal adenocarcinoma who underwent a staging FDG PET/CT study. The study demonstrates an intensely FDG-avid esophageal lesion (*arrow* in B) with an SUVmax of 25.8 and total lesion glycolysis of 258.9 and multiple, hypermetabolic, metastatic abdominal lymphadenopathy (*arrow* in C). Despite aggressive treatment, the patient died 10 months after the study.

accurate localization of the primary tumor and involved regional lymph nodes,[33] which in turn improves locoregional disease control and reduces radiation-induced complications. To intensify the role of PET/CT scan in radiation therapy, the time interval between relevant PET/CT scan and start of the radiotherapy should be minimized. In a prospective study, Muijs and colleagues[33] evaluated esophageal tumor progression within the time interval between the diagnostic PET/CT study and the PET/CT study performed for radiotherapy treatment planning. Despite the relatively short interval between two scans (median, 3 weeks), increased tumor length (31%), TNM progression (27%), and change in SUVmax values (67%) were observed, stressing the importance of re-evaluation of the tumor if the start of the treatment is delayed.

A systematic review that included 30 original studies showed that the use of ^{18}F-FDG PET/CT changes target volumes and consequently changes treatment planning in a considerable portion of patients. The authors, however, found limited evidence supporting the validity of ^{18}F-FDG PET/CT in precise tumor delineation.[20] Although some studies report a significant positive correlation between tumor lengths measured on ^{18}F-FDG PET and pathologic examination,[34–36] it

remains unknown whether ^{18}F-FDG PET/CT can precisely assess tumor extent.[20] The locoregional lymph node metastases, which should also be included in the radiation field, may be missed by ^{18}F-FDG PET/CT because of its wide variation in sensitivity demonstrated by different studies.[18,21,37] The systematic review mentioned previously by Muijs and colleagues[20] has shown a sensitivity of 30% to 93% for the detection of metastatic lymph nodes by ^{18}F-FDG PET/CT. Lastly, it has not been investigated yet whether the use of ^{18}F-FDG PET/CT for radiation planning improves locoregional control or survival compared with stand-alone CT.[20] There is also no uniform method of tumor volume delineation yet, which can either be done by visual interpretation or by (semi) automatic contouring with use of an SUV threshold. Further validation studies are required before implementing ^{18}F-FDG PET/CT for this purpose in routine patient care.

MONITORING OF RESPONSE TO NEOADJUVANT CHEMORADIOTHERAPY

Neoadjuvant chemotherapy has become an important treatment option in patients with esophageal cancer (**Fig. 3**). Patients who respond favorably benefit from it and surgery may be delayed or

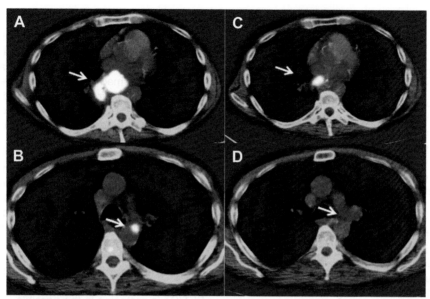

Fig. 3. Staging and neoadjuvant treatment response assessment. Axial fused PET/CT (*A, B*) images of a 57-year-old man with a new diagnosis of esophageal squamous cell carcinoma who underwent a staging FDG PET/CT study. The study demonstrates an intensely FDG-avid (SUVmax, 10.7) midesophageal mass (*arrow* in A) extending into the right lung with hypermetabolic (SUVmax, 4.4), metastatic left hilar lymphadenopathy (*arrow* in B). He underwent chemoradiation and posttreatment fused PET/CT. (*C, D*) Images demonstrate interval decrease in metabolic activity (SUVmax, 5.3) in the esophageal lesion (*arrow* in C) with resolution of the previously seen hilar lymphadenopathy (*arrow* in D), consistent with treatment response. Following the study he underwent transhiatal esophagectomy.

even refrained from. However, in patients who respond insufficiently, neoadjuvant chemotherapy should be discontinued and surgery should no longer be delayed. In the Chemoradiotherapy for Esophageal Cancer Followed by Surgery Study (CROSS) trial, 39% of patients showed no histopathologic tumor regression.[7] Toxicity caused by chemotherapy occurs in 11% to 90% and there is also a risk of radiation-induced complications.[7,38] Hence it is crucial to identify patients who respond to neoadjuvant therapy accurately and as early as possible. At present, however, there is no method yet that can reliably differentiate responders from nonresponders early in the course of neoadjuvant treatment.

Several studies have indicated the usefulness of ^{18}F-FDG PET/CT scan in the monitoring of therapeutic response in esophageal cancer.[39,40] A previous meta-analysis comprising 20 studies showed that diagnostic performance of ^{18}F-FDG PET in assessing tumor response to neoadjuvant chemotherapy or chemoradiotherapy ranged widely with the pooled estimates (95% CI) of 67% (62%–72%) and 68% (64%–73%) for sensitivity and specificity, respectively.[39] A more recent meta-analysis on 30 studies estimated slightly better sensitivity (70.3%; 95% CI, 64.4%–75.8%) and specificity (70.1%; 95% CI, 65.1%–74.8%) for

^{18}F-FDG-PET/CT in the evaluation of neoadjuvant therapy response in patients with esophageal cancer. They suggested a 50% reduction in the SUV between preneoadjuvant and postneoadjuvant therapy PET/CT scan (within 2 weeks) as an optimal cut-off for predicting response to neoadjuvant treatment.[40]

The accuracy of PET/CT metabolic changes for the prediction of treatment outcome was not significantly influenced by the timing of the scan.[23,41] A recent meta-analysis on 26 studies comprised of 1544 patients showed that ^{18}F-FDG-PET is a significant predictor of long-term survival in patients with esophageal cancers, whether it is performed during or after neoadjuvant therapy. The pooled HR (95% CI) of the complete metabolic response versus no response for overall survival and disease-free survival was 0.51 (0.40–0.64) and 0.47 (0.38–0.57), respectively.[23]

However, there are numerous criticisms to be considered and some studies emphasized that PET/CT is not sufficiently reliable in the individual patient for determining therapeutic response in the primary tumor.[18,42,43] In a well-designed prospective study in which ^{18}F-FDG PET/CT was performed 14 days after start of neoadjuvant chemoradiotherapy, Malik and colleagues[43] found no correlation between change in tumor SUV with either histopathologic response or survival. They concluded that, in contrast to published reports on neoadjuvant chemotherapy, combined chemoradiotherapy lowers the predictive accuracy of ^{18}F-FDG PET/CT below clinically applicable levels. Increased ^{18}F-FDG uptake by radiation-induced inflammation or esophagitis may be an important cause in this clinical setting.[43,44]

In another study, van Heijl and colleagues[42] showed that although an SUV decrease was found to be significantly associated with histopathologic tumor response, its predictive accuracy was too low to justify the clinical use of ^{18}F-FDG PET/CT for tumor response assessment. Furthermore, many technical and patient-related factors affect the quantification of FDG-uptake, and criteria developed in one center may not be applicable in other centers.[18] Thus, a more accurate and universal response evaluation criteria should be formulated. Yanagawa and colleagues[45] compared two current, widely used response evaluation criteria (PET response criteria in solid tumors versus response evaluation criteria in solid tumors) in patients with locally advanced esophageal cancer after neoadjuvant chemotherapy. They concluded that PET response criteria in solid tumors would be more suitable for evaluation of chemotherapeutic response to esophageal cancer than response evaluation criteria in solid tumors ($P<.0001$).

RESTAGING

Precise imaging after therapy is crucial to diagnose residual, recurrent, or interval metastatic disease. ^{18}F-FDG PET/CT after neoadjuvant therapy is mainly performed to assess for interval metastases, because their presence precludes surgical resection. ^{18}F-FDG PET/CT can detect interval metastases in up to 8% of patients, as has been demonstrated by several independent studies. Interval metastases may be detected in the liver, lungs, distant lymph nodes, and bone.[46,47] The presence of distant metastases at unusual sites, such as skeletal muscle, has also been reported.[46] Because the presence of distant metastases dramatically changes the treatment plan and some of them may be outside the visual range of routine stand-alone CT imaging, ^{18}F-FDG PET/CT is a preferred imaging modality of choice in this setting.[46,47] A concern of ^{18}F-FDG PET/CT in restaging is the possible identification of lesions that are false-positive for metastases but require further diagnostic work-up. However, the number of false-positive ^{18}F-FDG PET/CT results for distant metastases seems to be low.[47,48] A common cause for false-positive results is inflammation or infection. False-positive results have been encountered in up to 8% of the patients.[47]

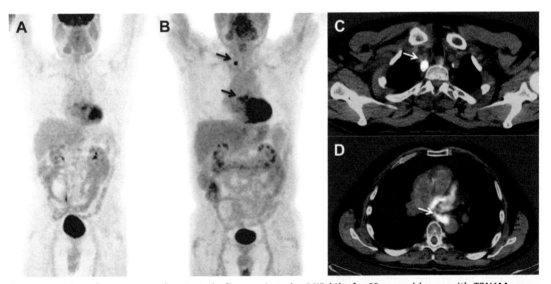

Fig. 4. Detection of recurrent and metastatic disease. Anterior MIP (*A*) of a 62-year-old man with T2N1Mo squamous cell carcinoma of the esophagus postchemoradiation who underwent a restaging FDG PET/CT study. The study demonstrated no evidence of metabolically active foci, consistent with complete response to treatment. However, the anterior MIP (*B*) axial fused PET/CT (*C, D*) images of the follow-up PET/CT study performed 18 months after the former study revealed recurrent, hypermetabolic (SUVmax, 4.1) disease in the distal esophagus (*arrows* in B, D) with a hypermetabolic (SUVmax, 6.4) metastatic cervical lymph node (*arrows* in B, C).

DETECTION OF RECURRENT DISEASE

The data of the CROSS I and II trials showed that after a minimum follow-up of 24 months after treatment, 34.7% of patients developed recurrent disease (Fig. 4).[49] Distant recurrences occurred in 59% and distant plus locoregional recurrences occurred in 31% of patients, whereas locoregional recurrences occurred in 9% of patients.[49] There is no proved benefit of routine imaging follow-up and it is also not clear yet whether this leads to prolonged survival. One retrospective, nonrandomized study investigating 174 patients with recurrent disease stated that patients who were treated for their recurrence had a significantly longer median survival.[50] ^{18}F-FDG PET/CT may have a role to diagnose and localize recurrent disease only in patients who are suspected on clinical grounds.

Guo and colleagues[51] studied 45 patients with esophageal squamous cell cancer who underwent ^{18}F-FDG PET/CT to detect a possible recurrence within a mean interval of 9.3 months after the initial treatment. They showed that overall sensitivity and specificity of ^{18}F-FDG PET/CT for detecting recurrent disease was 93.1% and 75.7%, respectively.[51] These values are comparable with those of Sun and colleagues,[52] who found a sensitivity of 100% and a specificity of 66.7% in 20 patients who underwent ^{18}F-FDG PET/CT for restaging within a mean of 20 months after initial treatment. These studies have also shown that ^{18}F-FDG PET/CT is highly sensitive and specific to detect metastases at distant sites. At local sites, sensitivity is high, but specificity is poor; false-positive findings are mostly caused by (radiation therapy and/or surgically induced) inflammatory changes. Chronic inflammation of mediastinal lymph nodes is another source of false-positive cases.[51,52] The time interval between treatment completion and the PET scan plays a significant role in the interpretation of these findings and clinical correlation with endoscopy and/or biopsy is often required to clarify the cause of these findings.

SUMMARY

^{18}F-FDG PET/CT has gained importance in the recent past in the evaluation of patients with esophageal cancer. It adds value to clinical evaluation by assisting in the accurate staging of patients, especially in the detection of distant disease and thereby having a significant impact on the treatment plan. It can provide valuable prognostic information by predicting survival. ^{18}F-FDG PET/CT improves target volume definition and adds important information that can be of value to radiation therapy planning. It can be used to assess treatment response to neoadjuvant chemoradiotherapy and can change subsequent treatment plans. In the follow-up period, ^{18}F-FDG PET/CT helps in accurate restaging of these patients, especially by detecting interval metastases. It also has value in detecting recurrent disease in patients with prior clinical suspicion.

REFERENCES

1. Tsuchiya T, Osanai T, Ishikawa A, et al. Hibernomas show intense accumulation of FDG positron emission tomography. J Comput Assist Tomogr 2006; 30:333–6.
2. Howlader N, Noone A,M Krapcho M, et al, editors. SEER cancer statistics review, 1975–2011. Bethesda (MD): National Cancer Institute. Available at: http://seer.cancer.gov/csr/1975_2011/. Accessed October 29, 2014.
3. Siegel R, Ma J, Zou Z, et al. Cancer statistics. CA Cancer J Clin 2014;64:9–29.
4. Enzinger PC, Mayer RJ. Esophageal cancer. N Engl J Med 2003;349:2241–52.
5. Lagergren J, Lagergren P. Recent developments in esophageal adenocarcinoma. CA Cancer J Clin 2013;63:232–48.
6. Sjoquist KM, Burmeister BH, Smithers BM, et al. Survival after neoadjuvant chemotherapy or chemoradiotherapy for resectable oesophageal carcinoma: an updated meta-analysis. Lancet Oncol 2011;12: 681–92.
7. van Hagen P, Hulshof MC, van Lanschot JJ, et al. Preoperative chemoradiotherapy for esophageal or junctional cancer. N Engl J Med 2012;366: 2074–84.
8. Dibble EH, Karantanis D, Mercier G, et al. PET/CT of cancer patients: part 1, pancreatic neoplasms. AJR Am J Roentgenol 2012;199:952–67.
9. Davison J, Mercier G, Russo G, et al. PET-based primary tumor volumetric parameters and survival of patients with non-small cell lung carcinoma. AJR Am J Roentgenol 2013;200:635–40.
10. Hadiprodjo D, Ryan T, Truong MT, et al. Parotid gland tumors: preliminary data for the value of FDG PET/CT diagnostic parameters. AJR Am J Roentgenol 2012;198:W185–90.
11. Davison JM, Subramaniam RM, Surasi DS, et al. FDG PET/CT in patients with HIV. AJR Am J Roentgenol 2011;197:284–94.
12. Agarwal A, Chirindel A, Shah BA, et al. Evolving role of FDG PET/CT in multiple myeloma imaging and management. AJR Am J Roentgenol 2013;200: 884–90.
13. Paidpally V, Tahari AK, Lam S, et al. Addition of 18F-FDG PET/CT to clinical assessment predicts overall

survival in HNSCC: a retrospective analysis with follow-up for 12 years. J Nucl Med 2013;54:2039–45.

14. Antoniou AJ, Marcus C, Tahari AK, et al. Follow-up or surveillance 18F-FDG PET/CT and survival outcome in lung cancer patients. J Nucl Med 2014;55(7): 1062–8.

15. Aoki J, Endo E, Watanabe H, et al. FDG-PET for evaluating musculoskeletal tumors: a review. J Orthop Sci 2003;8:435–41.

16. Hsu PK, Wu YC, Chou TY, et al. Comparison of the 6th and 7th editions of the American Joint Committee on Cancer tumor-node-metastasis staging system in patients with resected esophageal carcinoma. Ann Thorac Surg 2010;89:1024–31.

17. Talsma K, van Hagen P, Grotenhuis BA, et al. Comparison of the 6th and 7th editions of the UICC-AJCC TNM classification for esophageal cancer. Ann Surg Oncol 2012;19:2142–8.

18. Bruzzi JF, Munden RF, Truong MT, et al. PET/CT of esophageal cancer: its role in clinical management. Radiographics 2007;27:1635–52.

19. Walker AJ, Spier BJ, Perlman SB, et al. Integrated PET/CT fusion imaging and endoscopic ultrasound in the pre-operative staging and evaluation of esophageal cancer. Mol Imaging Biol 2011;13: 166–71.

20. Muijs CT, Beukema JC, Pruim J, et al. A systematic review on the role of FDG-PET/CT in tumour delineation and radiotherapy planning in patients with esophageal cancer. Radiother Oncol 2010;97: 165–71.

21. Shi W, Wang W, Wang J, et al. Meta-analysis of 18FDG PET-CT for nodal staging in patients with esophageal cancer. Surg Oncol 2013;22:112–6.

22. Barber TW, Duong CP, Leong T, et al. 18F-FDG PET/CT has a high impact on patient management and provides powerful prognostic stratification in the primary staging of esophageal cancer: a prospective study with mature survival data. J Nucl Med 2012; 53:864–71.

23. Schreurs LM, Janssens AC, Groen H, et al. Value of EUS in determining curative resectability in reference to CT and FDG-PET: the optimal sequence in preoperative staging of esophageal cancer? Ann Surg Oncol 2011. [Epub ahead of print].

24. Malik V, Johnston C, Donohoe C, et al. (18)F-FDG PET-detected synchronous primary neoplasms in the staging of esophageal cancer: incidence, cost, and impact on management. Clin Nucl Med 2012; 37:1152–8.

25. Brown C, Howes B, Jamieson GG, et al. Accuracy of PET-CT in predicting survival in patients with esophageal cancer. World J Surg 2012;36:1089–95.

26. Pan L, Gu P, Huang G, et al. Prognostic significance of SUV on PET/CT in patients with esophageal cancer: a systematic review and meta-analysis. Eur J Gastroenterol Hepatol 2009;21:1008–15.

27. Omloo JM, van Heijl M, Hoekstra OS, et al. FDG-PET parameters as prognostic factor in esophageal cancer patients: a review. Ann Surg Oncol 2011;18: 3338–52.

28. Hyun SH, Choi JY, Shim YM, et al. Prognostic value of metabolic tumor volume measured by 18F-fluorodeoxyglucose positron emission tomography in patients with esophageal carcinoma. Ann Surg Oncol 2010;17:115–22.

29. Soret M, Bacharach SL, Buvat I. Partial-volume effect in PET tumor imaging. J Nucl Med 2007;48: 932–45.

30. Wang WP, Wang KN, Chen LQ. PET could predict response to neoadjuvant therapy and long-term survival of patients with esophageal cancer. World J Surg 2013;37:930–1.

31. Foley KG, Fielding P, Lewis WG, et al. Prognostic significance of novel (1)(8)F-FDG PET/CT defined tumour variables in patients with oesophageal cancer. Eur J Radiol 2014;83:1069–73.

32. Boellaard R, O'Doherty MJ, Weber WA, et al. FDG PET and PET/CT: EANM procedure guidelines for tumour PET imaging: version 1.0. Eur J Nucl Med Mol Imaging 2010;37:181–200.

33. Muijs CT, Pruim J, Beukema JC, et al. Oesophageal tumour progression between the diagnostic (1)(8)F-FDG-PET and the (1)(8)F-FDG-PET for radiotherapy treatment planning. Radiother Oncol 2013;106: 283–7.

34. Mamede M, El Fakhri G, Abreu-e-Lima P, et al. Pre-operative estimation of esophageal tumor metabolic length in FDG-PET images with surgical pathology confirmation. Ann Nucl Med 2007;21:553–62.

35. Zhong X, Yu J, Zhang B, et al. Using 18F-fluorodeoxyglucose positron emission tomography to estimate the length of gross tumor in patients with squamous cell carcinoma of the esophagus. Int J Radiat Oncol Biol Phys 2009;73:136–41.

36. Han D, Yu J, Yu Y, et al. Comparison of (18)F-fluorothymidine and (18)F-fluorodeoxyglucose PET/CT in delineating gross tumor volume by optimal threshold in patients with squamous cell carcinoma of thoracic esophagus. Int J Radiat Oncol Biol Phys 2010;76: 1235–41.

37. Shimizu S, Hosokawa M, Itoh K, et al. Can hybrid FDG-PET/CT detect subclinical lymph node metastasis of esophageal cancer appropriately and contribute to radiation treatment planning? A comparison of image-based and pathological findings. Int J Clin Oncol 2009;14:421–5.

38. Malthaner RA, Collin S, Fenlon D. Preoperative chemotherapy for resectable thoracic esophageal cancer. Cochrane Database Syst Rev 2006:CD001556.

39. Kwee RM. Prediction of tumor response to neoadjuvant therapy in patients with esophageal cancer with use of 18F FDG PET: a systematic review. Radiology 2010;254:707–17.

40. Chen YM, Pan XF, Tong LJ, et al. Can (1)(8)F-fluoro-deoxyglucose positron emission tomography predict responses to neoadjuvant therapy in oesophageal cancer patients? A meta-analysis. Nucl Med Commun 2011;32:1005–10.

41. Zhu W, Xing L, Yue J, et al. Prognostic significance of SUV on PET/CT in patients with localised oesophagogastric junction cancer receiving neoadjuvant chemotherapy/chemoradiation: a systematic review and meta-analysis. Br J Radiol 2012;85:e694–701.

42. van Heijl M, Omloo JM, van Berge Henegouwen MI, et al. Fluorodeoxyglucose positron emission tomography for evaluating early response during neoadjuvant chemoradiotherapy in patients with potentially curable esophageal cancer. Ann Surg 2011;253:56–63.

43. Malik V, Lucey JA, Duffy GJ, et al. Early repeated 18F-FDG PET scans during neoadjuvant chemoradiation fail to predict histopathologic response or survival benefit in adenocarcinoma of the esophagus. J Nucl Med 2010;51:1863–9.

44. Wieder HA, Brucher BL, Zimmermann F, et al. Time course of tumor metabolic activity during chemoradiotherapy of esophageal squamous cell carcinoma and response to treatment. J Clin Oncol 2004;22:900–8.

45. Yanagawa M, Tatsumi M, Miyata H, et al. Evaluation of response to neoadjuvant chemotherapy for esophageal cancer: PET response criteria in solid tumors versus response evaluation criteria in solid tumors. J Nucl Med 2012;53:872–80.

46. Bruzzi JF, Swisher SG, Truong MT, et al. Detection of interval distant metastases: clinical utility of integrated CT-PET imaging in patients with esophageal carcinoma after neoadjuvant therapy. Cancer 2007;109:125–34.

47. Blom RL, Schreurs WM, Belgers HJ, et al. The value of post-neoadjuvant therapy PET-CT in the detection of interval metastases in esophageal carcinoma. Eur J Surg Oncol 2011;37:774–8.

48. Cerfolio RJ, Bryant AS, Ohja B, et al. The accuracy of endoscopic ultrasonography with fine-needle aspiration, integrated positron emission tomography with computed tomography, and computed tomography in restaging patients with esophageal cancer after neoadjuvant chemoradiotherapy. J Thorac Cardiovasc Surg 2005;129:1232–41.

49. Oppedijk V, van der Gaast A, van Lanschot JJ, et al. Patterns of recurrence after surgery alone versus preoperative chemoradiotherapy and surgery in the CROSS trials. J Clin Oncol 2014;32:385–91.

50. Abate E, DeMeester SR, Zehetner J, et al. Recurrence after esophagectomy for adenocarcinoma: defining optimal follow-up intervals and testing. J Am Coll Surg 2010;210:428–35.

51. Guo H, Zhu H, Xi Y, et al. Diagnostic and prognostic value of 18F-FDG PET/CT for patients with suspected recurrence from squamous cell carcinoma of the esophagus. J Nucl Med 2007;48:1251–8.

52. Sun L, Su XH, Guan YS, et al. Clinical usefulness of 18F-FDG PET/CT in the restaging of esophageal cancer after surgical resection and radiotherapy. World J Gastroenterol 2009;15:1836–42.

Role of 2-Deoxy-2-[18F]-fluoro-D-glucose-PET/Computed Tomography in Lymphoma

Sree Harsha Tirumani, MD[a,b], Ann S. LaCasce, MD[c,d], Heather A. Jacene, MD[a,b],*

KEYWORDS

- Lymphoma • Hodgkin lymphoma • Diffuse large B-cell lymphoma • FDG-PET/CT
- Interim PET/CT

KEY POINTS

- 2-Deoxy-2-[18F]-fluoro-D-glucose (FDG)-PET/computed tomography (CT) at the time of initial staging can help in appropriate staging of the patients.
- Both interim and end-of-therapy PETs have significant prognostic value in patients with Hodgkin lymphoma and aggressive non-Hodgkin lymphoma and more accurately assess for the presence of residual malignancy than anatomic imaging.
- Interim FDG-PET/CT and risk-adapted strategies are currently used in clinical trials but are an area of active investigation.
- Visual assessment based on Deauville criteria is recommended for interpretation of interim FDG-PET/CT.

INTRODUCTION

Lymphoma represents about half of all hematologic malignancies, with an estimated 79,990 new cases and 20,200 deaths in 2014.[1,2] The outcome for patients with lymphoma has significantly improved over the past few decades with 5-year survival rates (%) increasing from 72% in 1975 to 1977 to 87% in 2002 to 2008 for Hodgkin lymphoma (HL) and 47% in 1975 to 1977 to 71% in 2002 to 2008 for non-Hodgkin lymphoma (NHL).[3] This increase in survival is largely attributed to availability of newer chemotherapeutic regimens,

the introduction of anti-CD20 immunotherapy for NHL, and improvements in outcomes for patients undergoing stem cell transplantation. Major advances in the understanding of the molecular basis of lymphoma have also led to newer risk-stratification strategies as well as the development of targeted agents.

Functional imaging with combined PET/computed tomography (CT) using 2-deoxy-2-[18F]-fluoro-D-glucose (FDG) has evolved as the major work horse for imaging aggressive lymphomas in the past 15 years. FDG-PET/CT is now the cornerstone for the initial staging and

The authors have nothing to disclose.
[a] Department of Imaging, Dana-Farber Cancer Institute, Harvard Medical School, 450 Brookline Avenue, Boston, MA 02215, USA; [b] Department of Radiology, Brigham and Women's Hospital, Harvard Medical School, 75 Francis Street, Boston, MA 02115, USA; [c] Lymphoma Program, Dana-Farber Cancer Institute, Harvard Medical School, 450 Brookline Avenue, M227, Boston, MA 02215, USA; [d] Department of Medicine, Brigham and Women's Hospital, Harvard Medical School, 75 Francis Street, Boston, MA 02115, USA
* Corresponding author. Department of Imaging, Dana-Farber Cancer Institute, Harvard Medical School, 450 Brookline Avenue, Boston, MA 02215.
E-mail address: hjacene@partners.org

PET Clin 10 (2015) 207–225
http://dx.doi.org/10.1016/j.cpet.2014.12.005
1556-8598/15/$ – see front matter © 2015 Elsevier Inc. All rights reserved.

end-of-therapy treatment response assessment in aggressive lymphomas. The role of interim FDG-PET/CT, performed after a few cycles of chemotherapy, for risk-adapted therapy strategies is an area of active investigation in clinical trials.[4] In this article, the role of FDG-PET/CT at various time points in the course of lymphoma for guiding therapeutic management is reviewed.

CLINICAL BACKGROUND
Lymphoma Classifications

HL accounts for 12% of all lymphomas and is further classified as classic HL (CHL) (95%) or nodular lymphocyte-predominant HL (NLPHL) (5%).[2,5] CHL has 4 histologic subtypes: nodular sclerosis, mixed cellularity, lymphocyte-depleted, and lymphocyte-rich. The histologic hallmark of CHL is the multinucleated giant Reed-Sternberg cell, which accounts for ~1% of the tumor mass, in a background of inflammatory cells. NLPHL is characterized by the presence of Reed-Sternberg variants referred to as "popcorn or LP cells," which typically express CD20, in contrast with Reed-Sternberg cells, which express CD30 and CD15.[5]

NHL is a heterogeneous group of diseases further classified according to the cell of origin: B cell (85%), T cell (15%), and natural killer (NK) cell (rare).[5] NHL is further subdivided based on natural history into aggressive and indolent subtypes.[5–9] These subtypes are listed in **Box 1**.

Staging and Prognosis

Staging is an essential part of lymphoma management that acts as a guide for planning treatment strategies and for determining prognosis. Originally developed for HL, the Ann Arbor staging system with Cotswold modification has subsequently been used for staging both HL and NHL (**Table 1**) and is based on the number and location of nodal sites, extranodal site, and the presence or absence of B symptoms.[10,11]

The International Prognostic Score (IPS) is a strong predictor of outcome in HL and is based on the presence of unfavorable factors (**Table 2**).[12] The presence of more unfavorable factors is associated with a worse prognosis (eg, 5-year survival with an IPS of 5 is 67% versus 97% for an IPS of 1).[13] After initial diagnosis and staging, HL is further classified into early-stage favorable HL (stage I and II with no unfavorable factors), early-stage unfavorable HL with or without bulky disease (stage I and II with unfavorable factors), and advanced stage HL.[2]

The International Prognostic Index (IPI) is a similar 5-point scale used for assessment of prognosis in aggressive subtypes of NHL (see **Table 2**).[14] Several modifications of IPI have been proposed,

---

Box 1
Major subtypes of non-Hodgkin lymphoma

B cell (85%)

Aggressive

Diffuse large B-cell lymphoma (DLBCL)

Primary mediastinal large B-cell lymphoma

Intravascular large B-cell lymphoma

ALK+ large B-cell lymphoma

Plasmablastic lymphoma

Burkitt lymphoma

B-cell lymphoma, unclassifiable

Mantle cell lymphoma

Indolent

Small lymphocytic lymphoma/Chronic lymphocytic leukemia (CLL/SLL)

Follicular lymphoma

MZL (splenic, nodal, extranodal)

Hairy cell leukemia

Primary cutaneous B-cell lymphoma

Lymphoplasmacytic lymphoma

T-cell and NK cell (15%)

Aggressive

Extranodal NK/T-cell lymphoma, nasal type

Angioimmunoblastic T-cell lymphoma

Anaplastic large cell lymphoma, ALK+/−

Peripheral T-cell lymphoma (PTCL)

Enteropathy-associated T-cell lymphoma

Hepatosplenic T-cell lymphoma

Aggressive NK cell leukemia

Adult T-cell leukemia/lymphoma

Indolent

Primary cutaneous CD30+ T-cell lymphoproliferative disorder

T-cell large granular lymphocytic leukemia

T-cell prolymphocytic leukemia

Mycosis fungoides/Sezary syndrome

Adapted from Refs.[5–9]

---

including age-adjusted IPI, stage-adjusted IPI, National Comprehensive Cancer Network (NCCN)-IPI, and IPI for patients treated with rituximab.[14–18] Disease-specific prognostic scores are used for follicular lymphoma (FLIPI), mantle cell lymphoma (MIPI), T-cell lymphoma, and NK/T-cell lymphoma.[19,20] The prognosis of NHL also depends

Table 1
Ann Arbor staging of lymphoma

Stage	
I	Involvement of a single lymph node region (eg, cervical, axillary, inguinal, mediastinal) or lymphoid structure, such as the spleen, thymus, or Waldeyer ring
II	Involvement of 2 or more lymph node regions or lymph node structures on the same side of the diaphragm
III	Involvement of lymph node regions or lymphoid structures on both sides of the diaphragm
IV	Diffuse or disseminated involvement of one or more extranodal organs or tissue beyond that designated E, with or without associated lymph node involvement
A: No systemic symptoms	
B: Presence of systemic symptoms of significant unexplained fever, night sweats, or unexplained weight loss exceeding 10% of body weight during the 6 months before diagnosis	
E: Extranodal contiguous extension that can be encompassed within an irradiation field	
X: Bulky disease: mediastinal mass with a maximum width that is equal to or greater than one-third of the internal transverse diameter of the thorax at the level of T5/6 interspace or >10 cm maximum dimension of a nodal mass	

Adapted from Carbone PP, Kaplan HS, Musshoff K, et al. Report of the committee on Hodgkin's disease staging classification. Cancer Res 1971;31(11):1860–1; and Lister TA, Crowther D, Sutcliffe SB, et al. Report of a committee convened to discuss the evaluation and staging of patients with Hodgkin's disease: Cotswolds meeting. J Clin Oncol 1989;7(11):1630–6.

Table 2
International prognostic score and international prognostic index

International Prognostic Score[a]	International Prognostic Index[b]
Serum albumin <4 g/dL	Age >60 y
Hemoglobin <10.5 g/dL	Stage III or IV disease
Male gender	Elevated serum lactate dehydrogenase
Age >45 y	Eastern Cooperative Oncology Group (ECOG) performance status of 2, 3, or 4
Stage IV disease White blood cell count ≥15,000/μL Absolute lymphocyte count <600/μL and/or <8% of the total white blood cell count	More than 1 extranodal site

[a] One point is given for each of the characteristics listed that are present in the patient, for a total score ranging from 0 to 7.
[b] One point is given for each of the above characteristics present in the patient, for a total score ranging from 0 to 5.
Adapted from Hasenclever D, Diehl V. A prognostic score for advanced Hodgkin's disease. International Prognostic Factors Project on Advanced Hodgkin's Disease. N Engl J Med 1998;339(21):1510; and A predictive model for aggressive non-Hodgkin's lymphoma. The International Non-Hodgkin's Lymphoma Prognostic Factors Project. N Engl J Med 1993;329(14):991.

on the disease subtype as well as other molecular factors. For example, the outcome in diffuse large B-cell lymphoma (DLBCL) is less favorable for patients with the activated B-cell-type DLBCL compared with the germinal center B-cell subtype on gene expression profiling and for those with a c-myc translocation either alone or with a BCL-2 translocation ("double hit").[21–25]

ROLE AND IMPACT OF 2-DEOXY-2-[18F]-FLUORO-ᴅ-GLUCOSE-PET/COMPUTED TOMOGRAPHY

The role and impact of FDG-PET/CT in the management of patients with lymphoma vary depending on lymphoma subtype. Most of the literature focuses on HL and DLBCL and is growing for other subtypes. Subsequent sections of this article have been divided with this in mind as the currently available data allowed.

Diagnosis and Histologic Grading

Nearly all subtypes of lymphoma accumulate FDG.[26] The level of FDG uptake across the lymphoma subtypes varies along a continuum, with generally lower level uptake in indolent lymphomas and higher levels of uptake in aggressive lymphoma (**Fig. 1**).[27,28] In a retrospective study of 97 patients with NHL, indolent lymphomas had a maximum standardized uptake value (SUV_{max}) range of 2.3 to 13.0 compared with 3.2 to 43.0 in aggressive lymphomas. Using a SUV_{max} cutoff of 10, receiver operating characteristic analysis distinguished indolent and aggressive NHL with a sensitivity of 71% and a specificity of 81%.[28]

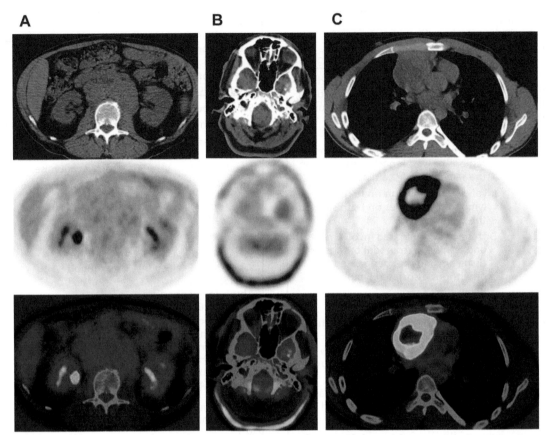

Fig. 1. Correlation of FDG uptake on FDG-PET/CT with histology (top row: CT; middle row: FDG-PET; bottom row: fused PET/CT). (*A*) A 65-year-old man with CLL. FDG-PET/CT demonstrates conglomerate retroperitoneal lymphadenopathy with low-level FDG uptake consistent with indolent lymphoma. (*B*) A 31-year-old man with cutaneous T-cell lymphoma. FDG-PET/CT images demonstrate diffuse FDG-avid skin thickening involving the occipital scalp as well as the rest of the body (not shown). (*C*) A 23-year-old man with DLBCL. FDG-PET/CT demonstrates an anterior mediastinal mass with intense peripheral FDG uptake and central photopenia consistent with necrosis.

Given the overlap of SUVs between the indolent and aggressive lymphomas, however, FDG-PET/CT cannot replace histologic evaluation, but rather can help guide biopsies (**Fig. 2**).

The utility of FDG-PET/CT for guiding biopsy is particularly true for patients with indolent NHL suspected to have transformation into a more aggressive histology. Transformation of indolent NHL can been seen on FDG-PET(/CT) as a disproportionately high accumulation of FDG in one area of disease compared with the others or a substantial increase in FDG uptake over serial scans. Several other cutoff levels of SUV, besides 10, have been used for suggesting transformation on FDG-PET/CT, leading to differences in reported sensitivities and specificities. In general, FDG-PET/CT is more specific for transformation in the presence of symptoms and as SUV or the difference in SUVs between areas of higher and lower uptake increase. FDG-PET/CT has a very high negative predictive value

(97%) for excluding transformation in patients with small lymphocytic lymphoma/chronic lymphocytic leukemia (SLL/CLL),[29] and higher cut thresholds are likely needed for follicular lymphoma (FL) versus SLL/CLL (**Fig. 3**).

Staging of Aggressive Lymphoma

Although it is the most widely available imaging modality, CT scan underestimates the presence of lymphoma in normal-sized lymph nodes as well as extranodal and bone marrow involvement. FDG-PET improves the accuracy of staging by detecting more disease sites and has been shown to have higher sensitivity and specificity compared with gallium scan or CT alone.[30–34]

Most studies assessing the role of FDG-PET for staging of lymphoma either included patients with both HL and NHL[32,34–37] or focused on

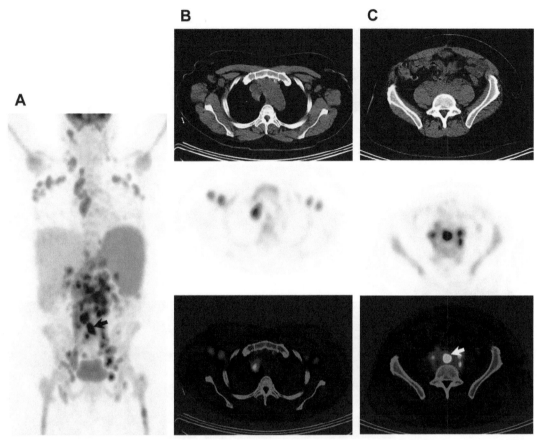

Fig. 2. A 52-year-old woman with grade 3 FL. Maximum intensity projection image (*A*) and axial FDG-PET/CT images (*B, C*) demonstrate moderately FDG-avid cervical thoracic, abdominopelvic, inguinal lymphadenopathy as well as increased FDG-uptake in the spleen and femur most consistent with metabolically active FL. Just distal to the level of the aortic bifurcation (*C*), there is more focal intense FDG uptake in a retroperitoneal lymph node (*arrows* in A and C), found to represent transformation to a higher grade lymphoma on pathology (top row: CT; middle row: FDG-PET; bottom row: fused PET/CT).

HL.[30,31,33,38,39] Overall, FDG-PET changed the clinical stage in 8% to 48% of patients, resulting in treatment changes in 3% to 45%. In these studies, upstaging was generally more common than downstaging. In a prospective study of 186 patients with HL,[39] CT and PET were concordant for stage in 156 (84%). In the 30 discordant cases (16%), 27 were upstaged because of detection of disease in normal-sized lymph nodes and extranodal sites on FDG-PET.[39] A change in treatment based on PET results occurred in 7% of patients in this study.

The major limitations of these initial studies investigating FDG-PET(/CT) for staging of lymphoma include mixed populations of patients, lack of biopsies confirming the PET/CT findings, and lack of correlation that changes in stage and treatment affects outcomes. Despite the limitations of these studies, FDG-PET/CT is considered an integral component of the initial workup for

patients with HL and DLBCL according to the NCCN guidelines.[1,2]

The coregistration of PET with CT has been shown to be more accurate than PET or CT alone for staging lymphoma.[32,39] However, the role of PET with contrast-enhanced CT (CECT) is still controversial.[40–42] In a study of 101 patients, both low-dose PET/CT and PET/CECT had similar sensitivity for detecting lymphoma in nodes (97%) and both were better than PET (82%) and CT (91%) alone.[41] In another recent study of 163 patients, CECT performed after low-dose PET/CT had no clinical impact in 92% cases and had clear clinical impact in 3% cases (upstaging in 2 patients and diagnosis of deep venous thrombosis in 5 patients), however, at the cost of increased radiation dose.[40] A debatable clinical impact was noted in 5% of cases that necessitated additional investigations that either delayed or did not influence treatment. Therefore, although the

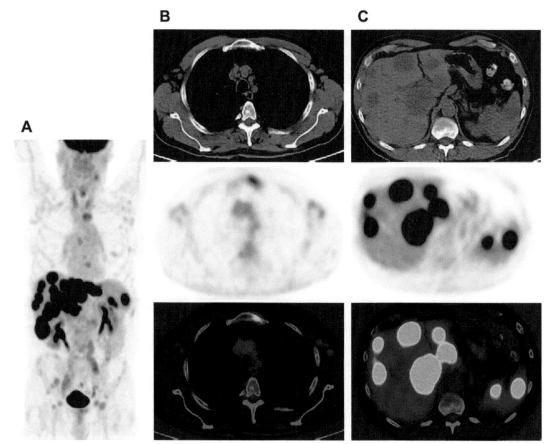

Fig. 3. A 68-year-old man with history of CLL. Maximum intensity projection image (*A*) and axial FDG-PET/CT images (*B, C*) demonstrate mildly FDG-avid axillary, mediastinal, retroperitoneal, and pelvic lymphadenopathy. There are, however, intense FDG-avid focal lesions in the liver and spleen found to represent transformation to a higher grade lymphoma on pathology (top row: CT; middle row: FDG-PET; bottom row: fused PET/CT).

administration of intravenous contrast may help in detecting additional clinically relevant findings in some patients and excluding false positive results due to bowel loops and vessels, this seems to be only in a small number of patients not mandating both FDG-PET/CT and CECT for all patients.

Assessment of Bone Marrow Involvement at Initial Staging

Bone marrow involvement occurs in 5% to 15% of patients with HL and 20% to 40% of patients with NHL and adversely affects 5-year overall survival.[43–47] Bone marrow biopsy (BMB) is a painful procedure and can be falsely negative in patients with focal involvement away from the standard iliac crest biopsy sites or can be inconclusive if the samples are inadequate.

Several studies have shown that FDG-PET/CT is the most accurate imaging modality for detecting bone marrow involvement in lymphoma.[27,48–51] In

a meta-analysis of 32 studies consisting of both NHL and HL, the pooled sensitivity of FDG-PET/CT (91.6%, 95% confidence interval [CI]: 85.1, 95.9) was statistically higher than for FDG-PET alone (81.5%, 95% CI: 77.3, 85.3) or MRI (90.3%, 95% CI: 82.4, 95.5). Pooled specificity was also higher for FDG-PET/CT (90.3%, 95% CI: 85.9, 93.7) versus FDG-PET alone (87.3%, 95% CI: 84.9, 89.5) and MRI (75.9%, 95% CI: 69.8, 81.2).[51]

FDG-PET/CT and BMB have a high concordance rate (~80%) for detecting bone marrow involvement.[48–50,52,53] In discordant cases of a positive PET scan and negative BMB, the most common causes are sampling error and diffuse uptake due to reactive marrow (**Fig. 4**).[48,50,54–56] In one study of 106 patients with HL, diffuse bone marrow uptake was often inflammatory while diffuse splenic uptake was more likely to be due to lymphoma.[56] A negative FDG-PET in the bone marrow and positive biopsy most commonly occur with less FDG-avid nodal disease (eg, lower-grade

A **B**

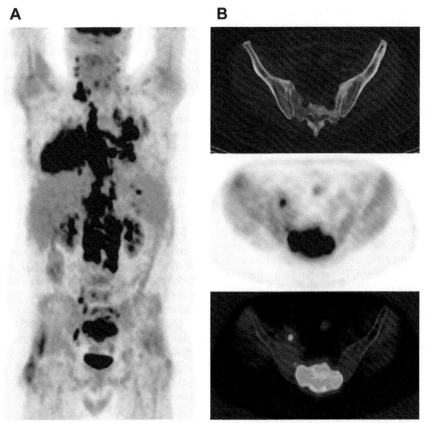

Fig. 4. A 39-year-old man with HL presents for initial staging. Maximum intensity projection (*A*) and axial FDG-PET/CT (*B*) images of the pelvis demonstrate intense FDG uptake in the sacrum, which was confirmed at biopsy as HL. BMB of the iliac crest was negative for lymphomatous involvement. There was normal marrow uptake in the iliac crests, which explains the discordant results between FDG-PET and BMB. There are numerous additional sites of lymphomatous involvement, including the lungs and lymph nodes above and below the diaphragm.

lymphomas) and less overall involvement in the marrow.[48,50,54]

Whether FDG-PET/CT should replace BMB remains controversial. The results of several recent studies have shown that FDG-PET/CT performs better than BMB in HL by detecting more patients with bone marrow involvement and upstaging more patients compared with BMB (see **Fig. 4**).[52,53,55–57] Some authors have concluded that BMB can be avoided in the workup of patients with HL.[57]

In patients with DLBCL, a few studies have similarly shown that FDG-PET/CT has better diagnostic performance than BMB for assessing bone marrow involvement. In a single-institution retrospective study of 133 patients, FDG-PET/CT had higher sensitivity (94%), negative predictive value (98%), and accuracy (98%) compared with BMB (24%, 80%, 81%, respectively) and in addition to IPI was the only independent predictor of progression-free survival (PFS) on multivariate analysis.[58] In another retrospective study of 130

patients, sensitivity of PET/CT for bone marrow involvement was 94% compared with 40% for BMB. Specificity was 100% for both. The authors concluded that routine BMB can be omitted in the staging of DLBCL except in patients with diffuse uptake in the bone marrow to differentiate reactive hematopoiesis from bone marrow involvement. In the authors' clinical experience, diffuse bone marrow uptake of FDG is oftentimes reactive, and it is helpful to consider the overall intensity of the uptake in relation to the uptake of the nodal disease as well as the heterogeneity of the uptake.

End-of-Therapy Response Assessment

Diagnostic and prognostic performance of end-of-therapy 2-deoxy-2-[18F]-fluoro-D-glucose-PET

Residual masses are seen on anatomic imaging in up to 80% of patients with HL and 40% with NHL.[59–62] Unlike CT, FDG-PET(/CT) at the end of therapy can differentiate residual malignant tumor from fibrosis.[63–66] In a meta-analysis of 15 studies, pooled sensitivity and specificity for detecting active malignancy in residual masses on FDG-PET(/CT) were 84% and 90% in HL and 72% and 100% in NHL.[66] In another meta-analysis of 19 studies (18 of which were PET-based whereas one was PET/CT-based), end-of-therapy FDG-PET had sensitivity and specificity of 50% to 100% and 67% to 100% for predicting relapse in HL. For aggressive NHL, this was 33% to 77% and 82% to 100%, respectively.[65] Overall, end-of-therapy FDG-PET has a high negative predictive value in HL and high positive predictive value in NHL for detecting residual lymphoma.[63] Nearly all studies of end-of-therapy FDG-PET(/CT) have shown that a positive scan is a poor prognostic factor in HL and NHL. However, a negative end-of-therapy FDG-PET(/CT) without a residual mass has better outcome than one with a residual mass because this does not exclude minimal residual disease.[64]

2-Deoxy-2-[18F]-fluoro-D-glucose-PET/computed tomography—based response criteria

In the pre-PET era, CT was routinely used for determining response based on changes in size of lymph nodal masses as defined in the 1999 International Working Group (IWG) response criteria for lymphoma.[67] Although retrospective, an important study of 54 patients with aggressive NHL showed that the combination of IWG criteria and end-of-therapy FDG-PET provided a more accurate response assessment than IWG criteria alone by identifying a subset of patients with FDG-PET negative residual masses and an excellent prognosis.[68]

These data led to the revision of the IWG response criteria in 2007, essentially converting the anatomic-based criteria to one primarily based on functional imaging.[69] A summary of the revised IWG criteria is shown in **Table 3**. The primary response assessment is based on a qualitative visual assessment of FDG uptake in tumor compared with mediastinal blood pool for residual masses greater than 2 cm and background activity for residual nodes less than 2 cm (**Fig. 5**). The revised IWG guidelines are accompanied by a consensus of the Imaging Subcommittee of the International Harmonization Project in Lymphoma, which provides more specific guidelines for FDG-PET(/CT) image acquisition and interpretation. Some additional important recommendations are shown in **Table 3**. The use of the semiquantitative-based SUV parameter may provide additional useful information, but this has

been primarily studied in the interim and not the posttherapy setting.

Interim PET/Computed Tomography: Risk-Adapted Strategies

Numerous studies have consistently demonstrated the prognostic value of FDG-PET(/CT) performed after 2 to 3 cycles of chemotherapy in patients with aggressive lymphoma despite variability in study designs, patient populations, and FDG-PET(/CT) scanning and assessment techniques.[70–73] Interim FDG-PET/CT scanning has also been shown to more strongly predict outcome compared with validated prognostic indices, IPS for HL,[74] which are population-based and have long been used for clinical trial design and patient management strategies. A plausible explanation for this is that interim FDG-PET/CT provides information about the chemosensitivity of an individual patient's tumor. Risk-adapted strategies for aggressive lymphomas based on interim FDG-PET/CT are an area of active investigation in clinical trials (**Tables 4** and **5**). The overall goals of the risk-adapted strategies include both minimizing long-term toxicities for good risk disease and maximizing effective therapy for poor risk disease.[75–77]

Deauville criteria for interpretation of interim 2-deoxy-2-[18F]-fluoro-D-glucose-PET/computed tomography

Several qualitative scales based on visual analysis have been used for the interpretation of interim FDG-PET/CT scans. Several criticisms with this method include interobserver variability in readings and use of the end-of-therapy IWG response criteria, which can result in false positive scans. As experience was gained interpreting FDG-PET(/CT) in the interim setting, it was realized that a higher threshold for "positive" was likely needed, possibly because of ongoing inflammation from treatment effects.

The Deauville criteria were proposed in 2009 and are now the most widely used in the interim setting.[78,79] The Deauville criteria are a qualitative 5-point scale with uptake in tumor scored in comparison with mediastinal blood pool or liver uptake (**Table 6**). In the Deauville criteria, the cutoff point for a positive versus negative scan is decided based on the risk of residual/recurrent disease and the specific question being asked in the clinical trial. For example, if the research question is withdrawing potentially curative treatment in patients with low-risk HL, interim FDG-PET/CT should be specific for the absence of disease and the cutoff point might be between Deauville scores 1 and 2 or 2 and 3 (see **Fig. 5**).

Table 3
Revised international working group criteria (international harmonization project)

Response	Criteria
CR	1. Disappearance of all evidence of disease 2. Nodal masses: FDG-avid or PET positive before therapy; mass of any size permitted if PET negative Variably FDG-avid or PET negative; regression to normal size on CT 3. Spleen and liver: not palpable, nodules disappeared 4. Bone marrow: infiltrate cleared on repeat biopsy; if indeterminate by morphology, immunohistochemistry should be negative
PR	1. Regression of measurable disease and no new sites 2. Nodal masses: ≥50% decrease in SPD of up to 6 largest dominant nodes or masses; no increase in size of the other nodes FDG-avid or PET positive before therapy; one or more PET positive at previously involved site Variably FDG-avid or PET negative; regression on CT 3. Spleen and liver: ≥50% decrease in SPD of nodules (for single nodule in greatest transverse diameter); no increase in size of liver or spleen 4. Bone marrow: irrelevant if positive before therapy; cell type should be specified Patients who achieve CR by the above criteria, but have persistent morphologic bone marrow involvement will be considered PR
SD	Failure to attain CR/PR or PD FDG-avid or PET positive before therapy; PET positive at prior sites of disease and no new sites on CT or PET Variably FDG-avid or PET negative; no change in size of previous lesions on CT
PD	1. Any new lesion or increase by >50% of previously involved sites from nadir 2. Nodal masses: appearance of a new lesion or lesions >1.5 cm in any axis, ≥50% increase in SPD of more than one node, or, ≥50% increase in longest diameter of a previously identified node >1 cm in short axis Lesions PET positive if FDG-avid lymphoma or PET positive before therapy 3. Spleen and liver: ≥50% increase from nadir in the SPD of any previous lesions 4. Bone marrow: new or recurrent involvement

Additional imaging considerations:
1. Posttherapy PET/CT after 6–8 wk of completion of chemotherapy and chemoimmunotherapy and 8–12 wk after radiotherapy and not before 3 wk to exclude posttreatment inflammatory changes
2. Visual inspection of the uptake rather than absolute SUV is sufficient for assessment.
3. In patients with no lung involvement at baseline and a good response at known sites of disease, new lung lesions on posttherapy PET/CT are often inflammatory.

Abbreviations: CR, complete remission; PD, progressive disease; PR, partial remission; SD, stable disease; SPD, sum of the product of the diameters.

Adapted from Cheson BD, Pfistner B, Juweid ME, et al. Revised response criteria for malignant lymphoma. J Clin Oncol 2007;25(5):579–86.

The prognostic value of interim PET/CT based on the Deauville criteria in HL and NHL has recently been established.[80–82] Biggi and colleagues[80] performed an international validation study of the Deauville criteria in 260 patients with HL who were treated with adriamycin, bleomycin, vinblastine, and dacarbazine (ABVD) and evaluated with interim FDG-PET/CT. Interim FDG-PET/CT was negative (Deauville score 1–3) in 83% and positive (Deauville score 4–5) in 17%. The 3-year failure-free survival was 95% for patients with a negative interim PET and 28% for patients with a positive interim PET. There was excellent interreader agreement in this study.[80]

The addition of semiquantitative parameters for analyzing changes in FDG uptake in tumor in the interim setting compared with baseline may be helpful to reduce interreader variability if PET is performed using standardized methods. Lin and colleagues[83] found that in patients with DLBCL a decline in maximum SUV of greater than 65.7% after 2 cycles of therapy better predicted outcomes versus visual assessment by reducing the number of false positive scans, but this was not true when the FDG-PET was performed after 4 cycles of therapy.[84] Further evaluations of the use of SUV in the interim setting would be helpful.[81,85] In addition, combining changes in quantitative

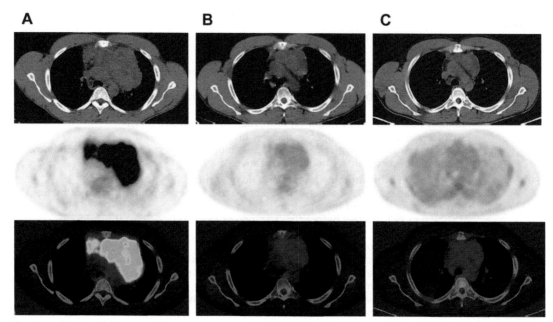

Fig. 5. A 23-year-old man with stage IIB HL. (*A*) Pretherapy FDG-PET/CT of the chest demonstrates a large intensely FDG-avid anterior mediastinal mass abutting the aortic arch and pulmonary artery, which is consistent with HL. (*B*) Interim FDG-PET/CT performed after 2 cycles of chemotherapy demonstrates complete metabolic response with residual anterior mediastinal mass. The mass has residual FDG uptake similar to the mediastinal blood pool (Deauville score: 2). (*C*) Posttherapy FDG-PET/CT performed after 4 cycles of chemotherapy and involved field radiotherapy demonstrates continued complete metabolic response based on the revised IWG response criteria for lymphoma. There is also mild diffusely increased FDG uptake through the lungs, which is most likely inflammatory in cause.

parameters from both anatomic and functional imaging in a multiparametric approach is also being investigated and has potential for improving the predictive value of interim FDG-PET/CT.[82]

Hodgkin lymphoma

The cure rate for early-stage (I/II) HL is 90% to 95%. The overall goal of risk-adapted strategies in this population is to minimize long-term toxicity

Table 4
Clinical trials evaluating interim FDG-PET in early-stage Hodgkin lymphoma

Trial	Phase	Standard Therapy
GHGS HD16	III	PET−: omit RT
EORTC/GELA/ FIL H10	III	PET−: omit RT PET+: BEACOPPesc
UK NCRI RAPID	III	PET−: RT vs no RT
CALGB 50604 (nonbulky)	II	PET−: total 4 cycles ABVD, no RT PET+: BEACOPPesc + RT
CALGB 50801 (bulky)	II	PET−: total 6 cycles ABVD, no RT PET+: BEACOPPesc + RT
ECOG 2410	II	PET+: BEACOPPesc + RT

Table 5
Clinical trials evaluating interim FDG-PET in advanced stage Hodgkin lymphoma

Trial	Phase	Standard Therapy
GITIL HD0607	II	PET+: BEACOPPesc
RATHL	III	PET−: ABVD vs AVD PET+: BEACOPPesc
Israel/Rambam	III	PET+: BEACOPPesc PET−: BEACOPP baseline
IIL HD0801	III	PET−: RT vs no RT PET+: salvage
GHSG HD18	III	PET−: 4 cycles vs 6 cycles BEACOPPesc
LYSA AHL2011	III	PET−: ABVD after BEACOPPesc
EORTC/PLRG H11	III	PET+: BEACOPPesc
SWOG S0816	II	PET+: BEACOPPesc

Table 6 Deauville 5-point scale	
1	No Uptake
2	Uptake ≤ mediastinal blood pool
3	Uptake > mediastinal blood pool but ≤ liver
4	Uptake moderate > liver
5	Uptake markedly > liver

NCCN modification: score 1–5a for sites that are initially involved and 5b for sites that are newly involved on the interim PET.[2]

Adapted from Meignan M, Gallamini A, Haioun C, et al. Report on the Second International Workshop on interim positron emission tomography in lymphoma held in Menton, France, 8–9 April 2010. Leuk Lymphoma 2010;51(12):2172; and Meignan M, Gallamini A, Itti E, et al. Report on the Third International Workshop on Interim Positron Emission Tomography in Lymphoma held in Menton, France, 26–27 September 2011 and Menton 2011 consensus. Leuk Lymphoma 2012;53(10): 1876–81.

from treatment by de-escalating therapy based on a negative interim FDG-PET(/CT) scan. Examples of ongoing clinical trials are shown in **Table 4** and some preliminary and interim analysis results have been reported in abstract form. In the EORTC/Lysa/Fil Intergroup H10 trial, patients in the control arm underwent interim FDG-PET/CT but received 2 to 4 cycles of ABVD chemotherapy and involved node radiation therapy (IN-RT) regardless of the result. Patients in the experimental arm received ABVD for 2 cycles and then either de-escalated to 2 more cycles of ABVD without IN-RT for a negative interim PET or escalated to bleomycin, etoposide, adriamycin, cyclophosphamide, oncovin (vincristine), procarbazine, and prednisone (BEACOPPesc) and radiation therapy (RT) for a positive interim PET. Preliminary reports showed a statistically higher number of events (relapses and recurrences) in the nonirradiated patients than in the patients who received combined modality treatment, and the chemotherapy arms of this study have subsequently been closed.[86] The interim report of the UK RAPID trial for nonbulky stage IA–IIA HL focused on the patients with a negative FDG-PET/CT after 3 cycles of chemotherapy. The 3-year PFS and overall survival were 95% and 97% for those randomized to receive involved-field radiation therapy (IFRT) compared with 91% and 99% for those randomized to no IFRT.[87] Longer-term follow-up and assessment of whether salvage rates are the same in both groups are needed to better understand the impact of these results.

The cure rate for advanced stage HL is 65% to 70% with 6 to 8 cycles of ABVD chemotherapy.[88–91] About one-third of patients with HL

is refractory to or relapses after initial therapy,[92] and for these patients, about one-third to two-thirds can be cured with high-dose chemotherapy (HDC) and blood or marrow transplant (**Fig. 6**). In this population, the goals of risk-adapted therapy using interim FDG-PET(/CT) are maximizing therapy for a positive interim PET and minimizing toxicity by de-escalating therapy for a negative interim PET. Tailored therapy based on interim scintigraphy or PET/CT has been shown to preserve fertility in female patients.[75] Examples of ongoing clinical trials are shown in **Table 5**. In the yet to be published GITIL/FIL HD0607 trial, after 2 cycles of ABVD, patients with a positive interim, PET2, were treated with BEACOPP escalated and BEACOPP baseline (4+4) without or with rituximab, whereas patients with a negative interim PET received 4 additional cycles of ABVD ± RT. Of the 446 patients enrolled in the study, PET2 was positive in 20%. Treatment efficacy was assessed in 187 patients who completed treatment and could be followed for 1 year. Of these 187 patients, 27 had a positive PET2. Escalated therapy in these 27 patients was associated with continued complete remission in 81% patients.[93]

Most experts agree that changing therapy based on interim FDG-PET(/CT) in HL is still best performed on clinical trials. The NCCN guidelines reiterate that the use of interim FDG-PET(/CT) in many scenarios remains unclear but provides some conservative guidelines, including biopsy for patients with a Deauville score of 5.

Non-Hodgkin lymphoma

The predictive value of interim FDG-PET/CT for treatment outcome in DLBCL is less defined than for HL. The results of most of the studies evaluating interim FDG-PET/CT in DLBCL have been inconsistent and inconclusive because of different patient selection criteria, different treatment strategies and duration, and different criteria for interpretation of the interim scans.[72] It is postulated that the routine use of rituximab increases false positive scans because of triggering of an inflammatory reaction.

In a large meta-analysis of 13 studies including 311 patients with DLBCL, no reliable conclusions were drawn about the role of interim FDG-PET/CT. The sensitivity and specificity were widely variable among the various studies with combined estimates of 78% and 87%, respectively.[72] In one study of a homogeneous cohort of 88 patients with newly diagnosed DLBCL, a positive interim FDG-PET/CT was not predictive of worse outcome.[94] In another study evaluating the role of interim FDG-PET(/CT) in a risk-adapted setting with a

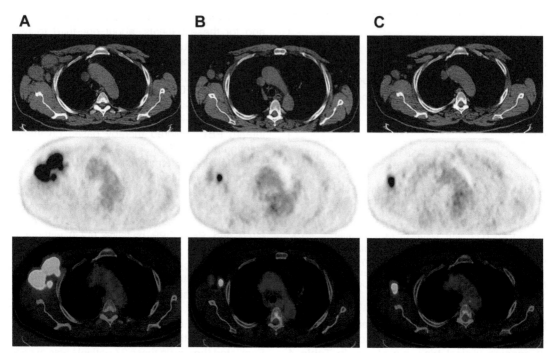

Fig. 6. A 52-year-old man with stage IIB HL. (*A*) Pretherapy FDG-PET/CT demonstrates intensely FDG-avid right axillary lymphadenopathy. There were also FDG-avid supraclavicular, subpectoral, and right hilar lymph nodes (not shown). (*B*) Interim FDG-PET/CT after 2 cycles of ABVD demonstrates interval decrease in the size and FDG avidity of the right axillary nodes as well as multiple right supraclavicular, subpectoral, and hilar lymph nodes (not shown). However, there remains intense FDG uptake (markedly more than liver) in one of the right axillary nodes (Deauville score: 5). (*C*) Posttherapy FDG-PET/CT after 4 cycles of ABVD shows new FDG uptake in another right axillary node with persistent uptake in the previously FDG-avid node (not shown). The remainder of the axillary nodes as well as nodes elsewhere showed continued remission. At the time of last follow-up, the patient was scheduled to receive additional chemotherapy and ASCT followed by RT for refractory disease.

dose-dense, sequential immunochemotherapy regimen, Moskowitz and colleagues[95] concluded that PFS was similar in patients with negative interim PET and positive interim FDG-PET(/CT) with negative biopsy. Interim FDG-PET/CT was positive in 38 of 98 patients (39%), but only 5 of these 38 (13%) had a positive biopsy result for residual lymphoma. Several reasons were postulated in this study for the high false positive rate of interim FDG-PET(/CT) in this study population, including the use of dose-dense immunochemotherapy and timing of the PET scan.

Data supporting risk-adapted strategies based on interim FDG-PET(/CT) in DLBCL are also fewer.[95–97] In the E3404 trial, patients with a positive interim FDG-PET after 3 cycles of rituximab, cyclophosphamide, doxorubicin, vincristine, and prednisone (R-CHOP), and one cycle of R-CHOP during central review were escalated to 4 cycles of rituximab ifosfamide, carboplatin, etoposide [R-ICE], whereas patients with negative interim PET received 3 more cycles of R-CHOP.[97] The 2-year PFS in the interim PET-positive group was 45% and the 3-year overall survival was

67%, which was better than historical controls.[98] The limitations of the study were lack of a control group and interobserver variability in the interpretation of the interim FDG-PET.[98] Given these results overall, interim FDG-PET(/CT) is not recommended outside the clinical trial setting in DLBCL.

Indolent Lymphomas

Indolent lymphoma is considered incurable by most and relapses are inevitable. As a result, the impact of FDG-PET/CT in the management of patients with indolent lymphomas has been less profound overall and depends more on the particular subtype. Of the low-grade lymphomas, FL is the most FDG-avid subtype, whereas SLL/CLL, marginal zone lymphoma (MZL), and peripheral T-cell lymphoma (PTCL) are least FDG-avid.[99] The sensitivity of PET for detecting FL is 94% and significantly drops to 71% and 53%, respectively, for MZL and SLL/CLL.[99]

Of the indolent NHLs, the impact of FDG-PET/CT has been the greatest in FL. The intrapatient and interpatient variability of FDG uptake in FL is considerable.[100] SUV$_{max}$ ranges have been reported from 1.7 to 41.2.[100] In patients with early-stage FL (stage I and stage II without bulky disease), treatment options include involved-site radiotherapy and immunotherapy with or without chemotherapy. FDG-PET/CT can help in proper selection of these patients by detecting additional sites of disease. In one study of 45 patients with biopsy-proven FL, FDG-PET/CT detected more nodal and extranodal disease sites, compared with CT alone, resulting in change of early-stage disease to advanced stage in 11% of patients.[101] In the FOLL05-phase III trial of 125 patients, FDG-PET/CT detected more nodal and extranodal sites upstaging 62% of patients with limited stage disease.[102]

In FL, postchemotherapy FDG-PET/CT has been shown to have better prognostic value than the FLIPI. In one study of 121 patients, FDG-PET performed at the end of treatment in 106 patients was negative in 83 (78%) patients and positive in 23 (22%) patients.[103] Using a Deauville score of 4 as a cutoff, 2-year PFS was 87% for patients with a negative PET and 51% for those with a positive PET at the end of therapy.[103] In a meta-analysis of 8 studies consisting of 577 patients with FL, FDG-PET(/CT) was more efficient than CT in identifying patients with complete response at the end of treatment.[104] Preliminary studies of interim FDG-PET performed in patients with FL have shown strong prognostic value.[103] In a prospective trial of 121 patients with FL treated with 6 cycles of R-CHOP, Dupuis and colleagues[103] demonstrated 2-year PFS of 86% for interim PET-negative patients compared with 61% for interim PET-positive patients. Because of the variability of FDG uptake that can be seen in FL and because FDG-PET/CT is more accurate than CT, a baseline scan is often helpful for establishing whether FDG-PET/CT will be useful in the evaluation of an individual patient with FL.

Posttherapy Surveillance

The relapse rate after first-line chemotherapy for patients with HL and NHL ranges from 20% to 50%. The risk is highest in the first 3 years after completion of treatment with most occurring in the first 12 months in HL and the first 18 months in NHL.[105] The role of routine surveillance imaging is controversial, particularly in the early-stage, low-risk patient. Clinical symptoms typically precede CT imaging findings of relapse[106,107] and most current clinical guidelines do not recommend routine surveillance imaging. However, FDG-PET/CT detects relapses before clinical symptoms

and CT scanning, by up to 9 months in one study.[108]

In a retrospective study of 125 patients (42 with HL; 83 with NHL), relapses were more often detected on imaging in HL, whereas most relapses in NHL (62%) were clinically detected.[109] The authors concluded that FDG-PET/CT has the potential for routine surveillance, at least in HL. In another study of 108 patients with relapsed NHL, relapse detected by imaging was found to have low risk compared with that detected clinically.[106]

Despite the potential advantage of earlier detection of recurrence, evidence is lacking that surveillance imaging leads to better disease eradication and outcomes. Additional drawbacks of FDG-PET(/CT) in the setting of surveillance are high reported false positive rates and high cost.[110–113] In one multicenter retrospective study, 161 patients with HL underwent 299 surveillance PET/CTs (either as routine surveillance [n = 211] or for clinical indication [n = 88]), about 2 per patient.[110] Twenty-two patients relapsed at a median follow-up of 34 months, and 10 were detected on FDG-PET/CT. The true positive rate of FDG-PET/CT was 5% to 13% and the false positive rate was 17% to 22%. The negative predictive value of PET/CT was 100%, whereas the positive predictive value was 22% to 37%. Factors like extranodal disease at presentation, positive interim, and end-of-therapy FDG-PET/CT were associated with higher detection of true positive relapses by surveillance PET/CT. The authors concluded that although routine surveillance is associated with low positive predictive value and high cost, it should be selectively used in high-risk patients.[110]

Few studies have suggested the selective use of FDG-PET surveillance in high-risk patients with HL[107] and DLBCL.[106] In a study of HL in first remission, more true positive recurrences were seen with increasing risk factors, including symptoms at the time of PET, residual mass on CT, and advanced stage disease. The authors concluded that asymptomatic patients with morphologic residual masses need follow-up PET/CT for 24 months, whereas those with advanced initial disease stage need follow-up PET/CT for more than 24 months.[107] In the DLBCL population, the PPV of FDG-PET/CT was 0.85 with higher true positive rates in patients older than 60 and with symptoms at the time of FDG-PET/CT. Based on these data, a risk-adapted approach to surveillance imaging seems reasonable, but demonstrating benefits on outcome, cost, and radiation exposure in a prospective manner is needed.

Stem Cell Transplantation in Aggressive Lymphoma

FDG-PET/CT can help in selecting patients for SCT because several studies have shown that a positive FDG-PET(/CT) before the SCT predicts poor outcome.[114–117] In a recent retrospective study of 55 patients with relapsed/refractory DLBCL who were treated with HDC and autologous stem cell transplant (ASCT), 19 prognostic factors were analyzed in an integrative model to predict the outcome of the treatment.[118] Only PET positivity before the ASCT and HDC was predictive of disease-specific events (hazards ratio [HR]: 3.9, $P = .01$) and deaths (HR: 3.4, $P = .04$) in multivariate analyses.[118] A similar study in 141 patients with refractory HL analyzed 21 prognostic factors and showed IPS 3 or more (HR: 3.7, $P = .001$) and positive pre-ASCT PET (HR: 3.4; $P = .011$) to be associated with higher hazard for disease-specific death.[119] In another study of patients with refractory HL, FDG-PET/CT allowed identification of high-risk patients who would benefit from tandem ASCT.[114] Overall, it appears that FDG-PET/CT provides prognostic information when performed before SCT, and different strategies, for example, additional different chemotherapy, may be beneficial in the case of residual PET positive malignancy.

SUMMARY

The role of PET and PET/CT has evolved significantly in the last one and half decades. FDG-PET/CT is now an integral part of the management of patients with lymphoma. This is reiterated in recent revisions to the 2007 IWG response criteria and imaging guidance, which were published since the initial submission of this manuscript and to which the reader is referred.[120,121] FDG-PET/CT at the time of initial staging can help in appropriate staging of the patients. Both interim and end-of-therapy PETs have significant prognostic value in patients with HL and aggressive NHL and more accurately assess for the presence of residual malignancy than anatomic imaging. The impact of interim FDG-PET/CT on risk-adapted strategies is an area of active investigation and the results of ongoing clinical trials will be informative. At various time points during its course, FDG-PET/CT can guide the oncologists in the best management strategies for patients with lymphoma.

REFERENCES

1. NCCN clinical practice guidelines in oncology non--Hodgkin's lymphoma version 2.2014. NCCN. 2014. Available at: http://www.nccn.org/professionals/physician_gls/f_guidelines.asp#site. Accessed March 27, 2014.
2. NCCN clinical practice guidelines in oncology Hodgkin lymphoma version 2.2014. NCCN. 2014. Available at: http://www.nccn.org/professionals/physician_gls/f_guidelines.asp#site. Accessed March 3, 2014.
3. Siegel R, Naishadham D, Jemal A. Cancer statistics, 2013. CA Cancer J Clin 2013;63(1):11–30.
4. Meignan M, Gallamini A, Haioun C. Report on the first international workshop on interim-PET-scan in lymphoma. Leuk Lymphoma 2009;50(8):1257–60.
5. Swerdllow S, Campo E, Harris NL. WHO classification of tumours of haematopoietic and lymphoid tissues. Lyon (France): IARC Press; 2008. p. 2008.
6. Gribben JG. How i treat indolent lymphoma. Blood 2007;109(11):4617–26.
7. Jaffe ES. The 2008 WHO classification of lymphomas: implications for clinical practice and translational research. Hematology Am Soc Hematol Educ Program 2009;523–31.
8. Jaffe ES, Pittaluga S. Aggressive B-cell lymphomas: a review of new and old entities in the WHO classification. Hematology 2011;2011:506–14.
9. Rezania D, Sokol L, Cualing HD. Classification and treatment of rare and aggressive types of peripheral T-cell/natural killer-cell lymphomas of the skin. Cancer Control 2007;14(2):112–23.
10. Carbone PP, Kaplan HS, Musshoff K, et al. Report of the committee on Hodgkin's disease staging classification. Cancer Res 1971;31(11):1860–1.
11. Lister TA, Crowther D, Sutcliffe SB, et al. Report of a committee convened to discuss the evaluation and staging of patients with Hodgkin's disease: Cotswolds meeting. J Clin Oncol 1989;7(11):1630–6.
12. Hasenclever D, Diehl V. A prognostic score for advanced Hodgkin's disease. International prognostic factors project on advanced Hodgkin's disease. N Engl J Med 1998;339(21):1506–14.
13. Moccia AA, Donaldson J, Chhanabhai M, et al. International prognostic score in advanced-stage Hodgkin's lymphoma: altered utility in the modern era. J Clin Oncol 2012;30(27):3383–8.
14. A predictive model for aggressive non-Hodgkin's lymphoma. The international non-Hodgkin's lymphoma prognostic factors project. N Engl J Med 1993;329(14):987–94.
15. Miller TP, Dahlberg S, Cassady JR, et al. Chemotherapy alone compared with chemotherapy plus radiotherapy for localized intermediate- and high-grade non-Hodgkin's lymphoma. N Engl J Med 1998;339(1):21–6.
16. Moller MB, Pedersen NT, Christensen BE. Factors predicting long-term survival in low-risk diffuse large B-cell lymphoma. Am J Hematol 2003;74(2):94–8.

17. Zhou Z, Sehn LH, Rademaker AW, et al. An enhanced international prognostic index (NCCN-IPI) for patients with diffuse large B-cell lymphoma treated in the rituximab era. Blood 2014;123(6):837–42.

18. Ziepert M, Hasenclever D, Kuhnt E, et al. Standard International prognostic index remains a valid predictor of outcome for patients with aggressive CD20+ B-cell lymphoma in the rituximab era. J Clin Oncol 2010;28(14):2373–80.

19. Lee J, Suh C, Park YH, et al. Extranodal natural killer T-cell lymphoma, nasal-type: a prognostic model from a retrospective multicenter study. J Clin Oncol 2006;24(4):612–8.

20. Solal-Celigny P, Roy P, Colombat P, et al. Follicular lymphoma international prognostic index. Blood 2004;104(5):1258–65.

21. Gascoyne RD, Adomat SA, Krajewski S, et al. Prognostic significance of Bcl-2 protein expression and Bcl-2 gene rearrangement in diffuse aggressive non-Hodgkin's lymphoma. Blood 1997;90(1):244–51.

22. Green TM, Young KH, Visco C, et al. Immunohistochemical double-hit score is a strong predictor of outcome in patients with diffuse large B-cell lymphoma treated with rituximab plus cyclophosphamide, doxorubicin, vincristine, and prednisone. J Clin Oncol 2012;30(28):3460–7.

23. Iqbal J, Meyer PN, Smith LM, et al. BCL2 predicts survival in germinal center B-cell-like diffuse large B-cell lymphoma treated with CHOP-like therapy and rituximab. Clin Cancer Res 2011;17(24):7785–95.

24. Johnson NA, Slack GW, Savage KJ, et al. Concurrent expression of MYC and BCL2 in diffuse large B-cell lymphoma treated with rituximab plus cyclophosphamide, doxorubicin, vincristine, and prednisone. J Clin Oncol 2012;30(28):3452–9.

25. Shipp MA, Ross KN, Tamayo P, et al. Diffuse large B-cell lymphoma outcome prediction by gene-expression profiling and supervised machine learning. Nat Med 2002;8(1):68–74.

26. Weiler-Sagie M, Bushelev O, Epelbaum R, et al. (18)F-FDG avidity in lymphoma readdressed: a study of 766 patients. J Nucl Med 2010;51(1):25–30.

27. Ngeow JY, Quek RH, Ng DC, et al. High SUV uptake on FDG-PET/CT predicts for an aggressive B-cell lymphoma in a prospective study of primary FDG-PET/CT staging in lymphoma. Ann Oncol 2009;20(9):1543–7.

28. Schoder H, Noy A, Gonen M, et al. Intensity of 18fluorodeoxyglucose uptake in positron emission tomography distinguishes between indolent and aggressive non-Hodgkin's lymphoma. J Clin Oncol 2005;23(21):4643–51.

29. Bruzzi JF, Macapinlac H, Tsimberidou AM, et al. Detection of Richter's transformation of chronic lymphocytic leukemia by PET/CT. J Nucl Med 2006;47(8):1267–73.

30. Hutchings M, Loft A, Hansen M, et al. Position emission tomography with or without computed tomography in the primary staging of Hodgkin's lymphoma. Haematologica 2006;91(4):482–9.

31. Munker R, Glass J, Griffeth LK, et al. Contribution of PET imaging to the initial staging and prognosis of patients with Hodgkin's disease. Ann Oncol 2004;15(11):1699–704.

32. Tatsumi M, Cohade C, Nakamoto Y, et al. Direct comparison of FDG PET and CT findings in patients with lymphoma: initial experience. Radiology 2005;237(3):1038–45.

33. Weihrauch MR, Re D, Bischoff S, et al. Whole-body positron emission tomography using 18F-fluorodeoxyglucose for initial staging of patients with Hodgkin's disease. Ann Hematol 2002;81(1):20–5.

34. Wirth A, Seymour JF, Hicks RJ, et al. Fluorine-18 fluorodeoxyglucose positron emission tomography, gallium-67 scintigraphy, and conventional staging for Hodgkin's disease and non-Hodgkin's lymphoma. Am J Med 2002;112(4):262–8.

35. Buchmann I, Reinhardt M, Elsner K, et al. 2-(fluorine-18)fluoro-2-deoxy-D-glucose positron emission tomography in the detection and staging of malignant lymphoma. A bicenter trial. Cancer 2001;91(5):889–99.

36. Pelosi E, Pregno P, Penna D, et al. Role of whole-body [18F] fluorodeoxyglucose positron emission tomography/computed tomography (FDG-PET/CT) and conventional techniques in the staging of patients with Hodgkin and aggressive non Hodgkin lymphoma. Radiol Med 2008;113(4):578–90.

37. Raanani P, Shasha Y, Perry C, et al. Is CT scan still necessary for staging in Hodgkin and non-Hodgkin lymphoma patients in the PET/CT era? Ann Oncol 2006;17(1):117–22.

38. Partridge S, Timothy A, O'Doherty MJ, et al. 2-Fluorine-18-fluoro-2-deoxy-D glucose positron emission tomography in the pretreatment staging of Hodgkin's disease: influence on patient management in a single institution. Ann Oncol 2000;11(10):1273–9.

39. Rigacci L, Vitolo U, Nassi L, et al. Positron emission tomography in the staging of patients with Hodgkin's lymphoma. A prospective multicentric study by the Intergruppo Italiano Linfomi. Ann Hematol 2007;86(12):897–903.

40. Chalaye J, Luciani A, Enache C, et al. Clinical impact of contrast-enhanced computed tomography combined with low-dose F-fluorodeoxyglucose positron emission tomography/computed tomography on routine lymphoma patient management. Leuk Lymphoma 2014;55:2887–92.

41. Pinilla I, Gomez-Leon N, Del Campo-Del Val L, et al. Diagnostic value of CT, PET and combined PET/CT performed with low-dose unenhanced CT and full-dose enhanced CT in the initial staging of lymphoma. Q J Nucl Med Mol Imaging 2011; 55(5):567–75.

42. Schaefer NG, Hany TF, Taverna C, et al. Non-Hodgkin lymphoma and Hodgkin disease: coregistered FDG PET and CT at staging and restaging–do we need contrast-enhanced CT? Radiology 2004; 232(3):823–9.

43. Brunning RD, Bloomfield CD, McKenna RW, et al. Bilateral trephine bone marrow biopsies in lymphoma and other neoplastic diseases. Ann Intern Med 1975;82(3):365–6.

44. Coller BS, Chabner BA, Gralnick HR. Frequencies and patterns of bone marrow involvement in non-Hodgkin lymphomas: observations on the value of bilateral biopsies. Am J Hematol 1977;3: 105–19.

45. Conlan MG, Bast M, Armitage JO, et al. Bone marrow involvement by non-Hodgkin's lymphoma: the clinical significance of morphologic discordance between the lymph node and bone marrow. Nebraska Lymphoma Study Group. J Clin Oncol 1990;8(7):1163–72.

46. Morra E, Lazzarino M, Castello A, et al. Bone marrow and blood involvement by non-Hodgkin's lymphoma: a study of clinicopathologic correlations and prognostic significance in relationship to the Working Formulation. Eur J Haematol 1989; 42(5):445–53.

47. Munker R, Hasenclever D, Brosteanu O, et al. Bone marrow involvement in Hodgkin's disease: an analysis of 135 consecutive cases. German Hodgkin's Lymphoma Study Group. J Clin Oncol 1995;13(2): 403–9.

48. Schaefer NG, Strobel K, Taverna C, et al. Bone involvement in patients with lymphoma: the role of FDG-PET/CT. Eur J Nucl Med Mol Imaging 2007; 34(1):60–7.

49. Moog F, Kotzerke J, Reske SN. FDG PET can replace bone scintigraphy in primary staging of malignant lymphoma. J Nucl Med 1999;40(9):1407–13.

50. Pakos EE, Fotopoulos AD, Ioannidis JP. 18F-FDG PET for evaluation of bone marrow infiltration in staging of lymphoma: a meta-analysis. J Nucl Med 2005;46(6):958–63.

51. Wu LM, Chen FY, Jiang XX, et al. 18F-FDG PET, combined FDG-PET/CT and MRI for evaluation of bone marrow infiltration in staging of lymphoma: a systematic review and meta-analysis. Eur J Radiol 2012;81(2):303–11.

52. Muzahir S, Mian M, Munir I, et al. Clinical utility of (1)(8)F FDG-PET/CT in the detection of bone marrow disease in Hodgkin's lymphoma. Br J Radiol 2012;85(1016):e490–6.

53. Weiler-Sagie M, Kagna O, Dann EJ, et al. Characterizing bone marrow involvement in Hodgkin's lymphoma by FDG-PET/CT. Eur J Nucl Med Mol Imaging 2014;41(6):1133–40.

54. Carr R, Barrington SF, Madan B, et al. Detection of lymphoma in bone marrow by whole-body positron emission tomography. Blood 1998;91(9): 3340–6.

55. Cortes-Romera M, Sabate-Llobera A, Mercadal-Vilchez S, et al. Bone marrow evaluation in initial staging of lymphoma: 18F-FDG PET/CT versus bone marrow biopsy. Clin Nucl Med 2014;39(1): e46–52.

56. Salaun PY, Gastinne T, Bodet-Milin C, et al. Analysis of 18F-FDG PET diffuse bone marrow uptake and splenic uptake in staging of Hodgkin's lymphoma: a reflection of disease infiltration or just inflammation? Eur J Nucl Med Mol Imaging 2009;36(11):1813–21.

57. El-Galaly TC, d'Amore F, Mylam KJ, et al. Routine bone marrow biopsy has little or no therapeutic consequence for positron emission tomography/ computed tomography-staged treatment-naive patients with Hodgkin lymphoma. J Clin Oncol 2012;30(36):4508–14.

58. Berthet L, Cochet A, Kanoun S, et al. In newly diagnosed diffuse large B-cell lymphoma, determination of bone marrow involvement with 18F-FDG PET/CT provides better diagnostic performance and prognostic stratification than does biopsy. J Nucl Med 2013;54(8):1244–50.

59. Canellos GP. Residual mass in lymphoma may not be residual disease. J Clin Oncol 1988;6(6):931–3.

60. Naumann R, Vaic A, Beuthien-Baumann B, et al. Prognostic value of positron emission tomography in the evaluation of post-treatment residual mass in patients with Hodgkin's disease and non-Hodgkin's lymphoma. Br J Haematol 2001;115(4): 793–800.

61. Radford JA, Cowan RA, Flanagan M, et al. The significance of residual mediastinal abnormality on the chest radiograph following treatment for Hodgkin's disease. J Clin Oncol 1988;6(6):940–6.

62. Surbone A, Longo DL, DeVita VT Jr, et al. Residual abdominal masses in aggressive non-Hodgkin's lymphoma after combination chemotherapy: significance and management. J Clin Oncol 1988;6(12): 1832–7.

63. Burton C, Ell P, Linch D. The role of PET imaging in lymphoma. Br J Haematol 2004;126(6):772–84.

64. Jerusalem G, Beguin Y, Fassotte MF, et al. Whole-body positron emission tomography using 18F-fluorodeoxyglucose for posttreatment evaluation in Hodgkin's disease and non-Hodgkin's lymphoma has higher diagnostic and prognostic value than classical computed tomography scan imaging. Blood 1999;94(2):429–33.

65. Terasawa T, Nihashi T, Hotta T, et al. 18F-FDG PET for posttherapy assessment of Hodgkin's disease and aggressive Non-Hodgkin's lymphoma: a systematic review. J Nucl Med 2008;49(1):13–21.

66. Zijlstra JM, Lindauer-van der Werf G, Hoekstra OS, et al. 18F-fluoro-deoxyglucose positron emission tomography for post-treatment evaluation of malignant lymphoma: a systematic review. Haematologica 2006;91(4):522–9.

67. Cheson BD, Horning SJ, Coiffier B, et al. Report of an international workshop to standardize response criteria for non-Hodgkin's lymphomas. NCI Sponsored International Working Group. J Clin Oncol 1999;17(4):1244.

68. Juweid ME, Wiseman GA, Vose JM, et al. Response assessment of aggressive non-Hodgkin's lymphoma by integrated International Workshop Criteria and fluorine-18-fluorodeoxyglucose positron emission tomography. J Clin Oncol 2005; 23(21):4652–61.

69. Cheson BD, Pfistner B, Juweid ME, et al. Revised response criteria for malignant lymphoma. J Clin Oncol 2007;25(5):579–86.

70. Markova J, Kahraman D, Kobe C, et al. Role of [18F]-fluoro-2-deoxy-D-glucose positron emission tomography in early and late therapy assessment of patients with advanced Hodgkin lymphoma treated with bleomycin, etoposide, adriamycin, cyclophosphamide, vincristine, procarbazine and prednisone. Leuk Lymphoma 2012;53(1):64–70.

71. Sher DJ, Mauch PM, Van Den Abbeele A, et al. Prognostic significance of mid- and post-ABVD PET imaging in Hodgkin's lymphoma: the importance of involved-field radiotherapy. Ann Oncol 2009;20(11):1848–53.

72. Terasawa T, Lau J, Bardet S, et al. Fluorine-18-fluorodeoxyglucose positron emission tomography for interim response assessment of advanced-stage Hodgkin's lymphoma and diffuse large B-cell lymphoma: a systematic review. J Clin Oncol 2009; 27(11):1906–14.

73. Zinzani PL, Rigacci L, Stefoni V, et al. Early interim 18F-FDG PET in Hodgkin's lymphoma: evaluation on 304 patients. Eur J Nucl Med Mol Imaging 2012;39(1):4–12.

74. Gallamini A, Hutchings M, Rigacci L, et al. Early interim 2-[18F]fluoro-2-deoxy-D-glucose positron emission tomography is prognostically superior to international prognostic score in advanced-stage Hodgkin's lymphoma: a report from a joint Italian-Danish study. J Clin Oncol 2007;25(24):3746–52.

75. Dann EJ, Blumenfeld Z, Bar-Shalom R, et al. A 10-year experience with treatment of high and standard risk Hodgkin disease: six cycles of tailored BEACOPP, with interim scintigraphy, are effective and female fertility is preserved. Am J Hematol 2012;87(1):32–6.

76. Gallamini A, Hutchings M, Avigdor A, et al. Early interim PET scan in Hodgkin lymphoma: where do we stand? Leuk Lymphoma 2008;49(4):659–62.

77. Gallamini A, Kostakoglu L. Interim FDG-PET in Hodgkin lymphoma: a compass for a safe navigation in clinical trials? Blood 2012;120(25):4913–20.

78. Meignan M, Gallamini A, Haioun C, et al. Report on the Second International Workshop on interim positron emission tomography in lymphoma held in Menton, France, 8-9 April 2010. Leuk Lymphoma 2010;51(12):2171–80.

79. Meignan M, Gallamini A, Itti E, et al. Report on the Third International Workshop on Interim Positron Emission Tomography in Lymphoma Held in Menton, France, 26-27 September 2011 and menton 2011 consensus. Leuk Lymphoma 2012;53(10):1876–81.

80. Biggi A, Gallamini A, Chauvie S, et al. International validation study for interim PET in ABVD-treated, advanced-stage Hodgkin lymphoma: interpretation criteria and concordance rate among reviewers. J Nucl Med 2013;54(5):683–90.

81. Itti E, Meignan M, Berriolo-Riedinger A, et al. An international confirmatory study of the prognostic value of early PET/CT in diffuse large B-cell lymphoma: comparison between Deauville criteria and DeltaSUVmax. Eur J Nucl Med Mol Imaging 2013;40(9):1312–20.

82. Kostakoglu L, Schoder H, Johnson JL, et al. Interim [(18)F]fluorodeoxyglucose positron emission tomography imaging in stage I-II non-bulky Hodgkin lymphoma: would using combined positron emission tomography and computed tomography criteria better predict response than each test alone? Leuk Lymphoma 2012;53(11):2143–50.

83. Lin C, Itti E, Haioun C, et al. Early 18F-FDG PET for prediction of prognosis in patients with diffuse large B-cell lymphoma: SUV-based assessment versus visual analysis. J Nucl Med 2007;48(10): 1626–32.

84. Itti E, Lin C, Dupuis J, et al. Prognostic value of interim 18F-FDG PET in patients with diffuse large B-cell lymphoma: SUV-based assessment at 4 cycles of chemotherapy. J Nucl Med 2009;50(4):527–33.

85. Casasnovas RO, Meignan M, Berriolo-Riedinger A, et al. SUVmax reduction improves early prognosis value of interim positron emission tomography scans in diffuse large B-cell lymphoma. Blood 2011;118(1):37–43.

86. Andre MP, Reman O, Federico M, et al. Interim analysis of the randomized eortc/lysa/fil intergroup H10 trial on early PET-scan driven treatment adaptation in stage I/II Hodgkin lymphoma. ASH Annual Meeting Abstracts 2012;120(21):549.

87. Radford J, Barrington S, Counsell N, et al. Involved field radiotherapy versus no further treatment in patients with clinical stages IA and IIA Hodgkin lymphoma and a 'negative' PET scan after 3 cycles

ABVD. Results of the UK NCRI RAPID trial. ASH Annual Meeting Abstracts 2012;120(21):547.

88. DeVita VT, Serpick A. Combination chemotherapy in the treatment of advanced Hodgkin's disease. Proc Am Assoc Cancer Res 1967;8:13.

89. Klimo P, Connors JM. MOPP/ABV hybrid program: combination chemotherapy based on early introduction of seven effective drugs for advanced Hodgkin's disease. J Clin Oncol 1985;3(9):1174–82.

90. Canellos GP, Anderson JR, Propert KJ, et al. Chemotherapy of advanced Hodgkin's disease with MOPP, ABVD, or MOPP alternating with ABVD. N Engl J Med 1992;327(21):1478–84.

91. Canellos GP, Niedzwiecki D. Long-term follow-up of Hodgkin's disease trial. N Engl J Med 2002; 346(18):1417–8.

92. Akpek G, Ambinder RF, Piantadosi S, et al. Long-term results of blood and marrow transplantation for Hodgkin's lymphoma. J Clin Oncol 2001; 19(23):4314–21.

93. Gallamini A, Rossi A, Patti C, et al. Early treatment intensification in advanced-stage high-risk Hodgkin lymphoma (HL) patients, with a positive FDG-PET scan after two ABVD courses - first interim analysis of the GITIL/FIL HD0607 clinical trial. ASH Annual Meeting Abstracts 2012; 120(21):550.

94. Pregno P, Chiappella A, Bello M, et al. Interim 18-FDG-PET/CT failed to predict the outcome in diffuse large B-cell lymphoma patients treated at the diagnosis with rituximab-CHOP. Blood 2012; 119(9):2066–73.

95. Moskowitz CH, Schoder H, Teruya-Feldstein J, et al. Risk-adapted dose-dense immunochemotherapy determined by interim FDG-PET in advanced-stage diffuse large B-cell lymphoma. J Clin Oncol 2010;28(11):1896–903.

96. Kasamon YL, Wahl RL, Ziessman HA, et al. Phase II study of risk-adapted therapy of newly diagnosed, aggressive non-Hodgkin lymphoma based on midtreatment FDG-PET scanning. Biol Blood Marrow Transpl 2009;15(2):242–8.

97. Swinnen LJ, Li H, Quon A, et al. Response-Adapted Therapy for diffuse large B-cell non-Hodgkin's lymphoma (DLBCL) based on early [18F] FDG-PET scanning: an Eastern Cooperative Oncology Group Study (E3404). ASH Annual Meeting Abstracts 2012;120(21):687.

98. Horning SJ, Juweid ME, Schoder H, et al. Interim positron emission tomography scans in diffuse large B-cell lymphoma: an independent expert nuclear medicine evaluation of the Eastern Cooperative Oncology Group E3404 study. Blood 2010; 115(4):775–7 [quiz: 918].

99. Karam M, Novak L, Cyriac J, et al. Role of fluorine-18 fluoro-deoxyglucose positron emission tomography scan in the evaluation and follow-up of patients with low-grade lymphomas. Cancer 2006;107(1):175–83.

100. Bodet-Milin C, Kraeber-Bodere F, Moreau P, et al. Investigation of FDG-PET/CT imaging to guide biopsies in the detection of histological transformation of indolent lymphoma. Haematologica 2008; 93(3):471–2.

101. Le Dortz L, De Guibert S, Bayat S, et al. Diagnostic and prognostic impact of 18F-FDG PET/CT in follicular lymphoma. Eur J Nucl Med Mol Imaging 2010; 37(12):2307–14.

102. Luminari S, Biasoli I, Arcaini L, et al. The use of FDG-PET in the initial staging of 142 patients with follicular lymphoma: a retrospective study from the FOLL05 randomized trial of the Fondazione Italiana Linfomi. Ann Oncol 2013;24(8):2108–12.

103. Dupuis J, Berriolo-Riedinger A, Julian A, et al. Impact of [(18)F]fluorodeoxyglucose positron emission tomography response evaluation in patients with high-tumor burden follicular lymphoma treated with immunochemotherapy: a prospective study from the Groupe d'Etudes des Lymphomes de l'Adulte and GOELAMS. J Clin Oncol 2012;30(35):4317–22.

104. Pyo J, Won Kim K, Jacene HA, et al. End-therapy positron emission tomography for treatment response assessment in follicular lymphoma: a systematic review and meta-analysis. Clin Cancer Res 2013;19(23):6566–77.

105. Luigi Zinzani P, Stefoni V, Tani M, et al. Role of [18F] fluorodeoxyglucose positron emission tomography scan in the follow-up of lymphoma. J Clin Oncol 2009;27(11):1781–7.

106. Liedtke M, Hamlin PA, Moskowitz CH, et al. Surveillance imaging during remission identifies a group of patients with more favorable aggressive NHL at time of relapse: a retrospective analysis of a uniformly-treated patient population. Ann Oncol 2006;17(6):909–13.

107. Petrausch U, Samaras P, Veit-Haibach P, et al. Hodgkin's lymphoma in remission after first-line therapy: which patients need FDG-PET/CT for follow-up? Ann Oncol 2010;21(5):1053–7.

108. Jerusalem G, Beguin Y, Fassotte MF, et al. Early detection of relapse by whole-body positron emission tomography in the follow-up of patients with Hodgkin's disease. Ann Oncol 2003;14(1):123–30.

109. Goldschmidt N, Or O, Klein M, et al. The role of routine imaging procedures in the detection of relapse of patients with Hodgkin lymphoma and aggressive non-Hodgkin lymphoma. Ann Hematol 2011;90(2):165–71.

110. El-Galaly TC, Mylam KJ, Brown P, et al. Positron emission tomography/computed tomography surveillance in patients with Hodgkin lymphoma in first remission has a low positive predictive value and high costs. Haematologica 2012;97(6):931–6.

111. Lee AI, Zuckerman DS, Van den Abbeele AD, et al. Surveillance imaging of Hodgkin lymphoma patients in first remission: a clinical and economic analysis. Cancer 2010;116(16):3835–42.

112. Levine JM, Weiner M, Kelly KM. Routine use of PET scans after completion of therapy in pediatric Hodgkin disease results in a high false positive rate. J Pediatr Hematol Oncol 2006; 28(11):711–4.

113. Rhodes MM, Delbeke D, Whitlock JA, et al. Utility of FDG-PET/CT in follow-up of children treated for Hodgkin and non-Hodgkin lymphoma. J Pediatr Hematol Oncol 2006;28(5):300–6.

114. Devillier R, Coso D, Castagna L, et al. Positron emission tomography response at the time of autologous stem cell transplantation predicts outcome of patients with relapsed and/or refractory Hodgkin's lymphoma responding to prior salvage therapy. Haematologica 2012;97(7):1073–9.

115. Dickinson M, Hoyt R, Roberts AW, et al. Improved survival for relapsed diffuse large B cell lymphoma is predicted by a negative pre-transplant FDG-PET scan following salvage chemotherapy. Br J Haematol 2010;150(1):39–45.

116. Schot BW, Zijlstra JM, Sluiter WJ, et al. Early FDG-PET assessment in combination with clinical risk scores determines prognosis in recurring lymphoma. Blood 2007;109(2):486–91.

117. Spaepen K, Stroobants S, Dupont P, et al. Prognostic value of pretransplantation positron emission tomography using fluorine 18-fluorodeoxyglucose in patients with aggressive lymphoma treated with high-dose chemotherapy and stem cell transplantation. Blood 2003;102(1):53–9.

118. Akhtar S, Al-Sugair AS, Abouzied M, et al. Pretransplant (18)F-fluorodeoxyglucose positron emission tomography-based survival model in patients with aggressive lymphoma undergoing high-dose chemotherapy and autologous SCT. Bone Marrow Transplant 2013;48(4):551–6.

119. Akhtar S, Al-Sugair AS, Abouzied M, et al. Pretransplant FDG-PET-based survival model in relapsed and refractory Hodgkin's lymphoma: outcome after high-dose chemotherapy and autoSCT. Bone Marrow Transplant 2013;48(12):1530–6.

120. Cheson BD, Fisher RI, Barrington SF, et al. Recommendations for initial evaluation, staging and response assessment of Hodgkin and non-Hodgkin lymphoma: the Lugano classification. J Clin Oncol 2014;32(27):3059–68.

121. Barrington SF, Mikhaeel NG, Kostakoglu L, et al. Role of imaging in the staging and response assessment of lymhpoma: consensus of the International Conference of Malignant Lymphomas Imaging Working Group. J Clin Oncol 2014;32(27):3048–58.

Multiple Myeloma

Patrick J. Peller, MD

KEYWORDS

- Fluorodeoxyglucose • PET • PET/CT • Multiple myeloma • Monoclonal gammopathy
- Plasmacytoma

KEY POINTS

- Multiple myeloma is a heterogeneous disease process exhibiting a wide range of biological behaviors.
- PET/computed tomography (CT) imaging is useful in identifying additional bone lesions in patients with a plasmacytoma, and it is an important adjunct in the risk assessment of patients with multiple myeloma.
- Active myeloma can be identified from its indolent precursor states, allowing appropriate initiation of therapy.
- In the evaluation of patients with multiple myeloma, PET/CT is highly sensitive and specific for the detection of extraosseous disease.
- PET/CT aids therapy assessment before and after stem cell transplantation.

INTRODUCTION

Multiple myeloma (MM) arises from a single clone of differentiated plasma cells and typically produces high levels of a monoclonal immunoglobulin. These malignant plasma cells proliferate primarily within the marrow space and commonly produce osseous lesions.[1,2] MM is the most common malignant bone neoplasm in adults and incidence increases with age. Most patients with myeloma are diagnosed initially at 50 to 70 years of age.[2,3] Patients with MM present with a variety of symptoms: bone pain, fatigue, and lethargy from anemia, renal failure, and hypercalcemia.[2,4,5] Many patients are detected incidentally with laboratory tests demonstrating a monoclonal protein in the serum or urine. The treatment of myeloma is continuously evolving and currently uses thalidomide, protease inhibitors, chemotherapy, and long-acting steroids. Stem cell transplantation plays an important role in a patient with aggressive and extensive disease.[6–8]

Diagnostic imaging plays a critical role in the evaluation of patients with known or possible hematologic malignancies. Skeletal surveys covering the axial and proximal appendicular skeleton have been traditionally used in the workup of MM.[1] Computed tomography (CT) and magnetic resonance (MR) play a large role in staging patients with extraosseous hematologic malignancies, but, until recently, were used in MM for problem-solving only. [18]F fluorodeoxyglucose (FDG) PET identifies tumor sites based on their elevated glucose metabolism.[9,10] With the integration of PET and CT into a single scanner, it has become the modality of choice for the assessment of patients with hematologic malignancies.[10,11]

This article reviews myeloma and other plasma cell dyscrasias. The use of FDG PET/CT at crucial junctures in patients with myeloma adds additional clinical information, which provides an opportunity to impact medical management positively and therefore impact patient outcomes.

PLASMA CELL DYSCRASIAS

MM is one of many plasma cell dyscrasias resulting from a proliferating clone of plasma cells typically secreting a paraprotein (**Table 1**). Monoclonal gammopathy of undetermined significance

Dr P.J. Peller is a consultant for GE Medical.
Eka Medical Center - Jakarta, Central Business District Lot IX, BSD City, Tangerang 15321, Indonesia
E-mail address: ppeller11@gmail.com

PET Clin 10 (2015) 227–241
http://dx.doi.org/10.1016/j.cpet.2014.12.008

Table 1
Plasma cell dyscrasias

	Incidence (%)
Common	
MGUS	59
MM	18
Uncommon/rare	<10
Solitary plasmacytoma	
SMM	
WM	
Plasma cell leukemia	
Nonsecretory myeloma	
Solitary plasmacytoma	
Primary amyloidosis	
Heavy chain disease	
POEMS	

Adapted from Kyle RA, Rajkumar SV. Monoclonal gammopathy of undetermined significance and smoldering multiple myeloma. Hematol Oncol Clin North Am 2007;21:1093.

Table 2
Progression to multiple myeloma

	Monoclonal Protein (g/dL)	Marrow Plasma Cells (%)	Annual MM Progression (%)
MGUS	<3	<10	1
SMM	≥3	or ≥10 to <60	10
SPB	<3	<10	15–20[a]

[a] Assessment without FDG PET/CT.
Adapted from Rajkumar SV, Dispenzieri A, Fonseca R, et al. Thalidomide for previously untreated indolent or smoldering multiple myeloma. Leukemia 2001;15:1274; and Rajkumar SV, Larson D, Kyle RA. Diagnosis of smoldering multiple myeloma. N Engl J Med 2011;365:474, with permission.

(MGUS) is a most frequent member of this group. MGUS occurs in 1% to 3% of adults over the age of 50 and is typically detected incidentally on screen laboratory studies. A serum monoclonal protein less than 3 g/dL, bone marrow containing less than 10% plasma cells, and no evidence of end-organ damage (**Box 1**) caused by the plasma cell clone defines MGUS. MGUS is a premalignant state and is a precursor for MM, primary amyloidosis, light chain deposition disease, Waldenström macroglobulinemia (WM), lymphoma, and other plasma cell dyscrasias. The annual rate of progression to MM is approximately 1% (**Table 2**). At 25 years, nearly 70% of patients with MGUS have remained stable with no symptoms or evidence of progression. MGUS must be differentiated from less common but far more aggressive plasma cell dyscrasias.[12–16]

Smoldering myeloma (SMM) is a premalignant plasma cell dyscrasia, which is intermediate between MGUS and MM. SMM is differentiated from MGUS by higher serum monoclonal protein levels (≥3 g/dL) and a greater percentage of plasma cells in the bone marrow (≥10% and <60%), but no evidence of myeloma end-organ damage.[17,18] SMM patients are at much higher risk of progressing to MM than MGUS patients (see **Table 2**). The annual rate of progression to symptomatic MM is about 10%, with more than 50% conversion in 5 years.[19,20] Significant research is currently underway in SMM patients to determine which factors are associated with a higher risk for progression to active MM. If the SMM patient is completely asymptomatic, close observation is preferred and treatment is restricted to enrollment in prospective clinical trials.[21]

Solitary plasmacytomas are composed of plasma cells, which on biopsy are histologically identical to those seen in MM. Solitary plasmacytomas most frequently occur in bone (SPB), but can also be found in soft tissues.[22–24] SBP is characterized by a biopsy-proven clone of plasma cells, bone survey evidence of no additional lesions, and no end-organ damage. A monoclonal protein is present in a highly variable percentage (30%–70%) of SBP patients. Radiation therapy (40–50 Gy) to the SPB is a very effective treatment. The distinction between SBP and MM is the number of lesions found; 3 or more plasmacytomas are treated systemically as MM. SPB patients are at high risk of progression to MM compared with MGUS or SMM patients, with 40% to 60% progression at 4 years.[22,25,26]

Box 1
End organ damage in multiple myeloma

C = elevated calcium level (Ca >11.5 mg/dL)

R = renal insufficiency (Cr >2.0 mg/dL)

A = anemia (Hgb <10 g/dL)

B = lytic bony lesions

Adapted from Kyle RA, Rajkumar SV. Criteria for diagnosis, staging, risk stratification and response assessment of multiple myeloma. Leukemia 2009;23:3.

PET/COMPUTED TOMOGRAPHY IMAGING

FDG PET/CT plays important clinical roles in the management of MM patients and in the evaluation of rare plasma cell dyscrasias (**Box 2**). The axial coverage in patients with known or suspected MM should be as high as to at least the knees. The CT acquisition parameters should allow for high-quality sagittal spine reformatted images. The integrated PET/CT scanners should leverage the high spatial resolution of CT, for small lytic bone lesions and high sensitivity of FDG for malignant cells in a focal, multifocal, or diffuse infiltrative pattern.[27–29] Durie[30] specifically added FDG PET/CT and MR to the established Durie-Salmon staging (DSS) system (**Table 3**). The new DSS PLUS emphasized functional identification of marrow tumor burden, allowing better delineation of premalignant states from advanced/aggressive disease.

CLINICAL ROLES OF PET/COMPUTED TOMOGRAPHY IN MYELOMA
Identifying Truly Solitary Solitary Plasmacytomas of Bone

An SPB is composed of malignant plasma cells, of which histology is virtually identical to MM. The major clinical question is whether this lesion is truly solitary or actually one of many lesions. Because the natural history of SPB patients is to develop MM over the next 10 years, clinicians have been using advanced imaging. MR of the entire spine and pelvis will detect evidence for MM in up to one-third of patients with an SPB on radiographic bone survey.[31,32]

FDG PET/CT is used as initial imaging to identify the presence of additional, often smaller, FDG avid lytic lesions in patients with an SPB (**Fig. 1**). Published studies show that 33% to 47% of patients with an SPB have multiple bony abnormalities that indicate MM.[33–36] Kim and colleagues[34] evaluated the impact of PET/CT on SPB patient management, identifying additional osseous and extraosseous myeloma that changed therapy in

---

Box 2
Clinical roles of PET/computed tomography in myeloma

- Identifying truly solitary SPB
- Distinguishing MGUS or SMM from active MM
- Assessing risk by measuring disease extent and biological aggressiveness
- Detecting extraosseous myeloma
- Identifying skeletal complications
- Therapy assessment
- Rare plasma cell dyscrasias

Table 3
Durie/Salmon plus staging

Classification	MR or PET/Computed Tomography
MGUS	All negative
Stage 1A (SMM)	Negative or single plasmacytoma
Stage 1B (MM)	<5 focal lesions/mild diffuse
Stage 2A/B (MM)	5–20 focal lesions/mod diffuse
Stage 3A/B (MM)	>20 focal lesions/severe diffuse

A, serum creatinine less than 2 mg/dL + no extramedullary disease; B, serum creatinine greater than 2 mg/dL or extramedullary disease.

Adapted from Durie BG. The role of anatomic and functional staging in myeloma: description of Durie/Salmon plus staging system. Eur J Cancer 2006;42:1539; with permission.

35% of patients. The combination of an FDG PET/CT negative for additional lesions and normal flow cytometry and immunohistochemistry yielded a small group of patients with 100% disease-free survival following definitive radiotherapy (**Fig. 2**).[33]

Distinguishing Monoclonal Gammopathy of Undetermined Significance or Smoldering Myeloma from Active Multiple Myeloma

At the time of initial evaluation, every patient exhibiting a monoclonal serum protein may have MM or one of its premalignant stages, MGUS or SMM. For patients with MGUS and SMM, the standard of care is observation, whereas chemotherapy, steroids, and transplantation are frequently required for MM.[16,17,20] The major dividing line between MGUS/SMM and MM is the presence of end-organ damage caused by the underlying plasma cell dyscrasia. In elderly patients, comorbidities such as diabetes, hypertension, and a prior cancer might produce anemia, hypercalcemia, lytic bone lesions, or renal dysfunction confounding the evaluation. Patients with MGUS or SMM can be misdiagnosed as MM.[21,37]

For most patients with MGUS and many with SMM, PET/CT has no role until there is clinical evidence for progression. The PET/CT in patients with stable MGUS and SMM will typically be normal or show nonspecific low-grade, diffuse marrow uptake (**Fig. 3**). PET/CT identifies FDG avid and/or lytic bone lesions to establish the diagnosis of MM, prompting therapy initiation.[29,38–40] In some patients, the progression from SMM to MM is heralded by minor symptoms (**Fig. 4**).[37]

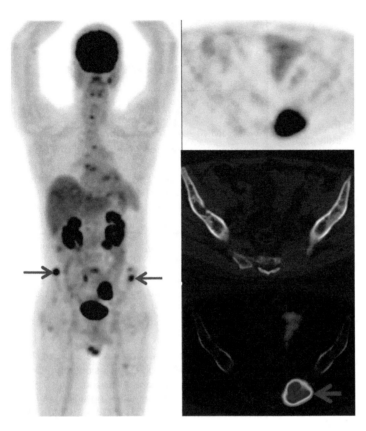

Fig. 1. A 59-year-old man who presented for sacral pain. Spine radiograph demonstrated a destructive lesion in the left sacrum (*arrows*, color PET/CT fused image) and a biopsy obtained clonal plasma cells. PET/CT scan showed multiple lesions with variable FDG uptake throughout the skeleton. Bone marrow biopsy of the posterior iliac crest showed more than 30% plasma cells. The patient was treated with systemic chemotherapy for MM in preparation for a stem cell transplant.

Assessing Risk by Measuring Disease Extent and Biological Aggressiveness

With the diagnosis of MM confirmed, initial therapy choice is driven by 2 main factors: risk assessment and eligibility of the patient to undergo autologous stem cell transplantation. MM risk stratification attempts to quantify disease extent and biological aggressiveness. There are 3 clinic systems for MM: the international staging system (ISS), the DSS system, and the Mayo Stratification of Myeloma and Risk-Adapted Therapy (mSMART) (**Table 4**). The ISS is simple, is easy to use provides a rough measure of disease extent, and is better at predicting group than individual patient risk.[41] DSS is predictive of disease extent and patient outcome with standard chemotherapy but may be less useful with newer treatment schemes.[42] The mSMART measures individual genetic risk profiles, which drive biological aggressiveness, but the pelvic marrow sample may not be the site of greatest disease activity.[43]

FDG PET/CT is used as a single procedure to measure disease extent and biological aggressiveness and to assist in clinical decision-making. MM is a very heterogeneous disease clinically, and this is reflected in the diversity of findings on PET/CT (**Fig. 5**). PET/CT interpretation should include the extent of marrow involvement, number of lesions, and the degree of FDG avidity (**Box 3**). Careful review of high-quality sagittal images is required to detect an infiltrative pattern of MM in the spine (**Fig. 6**). The high sensitivity of PET/CT can result in upstaging and more aggressive treatment in some patients, and individualized risk assessment is available on all patients.[28,29,43–47]

Detecting Extraosseous Myeloma

Extramedullary deposits of plasma cells are identified in 10% to 16% of MM patients, and the incidence has increased in the last 2 decades. The lymph nodes, spleen, and liver are most commonly involved, but extraosseous myeloma has been reported in every organ system. Extramedullary disease is a marker for more aggressive MM and is more common in younger patients. Patients with extraosseous disease respond less well to traditional myeloma treatment regimens, and sites outside the bone marrow may provide a sanctuary for myeloma cells during therapy. MM patients with extramedullary disease have shorter overall and disease-free survival.[47,48]

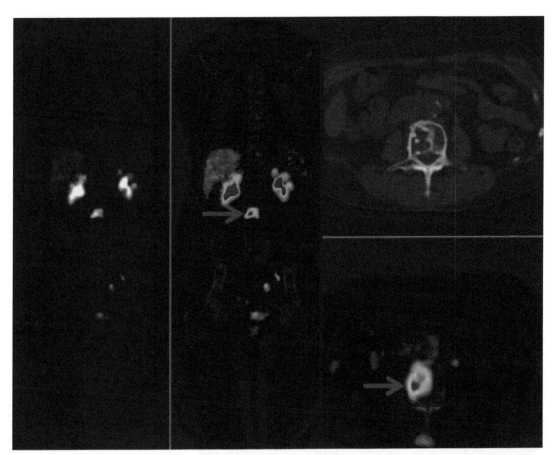

Fig. 2. A 67-year-old woman who presented with back pain; radiographs showed a lytic lesion in L2. The PET/CT demonstrates a single hypermetabolic focus (*arrows*), and biopsy confirmed solitary plasmacytoma. There was no evidence of end-organ damage, and the patient was observed without recurrence or progression to MM.

Myelomatous involvement produces bulky and intensely FDG avid lymph nodes on PET/CT that mimic a high-grade lymphoma. Involvement of multiple nodal stations is not uncommon.[49] Splenic and hepatic involvement can be focal, multifocal, or diffuse. The focal and multifocal patterns predominate in the liver and multifocal and diffuse patterns predominate in the spleen (**Fig. 7**). Extraosseous disease can occur with or without osseous disease.[38,43,49] Focal FDG avid disease can mimic a second primary malignancy and biopsy may be required to confirm myeloma. Careful review of areas with high physiologic uptake is necessary to detect extramedullary disease, especially in the brain and kidneys (**Fig. 8**).[49,50]

Identifying Skeletal Complications

Bone lesions are present in virtually all patients with advanced-stage MM and can result in substantial morbidity.[51,52] Increasing length of survival

with therapy advances increases the likelihood of skeletal complications. Severe bone pain and debilitating pathologic fractures complicate the care of MM patients. Hip fractures and vertebral collapse require stabilizing orthopedic surgery to preserve mobility and function.[53,54] In MM, lytic vertebral lesion places the patient at high risk for collapse, subsequent spinal cord compression, and paralysis. Early detection of skeletal complications can provide important clinical benefits for MM patients.[52,55,56]

Compression fractures in myeloma may be secondary to bone resorption and osteopenia or plasma cell tumor mass. Because MM bony lesions typically do not heal, patients remain at increased risk of compression fractures after treatment; this is especially true if the tumor mass supporting the cortex has been successfully treated. Review of high-quality sagittal PET, CT, and fused images in an MM patient allows for evaluation of structural integrity and degree of hypermetabolic myelomatous involvement of the spine.[6,56–58] MR

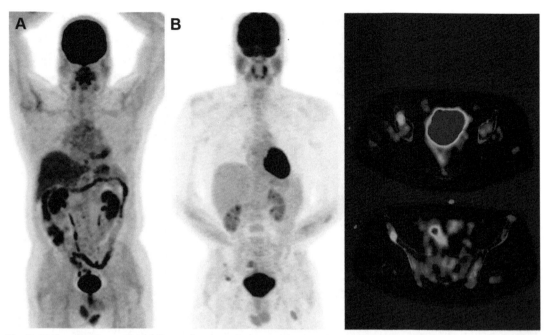

Fig. 3. Both patients presented for evaluation of abnormal monoclonal paraprotein (<3 g/dL), which was found on routine blood work as a trigger for anemia (patient A) and fatigue (patient B). No lytic lesions were reported on bony survey. A PET/CT scan was ordered to evaluate for possible MM. In patient A, the PET/CT revealed no FDG avid abnormalities and no lytic lesions within the skeleton. Patient A was diagnosed with MGUS. Patient B had 4 FDG avid skeletal lesions and was treated with systemic chemotherapy for MM.

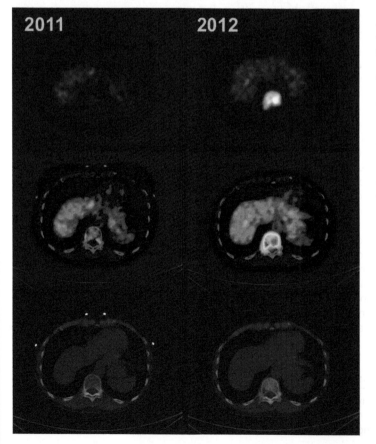

Fig. 4. This patient had elevated total protein level on routine chemistry tests in 1996. Her bone marrow showed 4% to 5% plasma cells, and her bone survey was negative. She was followed clinically with a diagnosis of MGUS for 15 years. In 2011, she was found to have increasing monoclonal protein levels. Bone marrow biopsy showed 15% plasma cells. Additional laboratory tests, bone survey, and PET/CT were normal. She was diagnosed with SMM. Six months later, in 2012, follow-up PET/CT revealed multiple FDG avid lesions throughout the spine, resulting in a diagnosis of MM.

Table 4
Clinical risk assessment

Staging System	Criteria
ISS	β-2 microglobulin and serum albumin
Durie/Salmon	Calcium, creatinine, hemoglobin, and M protein levels and skeletal radiographs
mSMART	Plasma cell fluorescence in situ hybridization, cytogenetics, plasma cell labeling index

Adapted from Refs.[41–43]

Box 3
PET/computed tomography assessment in multiple myeloma

Number and intensity of FDG avid foci

   Total number of foci, especially lesions > liver uptake

   Overall intensity of lesions, especially when ≥ cerebellum

Relative degree of marrow replacement

Extraosseous lesions

Number and extent of lytic lesions

Presence of significant osteopenia

Areas concerning for pathologic fracture

Spine abnormalities: collapse, epidural extension, cord compromise

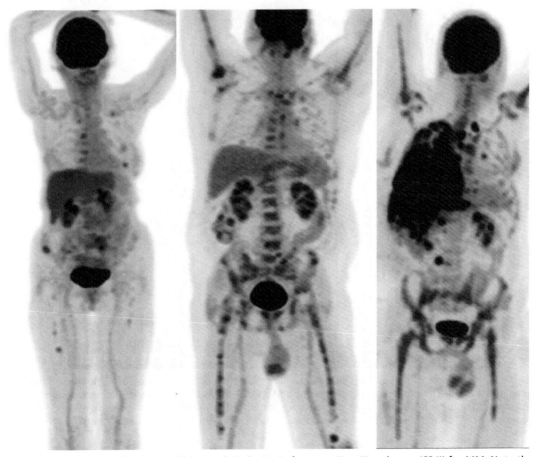

Fig. 5. These 3 patients all met Durie/Salmon clinical criteria for stage II or III and were ISS III for MM. Note the intrapatient and interpatient variation in the intensity of the lesions. The amount of marrow filling varies significantly from left to right. In the patient on the right, the osseous lesions in the thorax have extended outside of the skeleton. There is a wide spectrum of disease identified on PET/CT in MM patients.

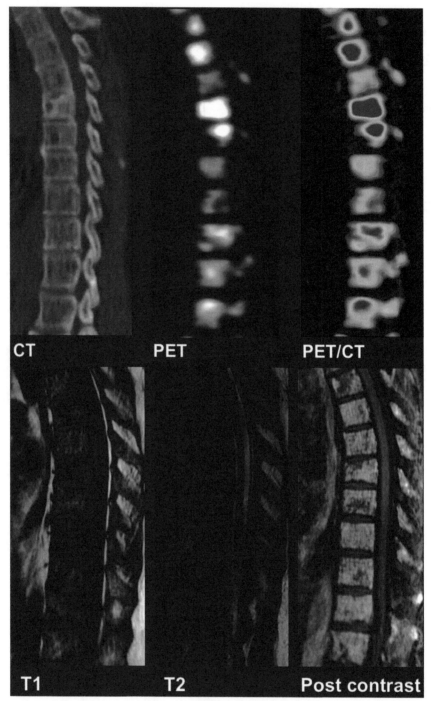

Fig. 6. Sagittal images of the spine provide an excellent evaluation of the bone marrow. This image is the initial imaging for a patient with genetically aggressive MM. PET/CT shows FDG avid myelomatous lesions of variable size and intensity. Sagittal MR images demonstrate abnormalities in the myeloma marrow lesions, which are commonly low T1 signal, high T2 signal, and associated enhancement in a variegated pattern.

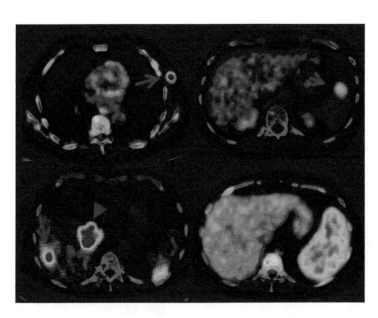

Fig. 7. Lymph nodes represent the most common extraosseous location of plasma cell tumors (*arrow, upper left*). The lymph nodes involved tend to be limited in number, but can be greater than 2 cm in size. Myeloma cells can spread directly from lymph nodes into surrounding tissues (*arrowhead*). Less commonly, the liver is involved and can be focal (*arrow, lower left*) or diffuse. Splenic involvement can be diffuse (*lower right*) or focal (*arrow, upper right*) in patients with MM.

is the imaging modality of choice to confirm cord compression (**Fig. 9**). Mulligan and colleagues[58] report the use of FDG PET/CT to characterize compression fracture as old or new. The combination of high FDG uptake (standardized uptake value >3.5) in a vertebral body and MR showing diffuse or multifocal vertebral body involvement correlated with an impending fracture.

Therapy Assessment

The treatment selection for newly diagnosed MM depends on the patient's comorbidities, ability to medically tolerate stem cell transplantation, and the presence of high-risk genetic characteristics.[6,42] Novel drugs, new combination therapy, and use of autologous stem cell transplantation have increased the frequency and duration of partial and complete responses. Still, few MM patients are cured and eventually most relapse. The current clinical staging systems have significant limitations when used to assess response to therapy. Measurement of monoclonal protein levels for assessment of disease response lacks sensitivity and specificity. Assessment of remission is most frequently performed with molecular biology techniques, polymerase chain reaction, and flow cytometry on marrow specimens, which are subject to sampling constraints.[59,60]

FDG PET/CT imaging is used to assess response to therapy to answer 3 important questions: (1) has this patient received sufficient therapy before initiating transplantation? (2) has all

evidence of MM been ablated by the transplant process? (3) what is the likelihood of relapse?

Patients for transplantation typically receive 3 to 4 months of combination chemotherapy to markedly decrease the number of myeloma cells residing within the bone marrow. Sager and colleagues[61] demonstrated that FDG uptake correlated with bone marrow cellularity and plasma cell infiltration following initial systemic therapy. In this study, the MM patients with biopsy-confirmed remissions had a negative follow-up PET/CT.[62] At this time point, the treatment response is evaluated with a goal of at least a 50% decrease in clinical, laboratory, and PET/CT measurements.[62,63] Patients with only mild decreased or increased laboratory or PET/CT data will require additional or alternative chemotherapy in preparation for transplantation. When assessing initial treatment, PET/CT is found to be more sensitive and specific than MR. PET/CT also demonstrates a much faster normalization of marrow lesions than MR.[45,51,64]

PET/CT is used to assess disease activity 90 to 100 days after transplantation. A normal PET/CT in the posttransplant setting not only provided diagnostic information but also provided valuable prognostic information. Prospective trials demonstrated that the absence of residual hypermetabolic abnormalities were predictive of a longer disease-free and overall survival (**Fig. 10**). Also, the converse was true: a positive PET/CT predicted an unfavorable outcome. The intensity of residual activity in MM lesions predicted the rapidity of clinical relapse.[62,65,66]

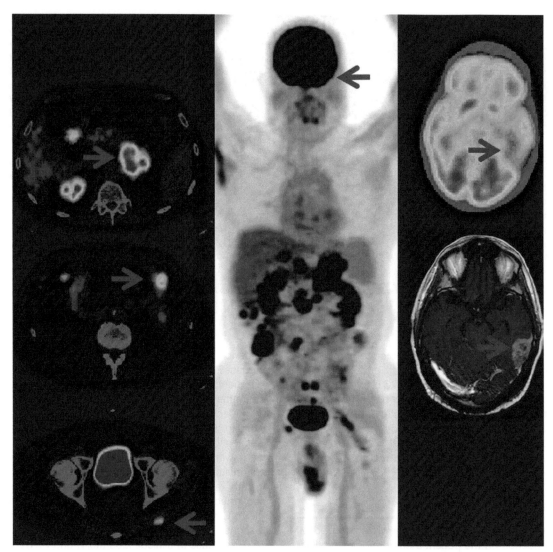

Fig. 8. 76-year-old man with numerous nonosseous plasmacytomas (*arrows*) and no significant osseous involvement at the time of his first recurrence of MM. On PET/CT, the intensely FDG avid plasmacytomas are seen in the retroperitoneal lymph nodes, small bowel, gluteus musculature, and soft tissues (*3 arrows in left panel*). The dural plasmacytoma is less active than the adjacent brain, which is better depicted on MR (*3 arrows in center and right panels*). The MR showed the dural enhancing plasmacytoma (*arrow*) surrounding cerebral edema and an absence of bone involvement.

RARE PLASMA CELL DYSCRASIAS

POEMS syndrome (polyneuropathy, organomegaly, endocrinopathy, monoclonal protein, skin changes) is a rare a paraneoplastic disorder produced by a plasma cell dyscrasia, which has sclerotic bone lesions. The diagnosis of this disorder requires a high degree of surveillance in all patients with polyneuropathy and monoclonal protein spike. The diagnosis of POEMS uses mandatory, major, and minor criteria codified by the Mayo Clinic.[67,68] No standard treatment of POEMS has been established. General practice is to irradiate patients with a limited number of bone lesions (≤4) and give systemic chemotherapy for widespread sclerotic bone disease and stem cell transplantation. Successful ablation of bone lesions often eliminates the polyneuropathy. Patients with POEMS syndrome have a much better prognosis than MM patients.[68,69]

Initial published data on PET/CT in POEMS syndrome suggest that bone lesions are typically FDG avid on PET and are usually sclerotic or mixed sclerotic and lytic on corresponding CT (**Fig. 11**). POEMS skeletal disease typically involves the

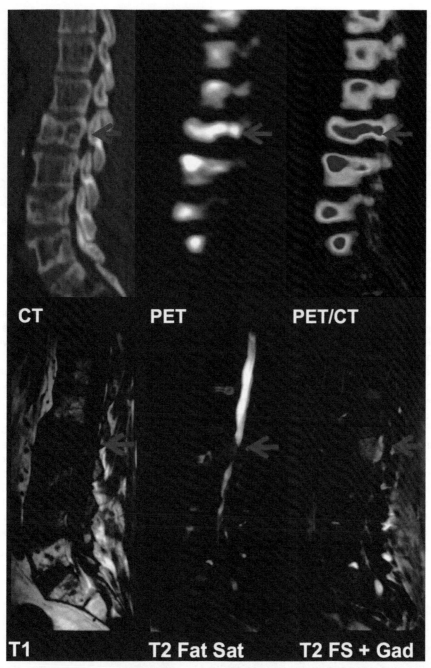

Fig. 9. A 77-year-old man who presented with back pain and prior treatment of multiple myeloma. Sagittal PET/CT images demonstrate diffuse myelomatous involvement of the thoracolumbar spine, including an L2 compression fracture. The intense FDG uptake extends posterior into the spinal canal (*arrow*). Sagittal MR images confirm pathologic compression of L2 with an associated soft tissue mass. Although there is retropulsion of the soft tissue mass into the spinal canal, no cord compression was present. MR is the imaging modality of choice in patients with suspected cord compression.

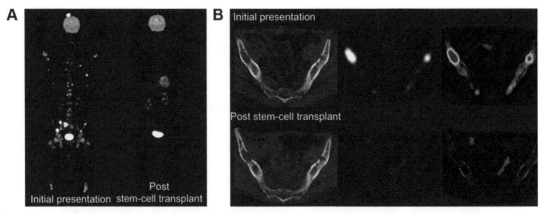

Fig. 10. The PET/CT maximum intensity projection images (A) show innumerable hypermetabolic marrow lesion throughout the axial and appendicular skeleton on initial evaluation. Biopsy confirmed MM. The posttransplant PET/CT images demonstrate complete resolution of all hypermetabolic lesions. Transaxial PET/CT images of the pelvis (B) show the resolution of FDG uptake on PET but persistence of the lytic bone lesions on CT.

pelvis, spine, ribs, and proximal long bones. FDG PET/CT can be useful in detecting unsuspected abnormalities and selecting the most accessible bone lesion and lymph node for biopsy. In patients with a limited number of osseous lesions, PET/CT can determine the number and be used for radiation therapy planning.[70–72] Recently, PET/CT has been used after transplantation to assess response.[69,73]

WM is uncommon plasma cell dyscrasia characterized by monoclonal immunoglobulin M (IgM) and lymphoplasmacytic cells infiltrating the bone marrow. Plasma cell infiltration in lymph nodes, liver, and spleen is seen in about 20% to 50% of WM patients. Similar to MM, the disease course is heterogeneous, with some patients progressing slowly and others more rapidly. Combination

therapy of bortezomib and rituximab has become the standard. Patients with WM have a median disease-free survival that is nearly twice that of MM patients.[74–77]

The triggers for therapy in WM patients are symptom severity, the serum monoclonal IgM levels, and the estimated percentage of marrow involvement. PET/CT is used to assess marrow tumor load and detect the presence of extramedullary disease. Elevated FDG uptake in the marrow is found in more than 40% of WM patients (Fig. 12). PET/CT identified nodal, splenic, and/or hepatic disease in about 80% of patients.[78,79] A prospective study of bortezomib and rituximab therapy showed that pretreatment and posttreatment PET/CT could be used to assess response.[80]

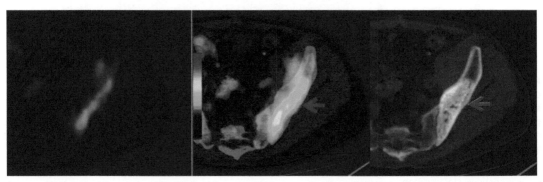

Fig. 11. A 52-year-old patient presented with a 2 year history of polyneuropathy of unknown cause. Additional workup demonstrated hypogonadotropic hypogonadism, a monoclonal M-spike, skin changes, and a hypermetabolic sclerotic lesion in his left iliac bone (arrow). This patient was diagnosed with POEMS, underwent localized radiation therapy to sclerotic lesion left pelvic lesions, and had substantial improvement in neuropathic symptoms.

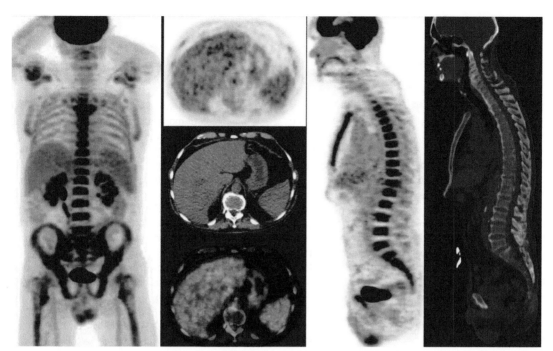

Fig. 12. A 72-year-old man who presented with anemia, weakness, headache, and a monoclonal IgM spike consistent with WM. PET/CT images demonstrate diffuse intense FDG uptake throughout the axial and proximal appendicular skeleton. Moderately increased, nodular FDG increased uptake is seen in the liver and spleen.

REFERENCES

1. Roodman GD. Skeletal imaging and management of bone disease. Hematology Am Soc Hematol Educ Program 2008;1:313.
2. Kyle RA, Therneau TM, Rajkumar SV, et al. Incidence of multiple myeloma in Olmsted County, Minnesota: trend over 6 decades. Cancer 2004;101:2667.
3. Siegel R, Naishadham D, Jemal A. Cancer statistics, 2012. CA Cancer J Clin 2012;62:10.
4. Kyle RA, Gertz MA, Witzig TE, et al. Review of 1027 patients with newly diagnosed multiple myeloma. Mayo Clin Proc 2003;78:21.
5. Turesson I, Velez R, Kristinsson SY, et al. Patterns of multiple myeloma during the past 5 decades: stable incidence rates for all age groups in the population but rapidly changing age distribution in the clinic. Mayo Clin Proc 2010;85:225.
6. Kumar SK, Dingli D, Lacy MQ, et al. Autologous stem cell transplantation in patients of 70 years and older with multiple myeloma: results from a matched pair analysis. Am J Hematol 2008;83:614.
7. Barlogie B, Jagannath S, Desikan KR, et al. Total therapy with tandem transplants for newly diagnosed multiple myeloma. Blood 1999;93:55.
8. Naumann-Winter F, Greb A, Borchmann P, et al. First-line tandem high-dose chemotherapy and autologous stem cell transplantation versus single high-dose chemotherapy and autologous stem cell transplantation in multiple myeloma, a systematic review of controlled studies. Cochrane Database Syst Rev 2012;(10):CD004626.
9. Gambhir SS. Molecular imaging of cancer with positron emission tomography. Nat Rev Cancer 2002;2:683.
10. Allen-Auerbach M, de Vos S, Czernin J. PET/computed tomography and lymphoma. Radiol Clin North Am 2013;51:833.
11. Beyer T, Townsend DW, Blodgett TM. Dual-modality PET/CT tomography for clinical oncology. Q J Nucl Med 2002;46:24.
12. Rajkumar SV, Kyle RA, Buadi FK. Advances in the diagnosis, classification, risk stratification, and management of monoclonal gammopathy of undetermined significance: implications for recategorizing disease entities in the presence of evolving scientific evidence. Mayo Clin Proc 2010;85:945.
13. Kyle RA, Rajkumar SV. Monoclonal gammopathy of undetermined significance. Br J Haematol 2006;134:573.
14. Kyle RA, Rajkumar SV. Monoclonal gammopathy of undetermined significance and smouldering multiple myeloma: emphasis on risk factors for progression. Br J Haematol 2007;139:730.
15. Bird J, Behrens J, Westin J, et al. UK Myeloma Forum (UKMF) and Nordic Myeloma Study Group (NMSG): guidelines for the investigation of newly detected M-proteins and the management of monoclonal gammopathy of undetermined significance (MGUS). Br J Haematol 2009;147:22.

16. Kyle RA, Durie BG, Rajkumar SV, et al. Monoclonal gammopathy of undetermined significance (MGUS) and smoldering (asymptomatic) multiple myeloma: IMWG consensus perspectives risk factors for progression and guidelines for monitoring and management. Leukemia 2010;24:1121.

17. Rajkumar SV, Larson D, Kyle RA. Diagnosis of smoldering multiple myeloma. N Engl J Med 2011; 365:474.

18. Kyle RA, Remstein ED, Therneau TM, et al. Clinical course and prognosis of smoldering (asymptomatic) multiple myeloma. N Engl J Med 2007;356:2582.

19. Rajkumar SV, Dispenzieri A, Fonseca R, et al. Thalidomide for previously untreated indolent or smoldering multiple myeloma. Leukemia 2001;15:1274.

20. Kyle RA, Rajkumar SV. Monoclonal gammopathy of undetermined significance and smoldering multiple myeloma. Hematol Oncol Clin North Am 2007;21:1093.

21. Gao M, Yang G, Tompkins VS, et al. Early versus deferred treatment for smoldering multiple myeloma: a meta-analysis of randomized, controlled trials. PLoS One 2014;9(10):e109758.

22. Soutar R, Lucraft H, Jackson G, et al. Guidelines on the diagnosis and management of solitary plasmacytoma of bone and solitary extramedullary plasmacytoma. Br J Haematol 2004;124:717.

23. Dimopoulos MA, Moulopoulos LA, Maniatis A, et al. Solitary plasmacytoma of bone and asymptomatic multiple myeloma. Blood 2000;96:2037.

24. Dores GM, Landgren O, McGlynn KA, et al. Plasmacytoma of bone, extramedullary plasmacytoma, and multiple myeloma: incidence and survival in the United States, 1992-2004. Br J Haematol 2009;144:86.

25. Dimopoulos MA, Goldstein J, Fuller L, et al. Curability of solitary bone plasmacytoma. J Clin Oncol 1992;10:587.

26. Tsang RW, Gospodarowicz MK, Pintilie M, et al. Solitary plasmacytoma treated with radiotherapy: impact of tumor size on outcome. Int J Radiat Oncol Biol Phys 2001;50:113.

27. Nanni C, Zamagni E, Farsad M, et al. Role of 18F-FDG PET/CT in the assessment of bone involvement in newly diagnosed multiple myeloma: preliminary results. Eur J Nucl Med Mol Imaging 2006;33:525–31.

28. Fonti R, Salvatore B, Quarantelli M, et al. 18F-FDG PET/CT, 99mTc-MIBI, and MRI in evaluation of patients with multiple myeloma. J Nucl Med 2008;49:195.

29. Zamagni E, Nanni C, Patriarca F, et al. A prospective comparison of 18F-fluorodeoxyglucose positron emission tomography-computed tomography, magnetic resonance imaging and whole-body planar radiographs in the assessment of bone disease in newly diagnosed multiple myeloma. Haematologica 2007;92:50.

30. Durie BG. The role of anatomic and functional staging in myeloma: description of Durie/Salmon plus staging system. Eur J Cancer 2006;42:1539.

31. Moulopoulos LA, Dimopoulos MA, Weber D, et al. Magnetic resonance imaging in the staging of solitary plasmacytoma of bone. J Clin Oncol 1993;11:1311.

32. Pertuiset E, Bellaiche L, Lioté F, et al. Magnetic resonance imaging of the spine in plasma cell dyscrasias. A review. Rev Rhum Engl Ed 1996;63:837.

33. Warsame R, Gertz MA, Lacy MQ, et al. Trends and outcomes of modern staging of solitary plasmacytoma of bone. Am J Hematol 2012;87:647.

34. Kim PJ, Hicks RJ, Wirth A, et al. Impact of 18F-fluorodeoxyglucose positron emission tomography before and after definitive radiation therapy in patients with apparently solitary plasmacytoma. Int J Radiat Oncol Biol Phys 2009;74:740.

35. Nanni C, Rubello D, Zamagni E, et al. 18F-FDG PET/CT in myeloma with presumed solitary plasmocytoma of bone. In Vivo 2008;22:513.

36. Salaun PY, Gastinne T, Frampas E, et al. FDG-positron-emission tomography for staging and therapeutic assessment in patients with plasmacytoma. Haematologica 2008;93:1269.

37. Rajkumar SV, Merlini G, San Miguel JF. Haematological cancer: redefining myeloma. Nat Rev Clin Oncol 2012;9:494.

38. Mulligan ME. Imaging techniques used in the diagnosis, staging, and follow-up of patients with myeloma. Acta Radiol 2005;46(7):716–24.

39. Mulligan ME, Badros AZ. PET/CT and MR imaging in myeloma. Skeletal Radiol 2007;36(1):5–16.

40. Durie BG, Waxman AD, D'Agnolo A, et al. Whole-body (18)F-FDG PET identifies high-risk myeloma. J Nucl Med 2002;43(11):1457–63.

41. Greipp PR, San Miguel J, Durie BG, et al. International staging system for multiple myeloma. J Clin Oncol 2005;23:3412.

42. Durie BG, Salmon SE. A clinical staging system for multiple myeloma. Correlation of measured myeloma cell mass with presenting clinical features, response to treatment, and survival. Cancer 1975;36:842.

43. Dispenzieri A, Rajkumar SV, Gertz MA, et al. Treatment of newly diagnosed multiple myeloma based on Mayo Stratification of Myeloma and Risk-adapted Therapy (mSMART): consensus statement. Mayo Clin Proc 2007;82:323.

44. Agarwal A, Chirindel A, Shah BA, et al. Evolving role of FDG PET/CT in multiple myeloma imaging and management. AJR Am J Roentgenol 2013;200:884.

45. Koppula B, Kaptuch J, Hanrahan CJ. Imaging of multiple myeloma: usefulness of MRI and PET/CT. Semin Ultrasound CT MR 2013;34:566.

46. Park S, Lee SJ, Chang WJ, et al. Positive correlation between baseline PET or PET/CT findings and clinical parameters in multiple myeloma patients. Acta Haematol 2014;131:193.

47. Dammacco F, Rubini G, Ferrari C, et al. (18)F-FDG PET/CT: a review of diagnostic and prognostic features in multiple myeloma and related disorders.

Clin Exp Med. 2014 Sep 14. [Epub ahead of print] PubMed PMID: 25218739.

48. Varettoni M, Corso A, Pica G, et al. Incidence, presenting features and outcome of extraosseous disease in multiple myeloma: a longitudinal study on 1003 consecutive patients. Ann Oncol 2010;21:325.

49. Wu P, Davies FE, Boyd K, et al. The impact of extra-medullary disease at presentation on the outcome of myeloma. Leuk Lymphoma 2009;50:230.

50. Hall MN, Jagannathan JP, Ramaiya NH, et al. Imaging of extraosseous myeloma: CT, PET/CT, and MRI features. AJR Am J Roentgenol 2010;195(5):1057–65.

51. Hur J, Yoon CS, Ryu YH, et al. Efficacy of multidetector row computed tomography of the spine in patients with multiple myeloma: comparison with magnetic resonance imaging and fluorodeoxyglucose-positron emission tomography. J Comput Assist Tomogr 2007;31:342–7. Ann Hematol 2009;88:1161.

52. Coleman RE. Skeletal complications of malignancy. Cancer 1997;80(8 Suppl):1588.

53. Kyle RA. Multiple myeloma: review of 869 cases. Mayo Clin Proc 1975;50:29.

54. Harrington KD. Orthopedic surgical management of skeletal complications of malignancy. Cancer 1997; 80:1614.

55. Manglani HH, Marco RA, Picciolo A, et al. Orthopedic emergencies in cancer patients. Semin Oncol 2000;27:299.

56. Hussein MA. Nontraditional cytotoxic therapies for relapsed/refractory multiple myeloma. Oncologist 2002;7(Suppl 1):20.

57. Yi J, Wang S, Ma S, et al. Disseminated plasmacytomas in multiple myeloma: atypical presentations on multimodality images, emphasized on PET/CT. Ann Hematol 2013;92:1421.

58. Mulligan M, Chirindel A, Karchevsky M. Characterizing and predicting pathologic spine fractures in myeloma patients with FDG PET/CT and MR imaging. Cancer Invest 2011;29:370.

59. Davies FE, Rawstron AC, Owen RG, et al. Minimal residual disease monitoring in multiple myeloma. Best Pract Res Clin Haematol 2002;15:197.

60. Sarasquete ME, García-Sanz R, González D, et al. Minimal residual disease monitoring in multiple myeloma: a comparison between allelic-specific oligonucleotide real-time quantitative polymerase chain reaction and flow cytometry. Haematologica 2005;90:1365.

61. Sager S, Ergül N, Ciftci H, et al. The value of FDG PET/CT in the initial staging and bone marrow involvement of patients with multiple myeloma. Skeletal Radiol 2011;40:843.

62. Bartel TB, Haessler J, Brown TL, et al. F18-fluoro-deoxyglucose positron emission tomography in the context of other imaging techniques and prognostic factors in multiple myeloma. Blood 2009;114:2068.

63. Dimitrakopoulou-Strauss A, Hoffmann M, Bergner R, et al. Prediction of progression-free survival in patients with multiple myeloma following anthracycline-based chemotherapy based on dynamic FDG-PET. Clin Nucl Med 2009;34:576–84.

64. Breyer RJ 3rd, Mulligan ME, Smith SE, et al. Comparison of imaging with FDG PET/CT with other imaging modalities in myeloma. Skeletal Radiol 2006;35:632.

65. Zamagni E, Patriarca F, Nanni C, et al. Prognostic relevance of 18-F FDG PET/CT in newly diagnosed multiple myeloma patients treated with up-front autologous transplantation. Blood 2011;118:5989.

66. Usmani SZ, Mitchell A, Waheed S, et al. Prognostic implications of serial 18-fluoro-deoxyglucose emission tomography in multiple myeloma treated with total therapy 3. Blood 2013;121:1819.

67. Dispenzieri A, Kyle RA, Lacy MQ, et al. POEMS syndrome: definitions and long-term outcome. Blood 2003;101:2496.

68. Dispenzieri A. POEMS syndrome. Blood Rev 2007; 21:285.

69. D'Souza A, Lacy M, Gertz M, et al. Long-term outcomes after autologous stem cell transplantation for patients with POEMS syndrome (osteosclerotic myeloma): a single-center experience. Blood 2012;120:56.

70. Albertí MA, Martinez-Yélamos S, Fernandez A, et al. 18F-FDG PET/CT in the evaluation of POEMS syndrome. Eur J Radiol 2010;76:180.

71. Montoriol PF, Cachin F, Michel JL, et al. Two more cases of evaluation of POEMS syndrome using 18-FDG PET/CT. Eur J Radiol 2011;80:861.

72. Minarik J, Scudla V, Bacovsky J, et al. Comparison of imaging methods in POEMS syndrome. Biomed Pap Med Fac Univ Palacky Olomouc Czech Repub 2012;156:52.

73. Stefanelli A, Treglia G, Leccisotti L, et al. Usefulness of F-18 FDG PET/CT in the follow-up of POEMS syndrome after autologous peripheral blood stem cell transplantation. Clin Nucl Med 2012;37:181–3.

74. Treon SP. How I treat Waldenstrom's macroglobulinemia. Blood 2009;114:2375.

75. Vijay A, Gertz MA. Current treatment options for Waldenstrom macroglobulinemia. Clin Lymphoma Myeloma 2008;8:219.

76. Ghobrial IM, Witzig TE. Waldenstrom macroglobulinemia. Curr Treat Options Oncol 2004;5:239.

77. Ghobrial IM, Gertz MA, Fonseca R. Waldenstrom macroglobulinaemia. Lancet Oncol 2003;4:679.

78. Walker RC, Brown TL, Jones-Jackson LB, et al. Imaging of multiple myeloma and related plasma cell dyscrasias. J Nucl Med 2012;53:1091.

79. Banwait R, O'Regan K, Campigotto F, et al. The role of 18F-FDG PET/CT imaging in Waldenstrom macroglobulinemia. Am J Hematol 2011;86:567.

80. Owen RG, Kyle RA, Stone MJ, et al. VIth International Workshop on Waldenström macroglobulinaemia. Response assessment in Waldenström macroglobulinaemia: update from the VIth International Workshop. Br J Haematol 2013;160:171.

PET/Computed Tomography and Patient Outcomes in Melanoma

Eric M. Rohren, MD, PhD[a,b,*]

KEYWORDS

- Melanoma • PET/CT • Outcomes • Surveillance

KEY POINTS

- Fludeoxyglucose F 18 (FDG)–PET/computed tomography (CT) has a high sensitivity and specificity for detection of distant metastatic disease from cutaneous malignant melanoma.
- Patients with melanoma are at risk for development of recurrence and metastases, and the risk increases with disease stage.
- Aggressive surgical intervention for resection of metastases has been shown to improve survival in patients with melanoma.
- FDG-PET/CT is superior to CT for detection of recurrence in the surveillance setting.
- The impact and cost-effectiveness of surveillance imaging in patients with melanoma has yet to be determined.

INTRODUCTION

Malignant melanoma is a tumor arising from melanocytes, which are neural crest–derived cells widely distributed throughout the tissues of the body, particularly the skin. Population statistics, such as Surveillance, Epidemiology, and End Results (SEER) data, have documented a rapid increase in the incidence of melanoma in the latter part of the twentieth century. Many factors are thought to contribute to this increase in melanoma diagnoses, including higher UV exposure and more prevalent screening programs. According to the 2014 statistics from the American Cancer Society SEER data, the number of new melanoma diagnoses in the United States is estimated to be 76,100, whereas the number of melanoma-related deaths is estimated to be 9710.[1]

Survival is closely linked to the extent of disease at the time of diagnosis. Localized melanoma is primarily a surgical disease, and complete resection of the tumor often results in a cure. The prospect of cure diminishes with more advanced disease. Although surgery can still play a significant role in such patients, locoregional and systemic therapies are usually added to improve outcome.

Traditional staging of melanoma takes into account features of the primary tumor as well as disease spread. The American Joint Committee on Cancer (AJCC) classifies melanoma according the standard TNM classification (**Table 1**). Unlike many tumors in which size is a major T determinant, melanoma T staging is based primarily on depth of invasion and the presence or absence of ulceration. N staging is based on the presence

The author has nothing to disclose.
[a] Department of Nuclear Medicine, The University of Texas MD Anderson Cancer Center, 1400 Pressler – Unit 1483, Houston, TX 77030, USA; [b] Department of Diagnostic Radiology, The University of Texas MD Anderson Cancer Center, 1400 Pressler – Unit 1483, Houston, TX 77030, USA
* Department of Nuclear Medicine, The University of Texas MD Anderson Cancer Center, 1400 Pressler – Unit 1483, Houston, TX 77030.
E-mail address: eric.rohren@mdanderson.org

PET Clin 10 (2015) 243–254
http://dx.doi.org/10.1016/j.cpet.2014.12.006
1556-8598/15/$ – see front matter © 2015 Elsevier Inc. All rights reserved.

or absence of metastatic disease (microscopic or macroscopic) in regional lymph nodes or in-transit disease, and M staging is based on distant metastases. A summary of TNM and staging of cutaneous malignant melanoma is presented in **Tables 1–5.**

As with many other malignancies, it is increasingly recognized that specific genetic alterations are associated with the development of malignant cutaneous melanoma. More than 70% of cutaneous melanomas have activating mutations in BRAF, NRAS, or KIT,[2,3] whereas uveal melanomas have been shown to have mutations in the GNAQ and GNA11 oncogenes.[4,5] Understanding these genetic events can aid in the prediction of response to targeted therapy and can help to develop novel targeted therapies in the treatment of advanced disease (**Fig. 1**).

To tailor the best therapy for a particular patient, accurate information is needed regarding the extent of disease and, if metastatic disease is present, the sites involved. A multimodality approach is often used in melanoma patients. PET/computed tomography (CT) using FDG has proved a valuable imaging method for evaluation of patients with melanoma.

NORMAL ANATOMY AND IMAGING TECHNIQUE
Fludeoxyglucose F 18–PET/Computed Tomography Imaging

FDG is a radioactive analog of glucose, transported across the cell membrane by glucose transporter molecules. Once intracellular, FDG is phosphorylated to FDG-6P but is then blocked from either further phosphorylation or dephosphorylation, leading to accumulation of FDG in the cell. Tissues in the body with increased glucose transporter expression, elevated hexokinase activity, and/or increased perfusion can all thereby show enhanced localization of FDG and are detected as areas of increased radioactivity on scanning. These criteria are characteristic of many malignancies, although other physiologic and pathologic processes can share these features.

Whereas a typical oncologic PET/CT is performed from the orbits to the proximal thighs, many institutions perform these true whole-body scans on melanoma patients. Although such an approach is mandatory in cases of a primary tumor located in the lower extremities, many institutions perform such whole-body scans on melanoma patients routinely. When a whole-body scan is performed, care must be taken to apply appropriate attenuation correction algorithms to avoid artifact

Table 2
N staging of melanoma

N Stage	Involvement	Extent
N0	No nodes	
N1	1 Node	a. Microscopic disease
		b. Macroscopic disease
N2	2–3 Nodes	a. Microscopic disease
		b. Macroscopic disease
		c. In-transit disease without nodal metastases
N3	4 or More nodes or Matted nodes or In-transit disease with nodal metastases	

Table 1
T staging of melanoma

T Stage	Thickness (mm)	Ulceration
T1	≤1.0	a. Without ulceration and Clark I/II
		b. With ulceration or Clark IV/V
T2	1.01–2.0	a. Without ulceration
		b. With ulceration
T3	2.01–4.0	a. Without ulceration
		b. With ulceration
T4	>4.0	a. Without ulceration
		b. With ulceration

Table 3
M staging of melanoma

M Stage	Site	Serum Lactate Dehydrogenase
M0	No distant metastases	
M1a	Distant skin, subcutaneous, or nodal metastases	Normal
M1b	Lung metastases	Normal
M1c	All other visceral metastases or Any distant metastasis	Normal / Elevated

Table 4
Staging of melanoma

Stage	TNM Categories	5-Year Survival (%)
Stage I	T1-2a, N0, M0	99
Stage II	T2b-4b, N0, M0	99
Stage III	Any T, N1-3, M0	65
Stage IV	Any T, Any N, M1a-c	15

Table 5
Detailed staging of melanoma: clinical versus pathologic staging

	Clinical Staging		
Stage	T	N	M
0	Tis	N0	M0
IA	T1a	N0	M0
IB	T1b	N0	M0
	T2a	N0	M0
IIA	T2b	N0	M0
	T3a	N0	M0
IIB	T3b	N0	M0
	T4a	N0	M0
IIC	T4b	N0	M0
III	Any T	N1	M0
IV	Any T	Any N	M1
	Pathologic Staging		
Stage	T	N	M
0	Tis	N0	M0
IA	T1a	N0	M0
IB	T1b	N0	M0
	T2a	N0	M0
IIA	T2b	N0	M0
	T3a	N0	M0
IIB	T3b	N0	M0
	T4a	N0	M0
	T4b	N0	M0
IIIA	T1-4a	N1a	M0
	T1-4a	N2a	M0
IIIB	T1-4b	N1a	M0
	T1-4b	N2a	M0
	T1-4a	N1b	M0
	T1-4a	N2b	M0
	T1-4a	N2c	M0
IIIC	T1-4b	N1b	M0
	T1-4b	N2b	M0
	T1-4b	N2c	M0
	Any T	N3	M0
IV	Any T	Any N	M1

at the margins of the body, in particular the skin surfaces (**Fig. 2**).

Although many PET/CT scans are performed without the use of oral or intravenous contrast, many facilities are increasingly using contrast enhancement on their scans for a variety of malignancies. Although no consensus exists on the usefulness or need for contrast enhancement in PET/CT, it can improve the CT visualization and characterization of lesions in some instances.

The goal of imaging with FDG-PET/CT in patients with melanoma is to detect foci of increased FDG localization, which may be an indicator of malignancy. In the setting of initial work-up and treatment planning, the goal is to provide disease staging information. In the post-therapy setting, the goal may be to detect disease recurrence at the primary site or to identify metastatic disease.

Imaging Findings/Pathology

The role of fludeoxyglucose F 18–PET/computed tomography in staging and detection of recurrence

Beginning with the primary tumor, FDG-PET/CT has little application in the assessment of lesion depth and/or ulceration, the major determinants of T stage. Although the primary lesion sometimes is visualized on PET/CT, this information is rarely impactful because the diagnosis is already established. Occasionally, incidental focal cutaneous activity is seen in PET/CT studies performed for other reasons, but such activity is often merely due to inflammatory conditions, such as folliculitis or an infected sebaceous cyst (**Fig. 3**). Conversely, the absence of activity in a site of known cutaneous melanoma (**Fig. 4**) imparts little in the way of prognostic or predictive information.

It is well established that FDG-PET/CT is not clinically useful in the evaluation of regional lymph node basins in patients with newly diagnosed melanoma. It has been found that the specificity for metastatic disease is high, up to 96% in some series,[6] and the presence of focal uptake in a regional lymph node is highly concerning for metastatic disease (**Fig. 5**). The sensitivity is correspondingly low, however. In a large patient series, when the results of FDG-PET/CT were correlated with the results of histopathology, the sensitivity of PET was between 15% and 49%.[7] In a large meta-analysis of the literature, the median sensitivity and specificity of FDG-PET/CT for regional lymph node staging were 11% and 97%, respectively.[8] Because of these data, FDG-PET/CT for evaluation of regional lymph nodes in patients with melanoma is a noncovered indication by the Centers for Medicare & Medicaid Services

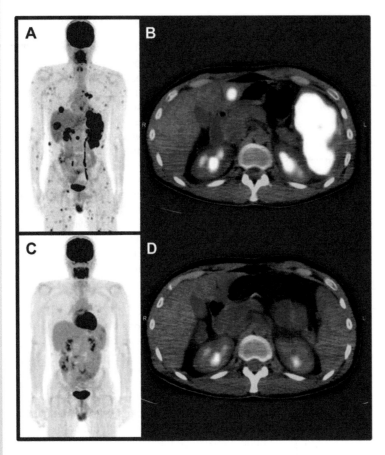

Fig. 1. Maximum intensity projection images and axial PET/CT images in a patient pre- and post-treatment with vemurafenib, an inhibitor of the BRAF enzyme. In (*A*) and (*B*), widespread FDG-avid metastatic disease is seen throughout the body, including bulky splenic disease. In (*C*) and (*D*), follow-up PET/CT performed approximately 2 months later shows near complete metabolic response.

(CMS). Lymphoscintigraphy and sentinel lymph node biopsy remain the recommended means of establishing early spread of disease to regional lymph nodes.

In patients with a positive sentinel lymph node, who by definition are at least stage III, the likelihood of additional sites of metastatic disease increases. Although there is ongoing debate regarding the usefulness of imaging in patients with stage IIIA versus IIIB disease, FDG-PET/CT is best utilized for the detection of unsuspected distant metastases.

One of the primary advantages of FDG-PET/CT compared with standard diagnostic CT and MR imaging is the ability to image the entire body from vertex to feet, with inclusion of the skin surfaces. In multiple studies, FDG-PET/CT has been shown an excellent imaging test for the detection of distant metastases. In a meta-analysis that pooled data from 14 separate studies of patients with advanced-stage melanoma (753 patients, 1948 lesions), PET was found to have a sensitivity of 88% and a specificity of 82% for metastatic disease.[9] A separate meta-analysis comparing CT and PET/CT found the median sensitivity and specificity of CT

for detection of distant metastases to be 51% and 69%, respectively, compared with values of 80% and 87% for PET/CT.[8]

In a study of 32 melanoma patients with suspected oligometastatic disease who were imaged with FDG-PET/CT in addition to standard clinical work-up (contrast-enhanced CT studies plus brain MR imaging), unexpected additional sites of metastatic disease were detected in 4 patients (12%), resulting in a change in management in all cases.[10]

As with any imaging study, FDG-PET/CT has its strengths and limitations.[11] Many sites of disease, in particular marrow disease, are often better identified with FDG-PET/CT than on CT alone (**Fig. 6**). CT may be superior, however, for detection of sub-centimeter pulmonary metastases (although the PET/CT technique can be modified to include full-inspiration, high-resolution images of the lungs), and MR imaging is conclusively more sensitive for the detection of cerebral metastases (**Fig. 7**). Detection of metastatic disease, even in the setting of other known distant metastasis, is important in patients with melanoma, because survival benefit may be gained by surgical excision of such metastases.[12–18]

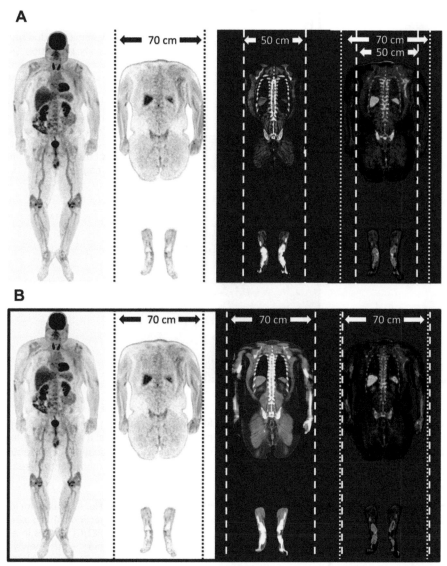

Fig. 2. (*A*) When performing FDG-PET/CT in patients with melanoma, it is important to match the axial field of view between the PET and CT components of the study. The PET is typically acquired at a wide field of view (eg, 70 cm) whereas CT is acquired at a narrower field of view (eg, 50 cm). Such disparity can result in incomplete attenuation correction and artifact at the skin surfaces and edges of the body. (*B*) By acquiring a CT scan at the same axial field of view as the PET study (eg, 70 cm), appropriate attenuation correction can be performed, eliminating truncation and attenuation artifacts at the periphery of the scan.

Although a majority of melanoma lesions are intensely hypermetabolic, some sites of melanoma may not show increased FDG uptake compared with regional background (**Fig. 8**). In a study of 124 patients with high-risk melanoma imaged with FDG-PET/CT, metastatic disease was detected in 53.[19] In 46 of these cases (87%), the sites of metastatic disease were visibly hypermetabolic on PET. In the remaining 7 cases (13%), the metastases were only minimally FDG avid and were detected and characterized only on CT. The

significance of such nonavid disease is debated. In 1 study,[20] low SUV in overt nodal metastases was associated with a better disease-free survival compared with high SUV. Such a relationship has not been demonstrated for distant metastatic disease, however.

Impact of fludeoxyglucose F 18–PET/computed tomography on patient outcome

Once a patient has been staged and has undergone primary therapy for malignant melanoma,

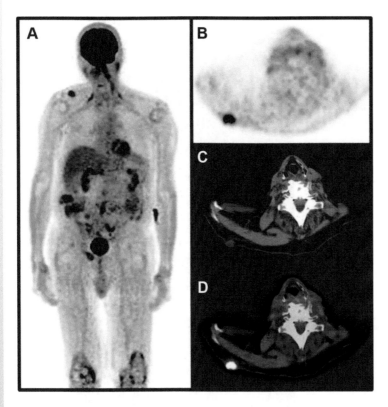

Fig. 3. FDG-PET/CT scan in a patient with previously treated melanoma, including maximum intensity projection (*A*) and axial images (*B-D*). An intensely hypermetabolic cutaneous/subcutaneous mass is seen in the right posterior shoulder, thought to represent metastatic melanoma. On visual inspection, this was an infected sebaceous cyst, which was treated with incision and drainage.

the emphasis turns toward follow-up and surveillance. Patients with melanoma are at risk for recurrent disease, with up to 33% of patients in some series developing metastatic disease during the follow-up period.[21,22] It has been shown in these patients that there is a survival benefit to early detection of both local/regional recurrence[13–15] as well as distant metastatic disease.[17,18] An

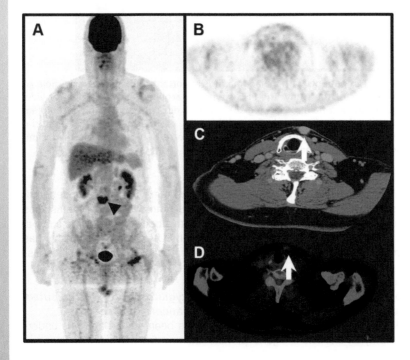

Fig. 4. Maximum intensity projection (*A*) and axial (*B-D*) FDG-PET/CT images in a 60-year-old man with newly diagnosed melanoma. Although the site of osseous metastatic disease in the L2 vertebral body is well visualized (*arrowhead*), the in situ primary melanoma in the anterior neck (*arrow*) shows no appreciable tracer uptake above regional background.

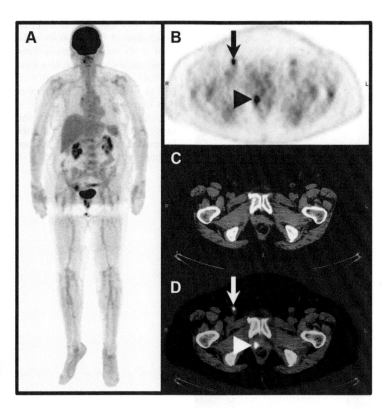

Fig. 5. Maximum intensity projection (A) and axial (B-D) images from a whole-body FDG-PET/CT scan in a 60-year-old woman with newly diagnosed vaginal melanoma. The primary lesion is identified as an intensely hypermetabolic focus along the right wall of the vagina (arrowhead). A 4-mm lymph node in the right inguinal fossa shows intense tracer uptake (arrow) and was proved on biopsy to be a site of metastatic disease.

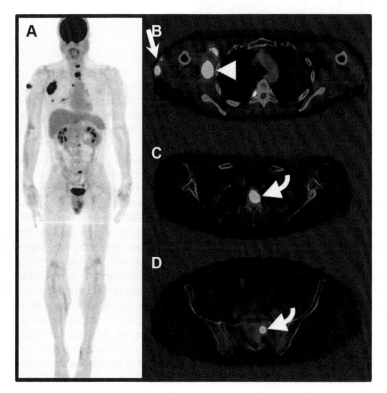

Fig. 6. Maximum intensity projection (A) and selected axial (B-D) images from an FDG-PET/CT scan in a 48-year-old man with newly diagnosed melanoma. The primary lesion is seen in the right upper arm (arrow) with an adjacent intransit metastasis. Bulky nodal metastatic disease in the right axilla also shows intense FDG uptake (arrowhead). PET/CT also demonstrates multiple unsuspected sites of marrow metastatic disease (curved arrows), not evident on CT imaging.

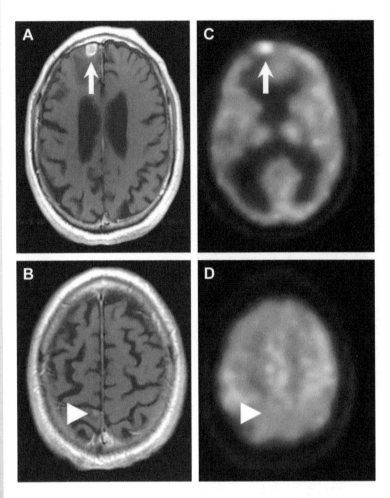

Fig. 7. Axial MR (*A, B*) and PET (*C, D*) images of the brain in a patient with recurrent melanoma. A cortical metastasis in the right frontal lobe (*arrows*) is visible on PET as a focus of hypermetabolism exceeding normal cortex in intensity. A smaller cortical metastasis in the right parietal lobe (*arrowhead*), however, is not visible on PET.

imaging strategy designed toward the early detection of recurrent disease, therefore, seem both appropriate and necessary in at-risk patients with malignant melanoma.

The need for imaging surveillance seems supported by a large meta-analysis performed by Xing and colleagues,[8] in which the summed data from 74 published studies were retrospectively analyzed. In total, 10,528 patients were represented by these trials. The investigators evaluated the relative performance characteristics of 4 imaging studies in the surveillance of patients with previously treated melanoma. Ultrasound was examined for detection of local and regional recurrence. For distant metastases, the study evaluated whole-body diagnostic CT (generally contrast-enhanced CT of the neck, chest, abdomen, and pelvis), PET, and PET/CT.

For detection of distant metastases, FDG-PET/CT was found to have the best performance, with a sensitivity of 86% and a specificity of 91%. The values for diagnostic CT were 63%

and 78%, respectively. Ultrasound performed best for detection of local recurrence and regional lymph node recurrence. The conclusion of the study was that PET/CT was superior for detection of distant metastases in both staging and surveillance.

In a separate meta-analysis, a study group in Belgium evaluated the role of FDG-PET/CT in the surveillance of melanoma patients for the development of pulmonary metastases.[23] The lung is a common site of metastatic disease from melanoma, and aggressive surgical approaches are pursued at many institutions based on an overall survival benefit. In patients with pulmonary metastatic disease, the 5-year survival is between 2% and 5%, whereas complete pulmonary metastasectomy can improve the 5-year survival to 21% to 39%. Patient selection is critical, however, to achieving a good outcome, and estimates are that only 10% to 35% of patients with pulmonary metastases would benefit from aggressive surgical intervention.

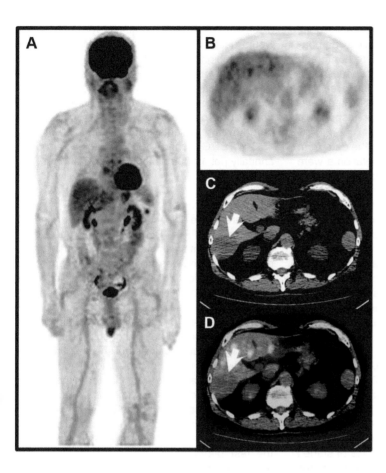

Fig. 8. Maximum intensity projection (*A*) and axial (*B-D*) images from an FDG-PET/CT scan in a 79-year-old man with previously treated melanoma. CT images show multiple large hepatic masses, including a 5-cm mass in the right lobe inferiorly (*arrow*). These masses have FDG uptake equivalent to normal liver but were proved on biopsy to be metastatic disease from melanoma.

In their study, the investigators reviewed published literature regarding surgical intervention of lung metastases and the use of imaging. They compared 2 strategies, defined as conventional imaging strategy (contrast-enhanced CT of the neck, chest, abdomen, and pelvis) and PET/CT strategy (whole-body FDG-PET/CT), and examined the estimated life-month gains (LMGs) and monetary costs for each. The results of their analysis showed that the conventional imaging strategy cost an average of €5022 for 86.08 LMGs whereas the PET/CT strategy cost an average of €3974 for 86.29 LMGs. Their conclusion was that the PET/CT strategy saved an average of €1048 for a small incremental benefit in LMGs. Importantly, by using the PET/CT strategy, up to 20% of surgeries could be avoided because they would be potentially futile for curative intent.

The role of FDG-PET/CT has been examined prospectively in specific clinical scenarios. In 1 such study,[24] 97 patients with in-transit or recurrent disease in a limb were enrolled in a multicenter prospective trial using isolated limb infusion (ILI) and screened for recurrence. The imaging strategy was to perform FDG-PET/CT at baseline, at 3-month intervals for the first year after treatment, and at 6-month intervals thereafter. As an imaging reference standard, CT and *Response Evaluation Criteria In Solid Tumors* guidelines were used.

The investigators found that for the assessment of residual tumor in the limbs treated with ILI, FDG-PET/CT was unable to reliably detect complete pathologic response. There was a high correlation of negative PET with complete response (CR), but 41% of patients with pathologic complete response (determined by biopsy) showed residual uptake in their tumors on PET. It did turn out, however, that this residual activity was a strong predictor of poor outcome, because the 3-year survival of patients with such residual FDG uptake was 29.4%, compared with a 3-year survival of 62.2% for those whose disease resolved completely on FDG-PET/CT. FDG-PET/CT was also useful for detection of distant metastatic disease outside the infused limb during the surveillance period, detecting disease in 52% of patients, approximately half of whom were judged candidates for surgical treatment of their metastatic disease.

Ultimately, the goal of any follow-up or surveillance strategy should be to improve patient outcome. Overall survival is a desirable goal, although this linkage is often difficult to demonstrate with imaging studies, which are not in and of themselves therapeutic. Other outcomes might be quality of life or disease-free survival, and certainly cost effectiveness and cost-benefit analyses are critical given the need for responsible use of health care dollars.

In a large single-institution study, the data from 1600 patients with stages I to III melanoma were used to develop models for melanoma natural history, including frequency of recurrence and surgical resectability of disease at the time of discovery.[25] The investigators then applied this model to a hypothetical group of 10,000 melanoma patients with stages I to III disease undergoing imaging surveillance with CT or FDG-PET/CT at 6-month and 12-month intervals. Results were parsed according to disease stage. As discussed previously, the driver of such surveillance imaging strategies is the data that indicate improvement in outcome when disease is detected early and can be treated aggressively.

In this model-based approach, FDG-PET/CT performed better than diagnostic CT for the detection of recurrence in all disease stages. As might be anticipated, the frequency of detection was related to disease stage. Using a 6-month surveillance interval, PET detected surgically treatable regional or distant recurrences in 6.4% of stage I patients. In patients with stage II disease, the detection rate increased to 18.5%, and for patients with stage III disease, the rate was 33.1%. When the surveillance interval was lengthened to every 12 months, fewer patients with surgically treatable disease were found, with rates of 3.0% for stage I, 7.9% for stage II, and 13.0% for stage III. Although both CT and PET/CT resulted in some false-positive studies, the frequency of this on PET was lower than on CT (9% vs 20%).

These data seem to support the use of surveillance imaging with FDG-PET/CT due to its ability to detect potentially curable recurrences and metastases at a rate higher than CT alone. Furthermore, patients imaged every 6 months were predicted to more often have surgically curable melanoma recurrence than when the surveillance interval was increased to 12 months.

In the final portion of their analysis, however, the investigators examined the overall survival of the patients. Despite the increased detection of surgically treatable recurrence or metastasis, the life expectancy gains for patients undergoing imaging surveillance were small, in the range of 2 months or less. Furthermore, when modeled to a population setting, the investigators estimated that to identify a single patient with potentially curable disease, 249 PET/CT scans or 362 CT scans would need to be performed on the population. Even for high-risk patients (stage IIIC), 26 PET/CT scans would need to be performed to detect a single treatable recurrence. Another way of expressing the impact of such a screening program is that to use a 12-month interval surveillance program for patients with stage I melanoma, 45,314 PET/CT scans would need to be performed annually per 10,000 patients with melanoma.

SUMMARY

There are ample data in the literature regarding the performance of FDG-PET and PET/CT in the evaluation of patients with cutaneous malignant melanoma. Melanoma was one of the earliest approved oncologic applications of FDG-PET imaging in the United States by CMS. It is well established that PET has good sensitivity and specificity values for the detection of disease in the staging and follow-up setting. The limitations of FDG-PET scanning are also well established, such as the insensitivity for small-volume regional nodal metastatic disease and the potential for false-positive scanning due to benign conditions.

What remains to be defined is what role FDG-PET/CT scanning is to play in the medical management of patients with melanoma. Although the test performance is good, there are costs associated with the imaging. Some of these costs are actual monetary costs (ie, the actual cost of the imaging test). Although traditionally considered an expensive imaging test, the costs to both the imaging facility and the health care system have declined. The widespread availability of FDG has brought down the per-dose cost of the radiopharmaceutical. Reimbursement for scans from payers has declined over time, and in many locations the charges for FDG-PET/CT approximate the summed charges for contrast-enhanced CT scans of the neck, chest, abdomen, and pelvis.

There are other less tangible costs of imaging, including PET/CT scanning. PET/CT makes use of ionizing radiation for both the PET portion of the study and the CT portion of the study. The dose delivered to the patient is lower than previously due to technical innovations, such as 3-D acquisition, time-of-flight PET, and CT dose reduction algorithms. Nevertheless, there is a radiation dose associated with the performance of PET/CT, carrying a theoretic risk to the patient.

So, too, there are risks associated with not imaging patients with cutaneous malignant melanoma. As put forward in the study by Rueth and colleagues[25], it is reasonable to conclude, based on tumor biology and imaging performance, that the avoidance of imaging surveillance (PET/CT or CT alone) would result in fewer opportunities to detect metastatic disease at a time when curative resection might be feasible. Even prolonging the surveillance interval from 6 months to 12 months was predicted to result in far fewer opportunities for surgical cure for patients. At the same time, however, their model did not substantiate a dramatic overall survival benefit as a result of imaging surveillance, and the anticipated costs to the health care system are high.

Given the somewhat conflicting conclusions of model-based studies and meta-analyses, what seems to be needed is an actual multicenter trial using variants of surveillance to truly determine the impact on both the patients and the health care system. Only with actual data can informed decisions be made on whether or not the inclusion of FDG-PET/CT has an impact on patient outcome and, if so, whether that change in outcome justifies the costs of such a surveillance program.

REFERENCES

1. American Cancer Society. Cancer facts & figures 2014. Atlanta (GA): American Cancer Society; 2014.
2. Curtin JA, Fridlyand J, Kageshita T, et al. Distinct sets of genetic alterations in melanoma. N Engl J Med 2005;353:2135–47.
3. Curtin JA, Busam K, Pinkel D, et al. Somatic activation of KIT in distinct subtypes of melanoma. J Clin Oncol 2006;24:4340–6.
4. Van Raamsdonk CD, Bezrookove V, Green G, et al. Frequent somatic mutations of GNAQ in uveal melanoma and blue naevi. Nature 2009;457:599–602.
5. Van Raamsdonk CD, Griewank KG, Crosby MB, et al. Mutations in GNA11 in uveal melanoma. N Engl J Med 2010;363:2191–9.
6. Wagner JD, Schauwecker D, Davidson D, et al. Prospective study of fluorodeoxyglucose-positron emission tomography imaging of lymph node basins in melanoma patients undergoing sentinel node biopsy. J Clin Oncol 1999;17(5):1508–15.
7. Mijnhout GS, Hoekstra OS, van Lingen A, et al. How morphometric analysis of metastatic load predicts the (un)usefulness of PET scanning: the case of lymph node staging in melanoma. J Clin Pathol 2003;56(4):283–6.
8. Xing Y, Bronstein Y, Ross MI, et al. Contemporary diagnostic imaging modalities for the staging and surveillance of melanoma patients: a meta-analysis. J Natl Cancer Inst 2011;103:129–42.
9. Ho Shon IA, Chung DK, Saw RP, et al. Imaging in cutaneous melanoma. Nucl Med Commun 2008; 10:847–76.
10. Bronstein Y, Ng CS, Rohren E, et al. PET/CT in the management of patients with stage IIIC and IV metastatic melanoma considered candidates for surgery: evaluation of the additive value after conventional imaging. AJR Am J Roentgenol 2012; 198:902–8.
11. Bastiaannet E, Wobbes T, Hoekstra OS, et al. Prospective comparison of [18F]fluorodeoxyglucose positron emission tomography and computed tomography in patients with melanoma with palpable lymph node metastases: diagnostic accuracy and impact on treatment. J Clin Oncol 2008;27:4774–80.
12. Zheng QY, Zhang GH, Zhang Y, et al. Adrenalectomy may increase survival of patients with adrenal metastases. Oncol Lett 2012;3:917–20.
13. Garbe C, Paul A, Kohler-Spath H, et al. Prospective evaluation of a follow-up schedule in cutaneous melanoma patients: recommendations for an effective follow-up strategy. J Clin Oncol 2003;21:520–9.
14. Benvenuto-Andrade C, Oseitutu A, Agero AL, et al. Cutaneous melanoma: surveillance of patients for recurrence and new primary melanomas. Dermatol Ther 2005;18:423–35.
15. Rhodes AR. Cutaneous melanoma and intervention strategies to reduce tumor-related mortality: what we know, what we don't know, and what we think we know that isn't so. Dermatol Ther 2006;19:50–69.
16. Petersen RP, Hanish SI, Haney JC, et al. Improved survival with pulmonary metastasectomy: an analysis of 1720 patients with pulmonary metastatic melanoma. J Thorac Cardiovasc Surg 2007;133:104–10.
17. Young SE, Martinez SR, Essner R. The role of surgery in treatment of stage IV melanoma. J Surg Oncol 2006;94:344–51.
18. Riker AI, Kirksey L, Thompson L, et al. Current surgical management of melanoma. Expert Rev Anticancer Ther 2006;6:1569–83.
19. Strobel K, Dummer R, Husarik DB, et al. High-risk melanoma: accuracy of FDG PET/CT with added CT morphologic information for detection of metastases. Radiology 2007;244:566–74.
20. Bastiaannet E, Hoekstra OS, de Jong JR, et al. Prognostic value of the standardized uptake value for (18)F-fluorodeoxyglucose in patients with stage IIIB melanoma. Eur J Nucl Med Mol Imaging 2012;39: 1592–8.
21. Balch CM, Soong SJ, Atkins MB, et al. An evidence-based staging system for cutaneous melanoma. CA Cancer J Clin 2004;54:131–49.
22. Lee ML, Tomsu K, Von Eschen KB. Duration of survival for disseminated malignant melanoma: results of a meta-analysis. Melanoma Res 2000;10:81–92.
23. Krug B, Crott R, Roch I, et al. Cost-effectiveness analysis of FDG PET-CT in the management of pulmonary metastases from malignant melanoma. Acta Oncol 2010;49:192–200.

24. Beasley GM, Parsons C, Broadwater G, et al. A multicenter prospective evaluation of the clinical utility of F-18 FDG-PET/CT in patients with AJCC stage IIIB or IIIC extremity melanoma. Ann Surg 2012;256:350–6.

25. Rueth NM, Xing Y, Chiang YJ, et al. Is surveillance imaging effective for detecting surgically treatable recurrences in patients with melanoma? A comparative analysis of stage-specific surveillance strategies. Ann Surg 2014;259:1215–22.

Prognostic Utility of PET in Prostate Cancer

Hossein Jadvar, MD, PhD, MPH, MBA

KEYWORDS

- Prostate • Cancer • PET • Imaging • Outcome

KEY POINTS

- Predictive tools are keys in clinical decision making and individualized management of patients with prostate cancer.
- Current nonimaging-based predictive tools may be limited in individual cases and need frequent updating.
- Novel platform of predictive tools that combine molecular, imaging, and clinical information are needed.

Prostate cancer is the second most common cancer and the sixth leading cause of cancer death in men worldwide, despite wide regional variation in incidence and mortality. This variation may be owing to the differences in biologic, socioeconomic, and diagnostic and therapeutic practices around the world.[1] In 2014, there is an estimated 233,000 new cases of prostate cancer representing 14% of all new cancer cases in the United States. The lifetime risk of prostate cancer developing in a man is approximately 15% (1 in 6). The estimated deaths from prostate cancer are 29,480, accounting for about 5% of all cancer deaths.[2] During 2004 to 2010, the percentages of cases by stage of disease at the time of initial presentation were 81% localized, 12% regional, 4% distant, and 3% unknown. The 5-year relative survival rate for the localized and regional stages is nearly 100%, but it decreases markedly to 28% in patients with metastatic disease.[2]

The natural history of disease is one of evolution from a clinically localized hormone-sensitive tumor to a castrate-resistant metastatic state.[3] Imaging plays an important current and emerging role in the evaluation of all the various clinical phases of this prevalent disease.[4–7] Transrectal ultrasound scan (which may include 3-dimensional, Doppler, use of contrast microbubbles, and shear wave sonoelastography techniques) is performed for guiding biopsy in men suspected of harboring prostate cancer, typically prompted by an elevated serum prostate-specific antigen (PSA) level or an abnormal digital rectal examination.[8–11] However such an approach in the post-PSA era has been associated with overdiagnosis of clinically insignificant tumors and overtreatment of these indolent tumors with its associated cost and morbidity.[12] Conversely, occasionally higher-grade tumors are missed on biopsy; therefore, an opportunity for delivering appropriate therapy may be lost. MR imaging with higher field strength, specialized coils, and multiparametric techniques (diffusion-weighted imaging, dynamic contrast imaging, elastography, spectroscopy) have also played an important role in the imaging evaluation of prostate cancer, which is anticipated to grow.[13–20] MR imaging may be useful in localization of lesions amenable to targeted biopsy (in addition to standard sites for biopsy) and for lesion characterization.[21] Real-time fusion of ultrasound

The author has nothing to disclose.
This work was supported by National Cancer Institute, National Institutes of Health, grants R01-CA111613, R21-CA142426, P30-CA014089.
Department of Radiology, Keck School of Medicine of USC, University of Southern California, 2250 Alcazar Street, CSC 102, Los Angeles, CA 90033, USA
E-mail address: jadvar@med.usc.edu

and MR images at the time of biopsy has been shown and may prove to be helpful in reducing the relatively high sampling error that is often associated with standard transrectal ultrasound–guided biopsy procedure.[22–25] Direct MR-guided biopsy procedures are also found to be feasible, although the technique is currently only performed at few specialized centers.[26–28]

When a diagnosis of prostate cancer is established, it is important to stage the disease accurately so that appropriate treatment can be delivered. In localized disease, the treatment with curative intent includes prostatectomy with pelvic lymph node dissection or radiation therapy. In some patients, active surveillance may also be a viable strategy. Unfortunately, up to 35% of patients (or higher in select high-risk groups) may experience biochemical recurrence (PSA relapse) within a decade of primary therapy. Stratification of patients with biochemical recurrence is crucial for prescribing and sequencing appropriate treatments. Such therapies may include salvage therapy (surgery or radiation) for local recurrence and systemic therapy for metastatic disease. When disease develops into a castrate-resistant state (defined as disease progression despite androgen deprivation), the prognosis is poor, and treatment is directed toward enhancing overall survival and comfort.[29–31]

Great recent strides have been made in treatment of metastatic castration-resistant prostate cancer and have been fueled by improved understanding the biology of the disease.[32,33] The US Food and Drug Administration has approved these treatments since the initial approval of docetaxel in 2004 based on the results of TAX-327 and SWOG 9916 clinical trials showing overall survival benefit.[34,35] The recently US Food and Drug Administration—approved agents include (1) cabazitaxel (Jevtana; Sanofi-Aventis, Paris, France), approved in 2010 as a second-line taxane therapy in patents who have not responded to docetaxel therapy (Treatment of Hormone-Refractory Metastatic Prostate Cancer Previously Treated with a Taxane-Containing Regimen [TROPIC]); (2) vaccine therapy with sipuleucel-T (Provenge; Dendreon, Seattle, WA), approved in 2010 for the treatment of asymptomatic or minimally symptomatic metastatic castration-resistant prostate cancer based on Immunotherapy for Prostate AdenoCarcinoma Treatment (IMPACT) trial; (3) the androgen synthesis inhibitor abiraterone acetate (Zytiga; Janssen Biotech, Horsham, PA), approved in 2011 for use in metastatic castration-resistant prostate cancer after docetaxel failure based on the COU-AA-301 trial; (4) androgen receptor blockade with enzalutamide (Xtandi; Medivation,

Inc [San Francisco, CA] and Astellas Pharma USA, Inc [Northbrook, IL]), approved in 2012 for treatment of patients with metastatic castration-resistant prostate cancer who were previously treated with docetaxel based on the clinical trial AFFIRM; and (5) radium-223 dichloride (Xofigo; Bayer Healthcare, Whippany, NJ) based on the Alpharadin in Symptomatic Prostate Cancer (AL-SYMPCA) clinical trial.[36–41]

Given the public health significance of prostate cancer and the ongoing accelerated targeted therapies, noninvasive imaging-based assessment of appropriateness for particular targeted treatments in individual patients and accurate predation of various relevant outcomes is considered clinically urgent.

OUTCOME MEASURES

Because prostate cancer is a remarkably heterogeneous disease, a personalized approach to patient care is most desired.[42] However, such approach will require identification of a combination of surrogate markers of disease that can portray the disease activity accurately before, during, and after biologically and clinically tailored treatment. To achieve this worthy goal, relevant endpoints will be needed to design and conduct trials for drug development that can have the most beneficial impact on a selected patient outcome at a minimal toxicity level. Such an approach may become reality as further understanding of the complex underlying biology of prostate cancer develops.

There is a plethora of outcome measures that can be selected for conducting clinical trials and ultimately for clinical decision making to select and sequence the most optimal management strategy to improve the selected outcome.[43] In the clinical setting of prostate cancer, these outcome measures include, but are not limited to, time to biochemical recurrence (time to PSA progression), time to first metastasis, time to symptomatic progression, time to initiation of cytotoxic chemotherapy, time to radiographic progression, time to castrate resistance state, progression-free survival (PFS), metastasis-free survival, disease-specific survival, and overall survival.

Even when a specific outcome measure is selected, there can be variability in interstudy design that makes comparison between the results of trials challenging. Gignac and colleagues[44] quantified the variability and the resultant error among phase II clinical trials of cystotoxic agents in metastatic castrate-resistant prostate cancer that used PFS as the outcome measure. There was heterogeneity in trial inclusion criteria and the type, timing, and frequency of disease assessment. In a simulation model, the investigators determined that there could be a significant difference between the trial detected and the true PFS that was directly related to variability in assessment schedules despite published standardization guidelines.[45] Such variability hinders effective comparison of reported outcomes among clinical trials and the comparative effectiveness of drug development process.

CURRENT PREDICTIVE TOOLS

Predictive tools help with the decision-making process for the clinician and the patients given the complex biology and clinical course of prostate cancer and the ever-changing landscape of treatment options at every phase of the natural history of the disease. The predictive tools include nomograms, propensity risk tables, artificial neural networks, and other methods.[45–49] Deciphering the exact utility of these tools may seem daunting for both the treating physician and the patient.

Nomogram is a graphic diagram that uses various clinical parameters to allow prediction of an outcome that can be useful for clinical management decisions. Many such nomograms exist in public domain for several cancers, including prostate cancer (http://www.nomogram.org/). Ross and colleagues[50] cataloged and evaluated the many nomograms that have been published between January 1966 and February 2000. The search produced 42 published nomograms that could be applied to various clinical phases of prostate cancer. It was interesting to note that only 18 (43%) of the nomograms had undergone validation and none had been compared with clinical judgment alone. In another study, the same group of investigators compared predictions of clinicians with prostate cancer nomograms.[50] They found that although nomograms did not generally extend clinician prediction accuracy (average doctor excess error, 1.4%; $P = .75$), nomograms could be beneficial in certain clinical decision-making situations.

Partin and colleagues[51,52] established the predictive nomogram tool in prostate cancer, which was updated in 2007 from its earlier versions in 2001 and 1997.[53,54] Partin tables use preoperative Gleason grade (which may differ from Gleason score of the surgical specimen), serum PSA level, and clinical stage to predict outcome after radical prostatectomy. Despite the updated versions, which included a multi-institutional dataset and accounted for the downward stage and Gleason score migration induced by PSA screening, the advantage of the newer versions over the initial version

of 1997 could not be shown.[55] This notion suggests that extensive validation may be needed before one predictive tool is hastily adopted over others. Others have argued that the nomograms may not be generalizable to all patients.[56,57] A group of investigators used the information from 44 published prostate cancer prediction tools to devise a "cancer metagram," which incorporated 16 treatment options and 10 outcomes (cancer control, morbidity, and survival). Despite limitations of noninclusion of all available treatment options and relevant outcomes, the authors contended that the metagram could provide easily understandable evidence-based and patient-specific outcome predictability for clinically localized prostate cancer.[58]

Shariat and colleagues[59] present an excellent critical review, including a comprehensive bibliography, of the prostate cancer predictive tools. They submit that prediction tools are generally more accurate at predicting risk than those assessed by the clinicians, who may be influenced by personal experiences or preferences in a setting of lack of consensus and conflicting or inconclusive data. They also list several criteria to evaluate these relatively numerous predictive tools. These criteria include discrimination (ability of the predictive tool to discriminate between patients with or without the outcome of interest), calibration (accuracy of prediction for the individual patient), generalizability (ability of the predictive tool for a specific outcome in setting of differing patient characteristics), level of complexity (too-complex tools may be of little utility in busy clinical practices), adjustment for competing risks (taking into account competing causes of morbidity and mortality), conditional probabilities (time-variability of individual patient's outcome), and head-to-head comparison (advantage of one predictive tool over another). The authors tabulate several prediction tools for prediction of prostate cancer on initial and repeat biopsy, prediction of pathologic state, prediction of biochemical recurrence before and after radical prostatectomy, prediction of biochemical recurrence after external beam radiation therapy or brachytherapy, prediction of metastatic progression, and prediction of survival and life expectancy. These investigators suggest that computational decision tool analysis may be helpful to compare the expected clinical consequences of various predictive tools in lieu of comparative randomized clinical trials, which are challenging to perform given the high cost, delay in attaining conclusive results, and practical limitations imposed by statistical power. They also submit rightfully that in this perplexing situation, incorporation of the newly emerging biomarkers, including imaging results, can add significant direct information about the tumor, which can then enhance the model's predictive power in comparison to the traditional use of clinical and pathologic parameters.

IMAGING AS A PROGNOSTIC TOOL

Imaging plays an important current and expanding role in the imaging evaluation of every phase of the natural history of prostate cancer.[60] Given the limitations of the current prediction tools, newer biomarkers, including circulating tumor cells, patient-reported outcomes, and imaging are of much interest for monitoring of clinical outcomes in specific groups of patients with prostate cancer.[61] Overall, relatively few studies have investigated the impact of imaging on patient outcome. This is partly because of the challenges that are associated with directly linking the results of an imaging study to an outcome given that many intervening events often occur that can also affect the outcome.

Bone scintigraphy has been a mainstay imaging in prostate cancer.[62] Bone scintigraphy has been demonstrated that a negative bone scan is associated with longer time to biochemical relapse.[63] Conversely, pretreatment percentage of the positive area on a bone scan may be an independent predictor of the disease death (relative risk ratio, 2.603; $P = .0155$).[64] Bone scintigraphy is typically analyzed visually. Computer-assisted quantitative assessment (bone scan index) has been attempted, which can diminish interobserver variability and aid with more robust longitudinal comparative studies.[65,66] Bone scan index captures the burden of osseous metastatic disease that has been shown to relate to outcome. Tait and colleagues[67] quantified the bone scan by simply counting the bone metastases in 561 men with metastatic castrate-resistant prostate cancer and correlating clinical outcome to thresholds of 1 to 4, 5 to 20 and greater than 20 detectable bone lesions. Patients with higher numbers of bone metastases had shorter PFS and overall survival. In fact, simply dichotomizing patients into groups with 1 to 4 (oligometastatic) and greater than 5 skeletal metastases provided significant prognostic information. In another similar study, a doubling of bone scan index was associated with a 1.9-fold increase in risk of death.[68]

PET is a sensitive quantitative molecular imaging tool for interrogation of the underlying tumor biology. Many radiotracers have been or are currently being investigated for imaging evaluation of prostate cancer with PET including, but not limited to, 18F-fluorodeoxyglucose (18F-FDG), 18F- and 11C-choline; 11C-acetate, 18F sodium fluoride, 16a-18F-fluoro-5a-dihydrotestosterone (18F-FDHT, targeted to the androgen receptor), anti-1-amino-3-18F-fluorocyclobutane-1-carboxylic acid (18F-FACBC, a synthetic L-leucine analog), and radiotracers targeted to the prostate-specific membrane antigen, prostate stem cell antigen, and gastrin-releasing peptide receptor.[69–71] Almost all the studies to date have focused on diagnostic (detection) utility of these radiotracers (ie, accumulation in tumor deposits and little or nonaccumulation in nontumor sites) either in comparison with defined reference standards or with other radiotracers. This focus is reasonable, as a potentially useful radiotracer needs first to be examined with regard to its biodistribution, in vivo stability, pharmacokinetics and pharmacodynamics, and ultimately its competitive advantage over other rival conventional and new PET and non-PET radiotracers and other imaging methods. Here we review the few published studies on the 2 major PET radiotracers (ie, FDG and 18F- or 11C-choline) that have reported specifically on the potential prognostic utility of these PET radiotracers in prostate cancer.

Few studies have examined the potential prognostic role of FDG PET/computed tomography (CT) in prostate cancer. Oyama and colleagues[72] from Japan investigated the prognostic value of glucose metabolism of the primary tumors in 42 patients with prostate cancer. The standardized uptake value (SUV) of the tumor was correlated to relapse-free survival after radical prostatectomy. Patients with tumors that displayed higher SUVs had a significantly poorer prognosis compared with those patients with tumors that showed lower SUVs. Despite this interesting result, FDG PET/CT is not expected to play a major role in the diagnosis and staging of primary prostate cancer in view of significant overlap that may occur among normal, benign, and malignant tissues. The researchers from the Memorial Sloan Kettering Cancer Center in New York tested the hypothesis that serial FDG PET (baseline and at 4 weeks and 12 weeks after chemotherapy) was useful as an outcome measure in men with metastatic castrate-resistant prostate cancer.[73] The maximum standardized uptake values of up to 5 lesions were averaged (SUVmaxavg). Changes in this imaging parameter were then correlated to changes in the serum PSA with greater than 25% PSA increase considered as progression (based on PSA Working Group Consensus Criteria Guideline). The authors noted that a greater than 33% increase in SUVmaxavg or the appearance of new lesions dichotomized patients as progressors and nonprogressors. In another report from the same group of investigators, the maximum SUV of the most active lesion in 43 patients with metastatic castrate-resistant prostate cancer was correlated with overall survival.[74] A maximum SUV threshold of 6.1 provided discriminatory information on prognosis with median survival of 14.4 months if maximum SUV was greater than 6.1 and 32.8 months if maximum SUV was $\leq$6.1 (P = .002). Jadvar and colleagues[75] from the University of Southern California in Los Angeles reported on a larger cohort of 87 patients with metastatic castrate-resistant prostate cancer who underwent FDG PET/CT and were followed up with prospectively for overall survival. PET parameters that were examined included not only the most metabolically active lesion, but also sum and average of up to 25 active lesions (including lymph nodes, bone, and soft tissue metastases). Comparison of overall survival was based on univariate and multivariate Cox regression analyses of continuous PET parameters adjusted for relevant standard clinical parameters including age, serum PSA level, serum alkaline phosphatase level, use of pain medication, prior chemotherapy, and Gleason score at initial diagnosis. The univariate analysis showed statistically significant hazard ratios of 1.01 (95% confidence interval [CI], 1.006–1.020; P = .002) for the sum of the maximum SUV of lesions and 1.11 (95% CI, 1.030–1.180; P = .010) for the most active lesion. However, in the multivariate analysis that adjusted for the potentially prognostic clinical parameters, only the sum of the maximum SUV remained significant with a hazard ratio of 1.01 (95% CI, 1.001–1.020; P = .053). Further grouping of this parameter into quartiles showed that the patients in the fourth quartile range had a significantly poorer survival than those patients in the

first quartile range with a univariate hazard ratio of 3.8 (95% CI, 1.80–7.90; **Figs. 1** and **2**). This and prior few studies suggest that there is indeed significant unique information provided by FDG PET/CT on the metabolic burden of disease that may be predictive of prognosis in men with metastatic castrate-resistant prostate cancer. This is an important notion that may be helpful in the objective assessment of the comparative effectiveness of various conventional and rapidly emerging treatments in this important clinical setting.

Systematic reviews with meta-analysis have summarized the diagnostic utility of 11C-choline or 18F-fluorocholine choline PET/CT in prostate cancer.[76–78] Despite the general notion of most utility of radiolabeled choline in disease restaging in patients with biochemical relapse after local primary treatment for prostate cancer, many analytical limitations have been identified that may hinder general applicability and will need attention in future investigations.[79–81]

A study reported on the comparative utility of 11C-choline PET/CT over clinical staging nomograms for preoperative staging of lymph nodes in intermediate-risk and high-risk prostate cancer.[82] The authors found that although in this clinical setting, 11C-choline PET/CT showed low sensitivity of 60% (at a specificity of 98%) for detection of lymph node metastases, but it performed better than clinical nomograms with equal sensitivity and better specificity.

PET with 18F-fluorocholine may have a role in predicting early progression in men with biochemical recurrence after primary treatment with curative intent. Gacci and colleagues[83] performed a longitudinal study of 103 consecutive patents who had 2 PET/CT scans, one at baseline and one after 6 months from the baseline scan. The

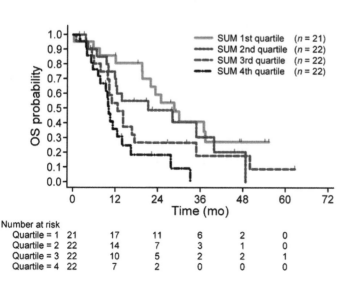

Number at risk

Quartile = 1	21	17	11	6	2	0
Quartile = 2	22	14	7	3	1	0
Quartile = 3	22	10	5	2	2	1
Quartile = 4	22	7	2	0	0	0

Fig. 1. Kaplan–Meier plot of overall survival (OS) probability against sum of SUVmax (SUM) grouped into quartiles. Patients in fourth-quartile group (*blue line*) have significantly poorer survival probability than reference first-quartile group (*green line*). SUM ranges: first-quartile, 0–4.6; second-quartile, 4.7–13.9; third-quartile, 14–28.6; fourth-quartile, 28.7–217.5. (*From* Jadvar H, Desai B, Ji L, et al. Baseline 18F-FDG PET/CT parameters as imaging biomarkers of overall survival in castrate-resistant metastatic prostate cancer. J Nucl Med 2013;54:1195–201; with permission.)

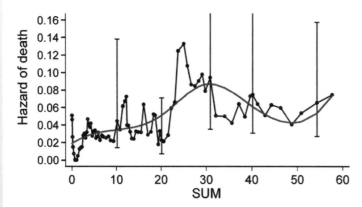

Fig. 2. Moving hazards of death (*blue line*) in relation to sum of SUVmax (SUM) interpreted as chance of death per person per month; cubic spline smoothed line (*red line*) is superimposed. There is upward shift of curve for SUM greater than 20. (*From* Jadvar H, Desai B, Ji L, et al. Baseline 18F-FDG PET/CT parameters as imaging biomarkers of overall survival in castrate-resistant metastatic prostate cancer. J Nucl Med 2013;54:1195–201; with permission.)

authors found that increase in serum PSA from baseline by greater than 5 ng/mL, decrease in PSA doubling time by less than 6 months, and increase in PSA velocity by greater than 6 ng/mL/mo were highly associated with the outcome of progression on the follow-up PET/CT. Studies have also reported on the use of 11C-choline PET/CT on the prediction of outcome after salvage radiation therapy after radical prostatectomy.[84] It is interesting that although initial tumor stage, risk profile, and serum PSA level before salvage radiation therapy were not different between responders and nonresponders, a positive 11C-choline was able to predict the treatment failure cases. However, other studies have found that the lower the serum PSA level at the beginning of salvage radiation therapy, the better the outcome after treatment and that the higher radiation doses are associated with greater PSA relapse-free rates.[85]

Breeuwsma and colleagues[86] correlated the findings on 11C-choline PET/CT with disease-specific survival in 64 men with biochemical recurrence after radical prostatectomy. The median serum PSA level was 1.4 ng/mL, and the median follow-up was 50 months. The investigators found that disease-specific survival was significantly higher in the negative PET/CT group than the group with positive PET/CT. In another similar but more comprehensive study, the Italian investigators evaluated retrospectively the potential utility of 11C-choline PET/CT in prediction of prostate cancer–specific survival in 195 patients who presented with biochemical failure (PSA >0.2 mg/mL during androgen deprivation therapy) after radical prostatectomy.[87] The median interval after radical prostatectomy and median follow-up after 11C-choline PET/CT were 8.9 years and 4.5 years, respectively. The median prostate cancer–specific survival in patients with positive and negative 11C-choline PET/CT was 11.2 years and 16.4 years,

respectively. Moreover, patients with positive prostatic bed or pelvic/retroperitoneal lymph nodes had longer median prostate cancer–specific survival of 12.1 years compared with patients with bone metastases who had a shorter median prostate cancer–specific survival of 9.9 years. Nomograms were constructed using age, serum PSA level, initial Gleason score, pathologic stage, additional therapy, and results of 11C-choline PET/CT for prediction of prostate cancer–specific survival at 5, 10, and 15 years after radical prostatectomy. The longer-term prediction at 15 years tended to overestimate the survival compared with the shorter-term predictions at 5 and 10 years.

Kwee and colleagues[88] from Hawaii investigated the prognostic significance of metabolically active tumor volume (MATV) as measured from 18F-fluorocholine PET/CT in 30 men with castrate-resistant prostate cancer. The MATV was calculated using a vendor-supplied algorithm that determined the SUVmax and volume (defined as region encompassing 40% of the SUVmax) of the lesions, multiplied the SUVmax of each lesion by the lesion volume and summed over all detected lesions, and then termed *net MATV*. A measure of activity distribution within the lesion volume, termed *total lesion activity* (TLA) was also obtained by multiplying the lesion mean SUV and MATV, then summed over all lesions and termed *net TLA*. The authors found that both net MATV and net TLA were significantly associated with overall survival, suggesting that PET-based assessment of metastatic burden provides important prognostic information.

SUMMARY

Predictive tools are keys in clinical decision making and individualized management of patients with prostate cancer. This report outlined the utility and limitations of the current non–imaging-based prognostic tools and then presented the published reports on the potential use of incorporating quantitative imaging data, particularly PET, in this important clinical arena.

REFERENCES

1. Center MM, Jemal A, Lortet-Tieulent J, et al. International variation in prostate cancer incidence and mortality rates. Eur Urol 2012;61:1079–92.
2. Surveillance, epidemiology, and end results program. National Cancer Institute. Available at: http://seer.cancer.gov/statfacts/html/prost.html. Accessed August 1, 2014.
3. Small EJ. Prostate cancer, incidence, management and outcomes. Drugs Aging 1998;13:71–81.
4. Outwater EK, Montilla-Soler JL. Imaging of prostate cancer. Cancer Control 2013;20:161–76.
5. Tabatabaei S, Saylor PJ, Coen J, et al. Prostate cancer imaging: what surgeons, radiation oncologists, and medical oncologists want to know. AJR Am J Roentgenol 2011;196:1263–6.
6. Lecouvert FE, Lhommel R, Pasoglou V, et al. Novel imaging techniques reshape the landscape in high-risk prostate cancers. Curr Opin Urol 2013;23:323–30.
7. Fox JJ, Shoder H, Larson SM. Molecular imaging of prostate cancer. Curr Opin Urol 2012;22:320–7.
8. Boczko J, Messing E, Dogra V. Transrectal sonography in prostate cancer. Radiol Clin North Am 2006; 44:679–87.
9. Good DW, Stewart GD, Hammer S, et al. Elasticity as a biomarker for prostate cancer: a systematic review. BJU Int 2014;113:523–34.
10. Smeenge M, de la Rosette JJ, Wijkstra H. Current status of transrectal ultrasound techniques in prostate cancer. Curr Opin Urol 2012;22:297–302.
11. Kundavaram CR, Halpern EJ, Trabulsi EJ. Value of contrast-enhanced ultrasonography in prostate cancer. Curr Opin Urol 2012;22:303–9.
12. Klotz L. Prostate cancer overdiagnosis and overtreatment. Curr Opin Endocrinol Diabetes Obes 2013;20:204–9.
13. Kirkham AP, Haslam P, Keanie JY, et al. Prostate MRI: who, when, and how? Report from a UK consensus meeting. Clin Radiol 2013;68:1016–23.
14. Sciarra A, Barentsz J, Bjartell A, et al. Advances in magnetic resonance imaging: how they are changing the management of prostate cancer. Eur Urol 2011;59:962–77.
15. Coakley FV, Qayyum A, Kurhanewicz J. Magnetic resonance imaging and spectroscopic imaging of prostate cancer. J Urol 2003;170(6 Pt 2):S69–75.
16. Yacoub JH, Oto A, Miller FH. MR imaging of the prostate. Radiol Clin North Am 2014;52:811–37.
17. Neto JA, Parente DR. Multiparametric magnetic resonance imaging of the prostate. Magn Reson Imaging Clin N Am 2013;21:409–26.
18. Hoeks CM, Barentsz JO, Hambrock T, et al. Prostate cancer: multiparametric MR imaging for detection, localization, and staging. Radiology 2011;261:46–66.
19. Dickinson L, Ahmed HU, Allen C, et al. Magnetic resonance imaging for the detection, localization, and characterization of prostate cancer: recommendations from a European consensus meeting. Eur Urol 2011;59:477–94.
20. Murphy G, Haider M, Ghai S, et al. The expanding role of MRI in prostate cancer. AJR Am J Roentgenol 2013;201:1229–38.
21. Turkbey B, Mena E, Aras O, et al. Functional and molecular imaging: applications for diagnosis and staging of localized prostate cancer. Clin Oncol (R Coll Radiol) 2013;25:451–60.
22. Ukimura O, Hirahara N, Fujihara A, et al. Technique for a hybrid system of real-time transrectal ultrasound with preoperative magnetic resonance imaging in the guidance of targeted prostate biopsy. Int J Urol 2010;17:890–3.
23. Ukimura O, Faber K, Gill IS. Intraprostatic targeting. Curr Opin Urol 2012;22:97–103.
24. Marks L, Young S, Natarjan S. MRI-ultrasound fusion for guidance of targeted prostate biopsy. Curr Opin Urol 2013;23:43–50.
25. Cornud F, Brolis L, Delongchamps NB, et al. TRUS-MRI image registration: a paradigm shift in the diagnosis of significant prostate cancer. Abdom Imaging 2013;38:1447–63.
26. Robertson NL, Emberton M, Moore CM. MRI-targeted prostate biopsy: a review of technique and results. Nat Rev Urol 2013;10:589–97.
27. Verma S, Bhavsar AS, Donovan J. MR imaging-guided prostate biopsy. Magn Reson Imaging Clin N Am 2014;22:135–44.
28. Futterer JJ, Barentsz JO. MRI-guided and robotic-assisted prostate biopsy. Curr Opin Urol 2012;22: 316–9.
29. Scher HI, Sawyers CL. Biology of progressive, castration-resistant prostate cancer: directed therapies targeting the androgen-receptor signaling axis. J Clin Oncol 2005;23:8253–61.
30. Petrylak DP. Current state of castration-resistant prostate cancer. Am J Manag Care 2013;19:S358–65.
31. Petrylak DP. Challenges in treating advanced disease. Am J Manag Care 2013;1:S366–75.
32. El-Amm J, Aragon-Ching JB. The changing landscape in the treatment of metastatic castration-resistant prostate cancer. Ther Adv Med Oncol 2013;5:25–40.
33. Gomella LG, Petrylak DP, Shayegan B. Current management of advanced and castration resistant prostate cancer. Can J Urol 2014;21(2 Suppl 1):1–6.
34. Petrylak D, Tangen C, Hussein M, et al. Docetaxel and estramustine compared with minxantrone and prednisone for advancer refractory prostate cancer. N Engl J Med 2004;351:1513–20.

35. Tannock L, de Wit R, Bery W, et al. Docetaxel plus prednision or mitxantrone plus prednisone for advance prostate cancer. N Engl J Med 2004;351:1502–12.

36. Kluetz PG, Ning YM, Maher VE, et al. Abiraterone acetate in combination with prednisone for the treatment of patients with metastatic castration-resistant prostate cancer: US Food and Drug Administration drug approval summary. Clin Cancer Res 2013;19: 6650–6.

37. de Bono J, Logothetis C, Molina A, et al. Abiraterone and increased survival in metastatic prostate cancer. N Engl J Med 2011;364:1995–2005.

38. de Bono J, Oudard S, Ozguroglu M, et al. Prednisone plus cabazitaxel or mixantrone for metastatic castration-resistant prostate cancer progressing after docetaxel treatment: a randomized open-label trial. Lancet 2010;376:1147–54.

39. Higano C, Schelhammer P, Small E, et al. Integrated data from 2 randomized, double-blind, placebo-controlled, phase 3 trials of active cellular immunotherapy with sipuleucel-T in advanced prostate cancer. Cancer 2009;115:3670–9.

40. Sternberg CN, de Bono JS, Chi KN, et al. Improved outcomes in elderly patients with metastatic castration-resistant prostate cancer treated with the androgen receptor inhibitor enzalutamide: results from the phase III AFFIRM trial. Ann Oncol 2014;25: 429–34.

41. Parker C, Nilsson S, Heinrich D, et al. Alpha emitter radium-223 and survival in metastatic prostate cancer. N Engl J Med 2013;369:213–23.

42. Armstrong AJ, Febbo PG. Using surrogate biomarkers to predict clinical benefit in men with castration-resistant prostate cancer: an update and review of the literature. Oncologist 2009;14:816–27.

43. Scher HI, Morris MJ, Basch E, et al. End points and outcomes in castrate-resistant prostate cancer: from clinical trials to clinical practice. J Clin Oncol 2011; 29:3695–704.

44. Gignac GA, Morris M, Heller G, et al. Assessing outcomes in prostate cancer clinical trials: a 21st century tower of babel. Cancer 2008;113:966–74.

45. Scher HI, Halabi S, Tannock I, et al. The Prostate Cancer Clinical Trials Working Group (PCCTWG) consensus criteria for phase II clinical trials for castration-resistant prostate cancer. J Clin Oncol 2007;25(18 Suppl):249s. ASCO Annual Meeting Proceedings. [abstract: 5057].

46. Donovan MJ, Costa J, Cordon-Carbo C. Personalized approach to prostate cancer prognosis. Arch Esp Urol 2011;64:783–91.

47. Shariat SF, Karakiewicz PI, Margulis V, et al. Inventory of prostate cancer predictive tools. Curr Opin Urol 2008;18:279–96.

48. Kattan MW, Scardino PT. Prediction of progression: nomograms of clinical utility. Clin Prostate Cancer 2002;1:90–6.

49. Matzkin H, Perito PE, Soloway MS. Prognostic factors in metastatic prostate cancer. Cancer 1993; 72(12 Suppl):3788–92.

50. Ross PL, Scardino PT, Kattan MW. A catalog of prostate cancer nomograms. J Urol 2001;165:1562–8.

51. Partin AW, Kattan MW, Subong EN, et al. Combination of prostate-specific antigen, clinical stage, and Gleason score to predict pathological stage of localized prostate cancer. A multi-institutional update. JAMA 1997;277:1445–51.

52. Partin AW, Mangold LA, I amm DM, et al. Contemporary update of prostate cancer staging nomograms (Partin Tables) for the new millennium. Urology 2001;58:843–8.

53. Ross PL, Gerigk C, Gonen M, et al. Comparisons of nomograms and urologists' predictions in prostate cancer. Semin Urol Oncol 2002;20:82–8.

54. Makarov DV, Trock BJ, Humphreys EB, et al. Updated nomogram to predict pathologic stage of prostate cancer given prostate-specific antigen level, clinical stage, and biopsy Gleason score (Partin tables) based on cases from 2000 to 2005. Urology 2007; 69:1095–101.

55. Augustin H, Isbarn H, Auprich M, et al. Head to head comparison of three generations of Partin tables to predict final pathological stage in clinically localized prostate cancer. Eur J Cancer 2010;46:2235–41.

56. Nguyen CT, Kattan MW. Development of a prostate cancer metagram. A solution to the dilemma of which prediction tool to use in patient counseling. Cancer 2009;115(13 Suppl):3039–45.

57. Turo R, Forster JA, West RM, et al. Do prostate cancer nomograms give accurate information when applied to European patients? Scand J Urol 2015; 49:16–24.

58. Penson DF, Grossfeld GD, Li YP, et al. How well does the Partin nomogram predict pathological stage after radical prostatectomy in a community based population? Results of the cancer of the prostate strategic urological research endeavor. J Urol 2002;167:1653–7 [discussion: 1657–8].

59. Shariat SF, Kattan MW, Vickers AJ, et al. Critical review of prostate cancer predictive tools. Future Oncol 2009;5:1555–84.

60. Akin O, Hricak H. Imaging of prostate cancer. Radiol Clin North Am 2007;45:207–22.

61. Morris MJ, Autio KA, Basch EM, et al. Monitoring the clinical outcomes in advanced prostate cancer: what imaging modalities and other markers are reliable? Semin Oncol 2013;40:375–92.

62. Dotan ZA. Bone imaging in prostate cancer. Nat Clin Pract Urol 2008;5:434–44.

63. Hori S, Jabbar T, Kachroo N, et al. Outcomes and predictive factors for biochemical relapse following primary androgen deprivation therapy in men with bone scan negative prostate cancer. J Cancer Res Clin Oncol 2011;137:235–41.

64. Noguchi M, Kikuchi H, Ischibashi M, et al. Percentage of the positive are of bone metastasis in an independent predictor of disease death in advanced prostate cancer. Br J Cancer 2003;88:195–201.

65. Ulmert D, Kaboteh R, Fox JJ, et al. A novel automated platform for quantifying the extent of skeletal tumor involvement in prostate cancer patients using the bone scan index. Eur Urol 2012;62:78–84.

66. Brown MS, Chu GH, Kim HJ, et al. Computer-aided quantitative bone scan assessment of prostate cancer treatment response. Nucl Med Commun 2012; 33:384–94.

67. Tait C, Moore D, Hodgson C, et al. Quantification of skeletal metastases in castrate-resistant prostate cancer predicts progression-free and overall survival. BJU Int 2014;114:E70–3.

68. Dennis ER, Jia X, Mezheritskiy IS, et al. Bone scan index: a quantitative treatment response biomarker for castration-resistant metastatic prostate cancer. J Clin Oncol 2012;30:519–24.

69. Jadvar H. Molecular imaging of prostate cancer with PET. J Nucl Med 2013;54:1685–8.

70. Mohsen B, Giorgio T, Rassoul ZS, et al. Application of C-11 acetate positron-emission tomography (PET) imaging in prostate cancer: systematic review and meta-analysis of the literature. BJU Int 2013;112: 1062–72.

71. Picchio M, Giovannini E, Messa C. The role of PET/computed tomography scan in the management of prostate cancer. Curr Opin Urol 2011;21:230–6.

72. Oyama N, Akino H, Suzuki Y, et al. Prognostic value of 2-deoxy-2-[F-18]fluoro-D-glucose positron emission tomography imaging for patients with prostate cancer. Mol Imaging Biol 2002;4:99–104.

73. Morris MJ, Akhurst T, Larson SM, et al. Fluorodeoxyglucose positron emission tomography as an outcome measure for castrate metastatic prostate cancer treated with antimicrotubule chemotherapy. Clin Cancer Res 2005;11:3210–6.

74. Meirelles GS, Schoder H, Ravizzini GC, et al. Prognostic value of baseline [18F]fluorodeoxyglucose positron emission tomography and 99mTc-MDP bone scan in progressing metastatic prostate cancer. Clin Cancer Res 2010;16:6093–6.

75. Jadvar H, Desai B, Ji L, et al. Baseline 18F-FDG PET/CT parameters as imaging biomarkers of overall survival in castrate-resistant metastatic prostate cancer. J Nucl Med 2013;54:1195–201.

76. Umbehr MH, Muntener M, Hany T, et al. The role of 11C-choline and 18F-fluorocholine positron emission tomography (PET) and PET/CT in prostate cancer: a systematic review and meta-analysis. Eur Urol 2013;64:106–17.

77. Bauman G, Belhocine T, Kovacs M, et al. 18F-fluorocholine for prostate cancer imaging: a systematic review of the literature. Prostate Cancer Prostatic Dis 2012;15:45–55.

78. von Eyben FE, Kairemo K. Meta-analysis of (11)C-choline and (18)F-choline PET/CT for management of patients with prostate cancer. Nucl Med Commun 2014;35:221–30.

79. Yu YC, Desai B, Ji L, et al. Comparative performance of PET tracers in biochemical recurrence of prostate cancer: a critical analysis of literature. Am J Nucl Med Mol Imaging 2014;4(6):580–601.

80. Jadvar H. Molecular imaging of prostate cancer - PET Radiotracers. AJR Am J Roentgenol 2012;199: 278–91.

81. Jadvar H. Prostate cancer: PET with 18F-FDG, 18F- or 11C-acetate, and 18F- or 11C-choline. J Nucl Med 2011;52:81–9.

82. Schiavina R, Scattoni V, Castellucci P, et al. 11C-choline positron emission tomography/computed tomography for preoperative lymph-node staging in intermediate-risk and high-risk prostate cancer: comparison with clinical staging nomograms. Eur Urol 2008;54:392–410.

83. Gacci M, Cai T, Siena G, et al. Prostate-specific antigen kinetics parameters are predictive of positron emission tomography features worsening in patients with biochemical relapse after prostate cancer treatment with radical intent: results from a longitudinal cohort study. Scand J Urol 2014; 48:259–67.

84. Reske SN, Moritz S, Kull T. [11C]Choline-PET/CT for outcome prediction of salvage radiotherapy of local relapsing prostate carcinoma. Q J Nucl Med Mol Imaging 2012;56:430–9.

85. Rischke HC, Knippen S, Kirste S, et al. Treatment of recurrent prostate cancer following radical prostatectomy: the radiation-oncologists point of view. Q J Nucl Med Mol Imaging 2012;56:409–20.

86. Breeuwsma AJ, Rybalov M, Leliveld AM, et al. Correlation of [11C]choline PET/CT with time to treatment and disease-specific survival in men with recurrent prostate cancer after radical prostatectomy. Q J Nucl Med Mol Imaging 2012;56:440–6.

87. Giovacchini G, Picchio M, Garcia-Parra R, et al. 11C-Choline PET/CT predicts cancer-specific survival in patients with biochemical failure during androgen-deprivation therapy. J Nucl Med 2014; 55:233–41.

88. Kwee SA, Lim J, Watanabe A, et al. Prognosis related to metastatic burden measured by 18F-fluorocholine PET/CT in castration-resistant prostate cancer. J Nucl Med 2014;55:905–10.

Value of Fluorodeoxyglucose PET/Computed Tomography Patient Management and Outcomes in Thyroid Cancer

Anthony Ciarallo, MD[a],*, Charles Marcus, MD[a], Mehdi Taghipour, MD[a], Rathan M. Subramaniam, MD, PhD, MPH[a,b,c]

KEYWORDS

- FDG • PET/CT • Thyroid cancer • Prognosis • Outcome

KEY POINTS

- Fluorodeoxyglucose (FDG) PET/computed tomography (CT) changes the clinical management in 14% to 78% of patients with suspected differentiated thyroid cancer recurrence.
- A positive FDG-PET/CT scan correlates with reduced survival in differentiated thyroid cancer. Other suggested prognostic factors include the time from the initial diagnosis to the restaging FDG-PET/CT and the functional tumor volume.
- The use of FDG-PET/CT in anaplastic thyroid cancer changes management in up to 50% of cases. A positive scan seems to carry a worse prognosis than a negative scan.
- FDG uptake in medullary thyroid cancer is variable, but some investigators have shown that FDG-PET/CT still has an advantage compared with conventional imaging and a positive FDG-PET/CT scan seems to be associated with poorer survival.
- Approximately one third of patients with incidental focal thyroid hypermetabolism on FDG-PET are found to have thyroid cancer, most commonly the papillary histologic subtype.

INTRODUCTION

Radioiodine has been applied in the diagnostic evaluation and therapeutic management of differentiated (papillary and follicular) thyroid carcinoma (DTC) for more than half a century. Nevertheless, not all thyroid cancers are iodine avid. Some variants of papillary thyroid cancers (PTCs) and occasionally recurrent DTC fail to take up iodine, as well as other histologic subtypes such as anaplastic thyroid carcinoma (ATC) and medullary thyroid carcinoma (MTC). Consequently, investigators have looked to other radiotracers in attempts to better characterize these types of thyroid cancers using functional imaging. Fluorodeoxyglucose (FDG) PET/computed tomography (CT) is useful in the management of many human solid tumors.[1–10] The potential of PET and PET/CT has gained the interest of many clinicians as a viable alternative for radioiodine imaging for iodine-refractory cases. In particular, multiple investigators have studied the use of 18F-FDG in thyroid

Disclosure: The Authors have nothing to disclose.
[a] Russell H Morgan Department of Radiology and Radiological Sciences, Johns Hopkins School of Medicine, 601 N Caroline Street, Baltimore, MD 21287, USA; [b] Sidney Kimmel Comprehensive Cancer Center, Johns Hopkins School of Medicine, 601 North Caroline Street, Baltimore, MD, USA; [c] Department of Health Policy and Management, Johns Hopkins Bloomberg School of Public Health, Johns Hopkins University, 624 North Broadway, Baltimore, MD 21205, USA
* Corresponding author. Division of Nuclear Medicine, Russel H Morgan Department of Radiology and Radiological Sciences, 601 North Caroline Street, Baltimore MD 21287.
E-mail address: aciaral1@jhmi.edu

cancer over the last couple of decades. Other PET tracers such as I-124 and, more recently, 18F-di-hydroxyphenylalanine (DOPA) have also been studied in thyroid cancer; however, this is beyond the scope of this article. Many investigators have shown that thyroid cancer can take up FDG to varying degrees, with or without concurrent radio-iodine uptake. Ultimately, the value of PET/CT is measured by its impact on clinical management and its ability to predict patient outcome. To that end, this article reviews the effect on management and the prognostic implications of FDG-PET(/CT) in thyroid cancer.

DIFFERENTIATED THYROID CANCER

Differentiated thyroid cancer is the most common of all histologic subtypes, accounting for 80% to 85% of all thyroid cancers, whereas about 5% to 10% are the medullary subtype and less than 5% are anaplastic.[11–13] About 20% to 30% of DTC recur, and of these patients 7% die within 10 years of initial diagnosis.[14] Initial treatment, namely complete resection and I-131 therapy, in-fluences the outcome of DTC.[15–18] Advanced tumor stage or metastasis at presentation has been shown to carry a worse prognosis.[15,19–21] In a study at the Mayo clinic, overall survival of metastatic PTC at 15 years was 20%.[22] Older age, extrathyroidal extension at initial surgery, and extrapulmonary distant metastasis had a negative prognosis. Among patients with iodine-avid lesions, those who received radioiodine ther-apy (RIT) had better survival than patients who did not. Furthermore, certain patterns of distant metastasis have a more indolent course, such as micronodular lung metastasis in younger individ-uals and isolated FDG-avid bone metastasis.[23]

In general, serum thyroglobulin (Tg) is used for the posttherapy surveillance of DTC. An increasing Tg level following total thyroidectomy suggests residual or recurrent disease.[24] Conven-tional imaging such as ultrasonography, CT, and magnetic resonance (MR) imaging are often inconclusive in the evaluation of the postsurgical neck.[25,26] Radioiodine imaging may fail to detect dedifferentiated recurrence because of the loss of its ability to trap iodine.[25] Thus, the role of RIT in these circumstances is less certain. Loss of iodine uptake by metastatic PTC is associated with worse survival.[27] Between 10% and 30% of I-131 scans are negative in patients with recurrent differentiated thyroid cancer and increased Tg level.[27–29] Localization of iodine-negative lesions is essential because surgery is the most effective curative option. Other therapeutic possibilities for recurrent DTC with negative iodine scans

(NIS) include radiotherapy and embolization. For patients with NIS and increased Tg level, alterna-tive imaging modalities are required for diagnostic evaluation. At the moment, there is no consensus for work-up or management of NIS with increased Tg level. Empiric I-131 therapy may be justified in high-risk patients when Tg level greater than 10 ng/mL.[30] Nonetheless, there is a significant reduction of Tg in 44% of patients with DTC with NIS in the absence of treatment.[31–33] Multiple publications have been produced on FDG-PET/CT in the work-up of thyroid cancer. Some inves-tigators have shown a correlation between increased glucose transporter 1 (GLUT1) expres-sion and dedifferentiation of thyroid cancer.[34] Nonetheless, coexistence of iodine trapping and FDG uptake has also been described.[35,36] Ac-cording to a meta-analysis by Leboulleux and col-leagues[37] (2007), the sensitivity and specificity of FDG-PET for localization of recurrent DTC ranges from 45% to 100% and 42% to 90%, respectively.

At the moment, there is no consensus for the use of FDG-PET/CT in DTC. According to the revised American Thyroid Association (ATA) guidelines for patients with DTC,[17] FDG-PET im-aging may be used (1) as part of initial staging in poorly differentiated thyroid cancers and invasive Hürthle cell carcinomas, especially those with other evidence of disease on imaging or because of increased serum Tg levels (Fig. 1); (2) as a prog-nostic tool (Fig. 2) in patients with metastatic dis-ease to identify those patients at highest risk for rapid disease progression and disease-specific mortality; and (3) as an evaluation of posttreatment response following systemic or local therapy for metastatic or locally invasive disease. This recom-mendation is based on expert opinion (ie, rating C).

The accuracy of FDG-PET/CT varies between studies, depending on the study design and pa-tient population. A more pertinent question is whether FDG-PET/CT significantly affects clinical management and patient survival. A literature review reveals that FDG-PET/CT changes the management of DTC in 14% to 78% of patients (Table 1).[38–47] The percentages indicated are relative to all patients who were scanned, not only those with FDG positivity. In order to limit the effect of chance, only studies with 30 or more patients are included in Table 1. Several smaller studies have reported data on the impact of PET on patient management in DTC, but are not reviewed here.[36,48–50] Among the studies under consideration, both prospective and retro-spective designs were used, and most patients had NIS and increased thyroglobulin level. Changes of management included, but were not limited to, guided surgery for resection of

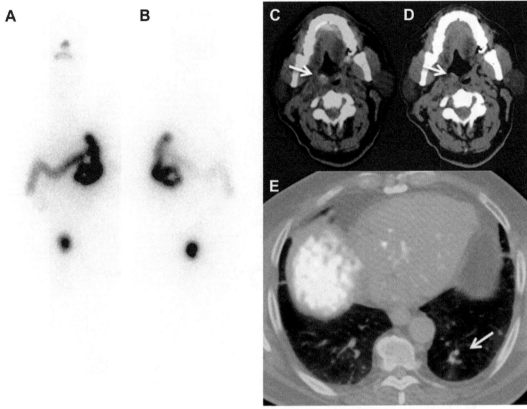

Fig. 1. DTC. Negative iodine scan with increased thyroglobulin level. Anterior (*A*) and posterior (*B*) planar I-123 whole-body scintigraphy images of a 78-year-old woman who underwent surgical excision and neck dissection for papillary carcinoma of the thyroid, during the follow-up period. The planar images show normal physiologic radiotracer uptake in the small bowel and urinary bladder, with no evidence of abnormal radiotracer accumulation to suggest active disease. However, her thyroglobulin level at that time was 751 ng/mL. Axial fused FDG-PET/CT (*C, E*) and CT (*D*) images of an FDG-PET/CT study done for evaluation revealed a moderately FDG-avid (SUV$_{max}$, 3.8) parapharyngeal lymph node (*arrow*, panels C, D) and multiple FDG-avid (SUV$_{max}$, 2.7) pulmonary nodules (*arrow*, panel E), consistent with metastatic disease.

oligometastasis, avoidance of futile surgery, radiotherapy planning, and implementation of redifferentiation therapy.

PET/CT provides important prognostic information for many malignancies, including breast cancer,[51] gastric cancer,[52] brain tumors,[53] prostate cancer,[54] esophageal cancer,[55] and lung cancer.[56] A few studies have published survival data on thyroid cancer but these studies were conducted retrospectively. No prospective studies have yet been performed to evaluate FDG-PET/CT prognostication for thyroid cancer. The survival data from 3 studies are summarized in **Table 2**.[11,57,58]

Robbins and colleagues[57] (2006) conducted the largest study to date of the survival of patients with DTC following FDG-PET/CT. Four hundred patients were retrospectively reviewed. Multivariate analysis revealed that age greater than 45 years, FDG positivity, and the number of FDG-avid lesions significantly correlated with survival. The maximum standard uptake value (SUV$_{max}$) also correlated significantly when substituted for number of FDG lesions. The 2-year survival was 52% in the quartile with the highest SUV$_{max}$ compared with 98% in the quartile with the lowest SUV$_{max}$. The median survival of patients with FDG-avid lesions was 53 months (ie, 89 of 221 patients died). These patients had 7.3 times higher risk of dying than patients with a negative scan. In contrast, only 2 thyroid cancer–related deaths were observed in patients with negative PET/CT scans. There was no difference in survival between patients with and without metastasis if their initial PET/CT scan was negative. For patients with positive PET/CT scans, survival varied based on the site of metastasis. Local lymph node metastasis to the neck had a more favorable prognosis than regional nodal metastasis (ie, supraclavicular and mediastinal). Patients with FDG-avid distant metastasis had the worst survival.

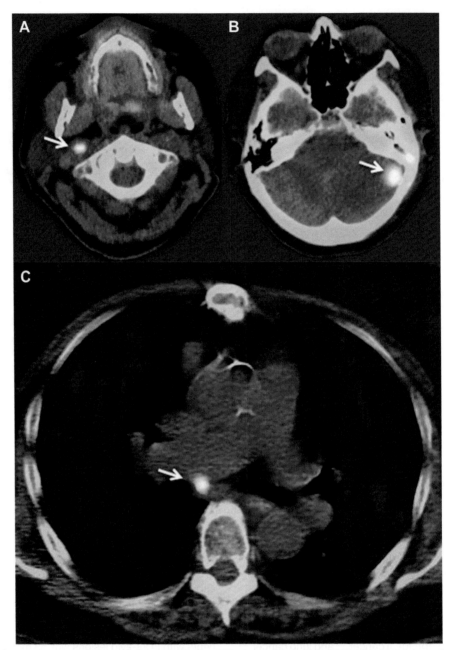

Fig. 2. Change in management and prognosis for PTC. Axial fused FDG-PET/CT (*A–C*) images of a 67-year-old woman with a history of PTC, after thyroidectomy, neck dissection, and radioiodine ablation, who underwent a restaging PET/CT study. The study shows hypermetabolic cervical lymphadenopathy with SUV_{max}, 3.9 (*arrow,* panel A), left cerebellar metastasis with SUV_{max}, 11.4 (*arrow,* panel B), and mediastinal lymphadenopathy with SUV_{max}, 4.0 (*arrow,* panel C). Following the study the patient underwent craniotomy and excision of cerebellar lesion, neck dissection, and chemotherapy. Despite aggressive management, there was significant disease progression resulting in death 2 months after the study.

In a smaller study, Schreinemakers and colleagues[11] (2012) showed that patients with FDG-avid lesions were significantly older and had higher median thyroglobulin levels, higher TNM (tumor, node, metastasis) stage, and larger tumors at the time of initial treatment. Disease-free survival was 15 months in the FDG-positive group and 41 months in the FDG-negative groups; however, no statistical significance was found, which is most likely secondary to insufficient power.

Table 1
FDG-PET/CT changes the management of DTC in 14% to 78% of patients

Author, Year	Design	Modality	Size	FDG+	RAI+	Tg (ng/mL)	Management Change, n (%)
Bannas et al,[38] 2012	Retro	PET/CT	30	19	—	2.2–8663	17 (57)
Giammarile et al,[39] 2003	Pros	PET	51	35	—	0.7–11,617	7 (14)
Helal et al,[40] 2001	Pros	PET	37	28	—	1.5–2800	29 (78)
Leboulleux et al,[41] 2009	Pros	PET/CT	63	40	—	<1–538	12 (19)
Nahas et al,[42] 2005	Retro	PET/CT	33	22	8 (24%)	1.2–629	13 (39)
Palmedo et al,[43] 2006	Pros	PET/CT	40	20	—	6.4 ± 3.1[a]	13 (33)
Rosenbaum et al,[44] 2012	Pros	PET/CT	90	26	32 (36%)	0.3–227210	19 (21)
Schluter et al,[45] 2001	Retro	PET	64	44	16 (25%)	<10 to >100	21 (33)
van Dijk et al,[46] 2013	Retro	PET[b]	52	12	—	0.18–1870	7 (13)
Zoller et al,[47] 2007	Retro	PET/CT	33[c]	35/47	5 (15%)	1.8–7712300	8 of 47 (17)

Abbreviations: FDG+, number of patients with positive FDG-PET or PET/CT; Pros, prospective; RAI+, number of patients with a positive radioactive iodine scan; Retro, retrospective.
[a] Mean Tg ± standard deviation. Thyroglobulin range not provided.
[b] Seven of 52 scans were performed as PET/CT.
[c] The data were reported according to the number of PET/CT scans (ie, 47) performed on 33 patients.
Data from Refs.[38–47]

Among the 22 patients with positive PET scans, 5 died but only 3 of these died of metastatic PTC. No deaths were observed in the 17 patients with negative PET scans. The follow-up period after PET scan was not specified. Nonetheless, these findings support a negative prognostication with a positive PET scan.

Creach and colleagues[58] (2013) presented more recent survival data on 76 patients with DTC, NIS, and increased thyroglobulin level of more than 3 ng/mL. They showed that the time to PET after initial diagnosis is a predictor of survival (median 3.5 years, ranging from 7 months to 28 years) in both univariate and multivariate analyses. Similar to the 2 previously mentioned articles, Creach and colleagues (2013) also found that PET positivity predicts death. The 5-year cause-specific survival was 63% in the FDG-positive group. Median follow-up after PET scanning was 2.7 years. No deaths were observed in 25 patients with a negative scan despite 4 patients progressing on follow-up and 1 false-negative case from local nodal metastasis detected by neck ultrasonography.

There are numerous criticisms to be considered. First, most study designs under review are retrospective, which raises concern for referral bias because there is no firm indication for FDG-PET/CT in DTC. The resulting patient population is heterogeneous, including some without clear indication for PET/CT, whereas others had a documented history of metastatic DTC with NIS. Furthermore, a subset of PET scans was performed while under thyroxine (T4) suppression, whereas others were stimulated, either endogenously by T4 withdrawal or exogenously with recombinant human thyroid-stimulating hormone (TSH). Some investigators included all variants of DTC, whereas others only analyzed PTC. Many studies had small patient populations that may have been underpowered. Multiple studies failed to have a definite reference standard, relying on multimodality imaging and clinical follow-up given that histopathologic correlation is not typically feasible for every patient. Some investigators used negative serum Tg to exclude recurrence on follow-up, but not all DTC recurrences express thyroglobulin. In general, the follow-up after PET scan was short. DTC can be indolent, requiring longer periods of follow-up, but the investigators argue that dedifferentiated recurrence, such as in NIS with increased thyroglobulin level, is more aggressive and is expected to recur earlier than iodine-avid disease. Some investigators included patients with NIS with detectable thyroglobulin as low as 0.2 ng/mL in their inclusion criteria, even though it has been shown that patients with increased serum thyroglobulin greater than 10 ng/mL are more likely to be PET positive. Inclusion of patients with low pretest probability would falsely diminish the proportion of cases in which FDG-PET/CT is found to be clinically useful. Variations of technical factors such as dose injected per body weight, time to imaging, type of PET crystal, and experience of the reader are also potential sources of error.

Table 2
Survival data on thyroid cancer

Author, Year	Robbins et al,[57] 2006		Schreinemakers et al,[11] 2012		Creach et al,[58] 2013	
Design	Retro		Retro		Retro	
Study Size (N)	400		41		76	
FDG-PET (n)	NS		11		15	
FDG-PET/CT (n)			30		61	
Mean Age ± SD	54 ± 16		46 ± 20		49[a]	
Female (%)	0.56		0.56		0.63	
Histology						
Papillary	201		41		52	
Follicular Variants	—		—		9	
Other Variants	76		—		12	
Follicular	31		—		2	
Hürthle	36		—		—	
Poorly Differentiated	45		—		1	
Anaplastic	11		—		—	
Initial Stage	AJCC	N	AJCC	N	AJCC	N
	I	139	I	13	I	28
	II	56	II	1	II	12
	III	133	III	11	III	34
	IV	62	IV	7	IV	3
	—	—	X[b]	7	—	—
FDG-PET						
Positive	221 of 400		22 of 41		51 of 76	
Negative	179 of 400		17 of 41		25 of 76	
Indeterminate	—		2 of 41[c]		—	
Positive Iodine scans						
I+/FDG+	158 of 221		5 of 22		Negative iodine scan	
I+/FDG−	90 of 179		8 of 17		N/A	
TSH						
Unstimulated	148		NS		16	
Stimulated	252				60	
Median Tg (ng/mL)						
FDG+	44 (0.3–214,000)		33 (0.9–1500)		42 (3.3–5015)	
FDG−	1.0 (0.3–128)		3.1 (0.3–300)		13 (3.7–193)	
Median Follow-up (y)						
Initial diagnosis	7.9 (0.15–39.7)		NS		7 (1.3–30)	
After PET	3.0 (0–6.9)				2.7 (0.1–10.5)	
Outcome	2-y OS[d]		Median DFS		5-y CSS	
FDG+	Q1 98%, Q2 73%, Q3 70%, Q4 52%		15 mo		63%	
FDG−	99%		41 mo		100%	
Predictors of Death	Positive PET # of FDG-avid lesions, or SUV$_{max}$ Age>45 y		Positive PET — —		Positive PET Time to PET[e] —	

Abbreviations: AJCC, American Joint Commission for Cancer; CSS, cause-specific survival; DFS, disease-free survival; I+/FDG+, iodine and FDG avid; I+/FDG−, iodine avid, FDG negative; N/A, not applicable; NS, not specified; OS, overall survival; Q1–4, first to fourth quartiles of FDG intensity, measured in SUV$_{max}$; SUV$_{max}$, maximum standard uptake value; TSH, thyroid-stimulating hormone.
[a] Median age is indicated. No mean age or standard deviation provided. Age range was 5–78 years.
[b] The letter X denotes unknown AJCC staging.
[c] Malignancy confirmed in both patients.
[d] Overall 2-year survival divided into quartiles of SUV$_{max}$, with Q1 representing the least metabolically active quartile and Q4 the most.
[e] Median time to PET scan from initial diagnosis was 3.5 years (range, 0.6–28 years).

ANAPLASTIC THYROID CARCINOMA

ATC occurs in an older demographic or as the result of dedifferentiation of DTC. It is the most aggressive histologic subtype of thyroid cancer. The median survival of ATC is about 6 to 8 months.[12] The ATA strongly recommends FDG-PET/CT as part of initial staging and follow-up evaluation at 3 to 6 months after therapy.[59]

Poisson and colleagues[60] (2010) retrospectively reviewed 20 (2 excluded) consecutive patients with ATC with FDG-PET/CT at initial staging and at follow-up. The patients were treated with surgery when feasible and with 6 cycles of a doxorubicin/cisplatin regimen followed by bifractionated and accelerated radiotherapy to the neck and mediastinum after 2 cycles of chemotherapy. Follow-up PET/CT was performed after 2 cycles and/or after completion of chemotherapy and/or after radiotherapy. PET/CT outperformed CT in organ-based and lesion-based analysis, detecting 62 of 63 (98.4%) involved organs and 264 of 265 (99.6%) lesions compared to 41 of 63 (65.1%) and 165 of 265 (62.3%) with CT, respectively.

Management was altered by FDG-PET/CT in 5 cases (25%). SUV_{max} and the volume of FDG uptake were predictive of survival by univariate analysis, although only the latter was predictive on bivariate analysis.

Bogsrud and colleagues[61] (2008) retrospectively reviewed 16 patients with ATC with FDG-PET/CT at initial staging and/or restaging (**Fig. 3**). FDG-PET/CT affected the management of 8 of 16 patients (50%). Due to the small size of the study it is difficult to interpret the prognostic value of FDG-PET.

MEDULLARY THYROID CARCINOMA

MTC is a rare endocrine tumor that, when confined to thyroid capsule, carries a good prognosis. The prognosis is significantly poorer when capsular invasion or metastatic spread is present at the time of diagnosis.[62,63] Surgery is the mainstay of treatment because neither chemotherapy nor external beam radiotherapy has proved effective for disease control.[64]

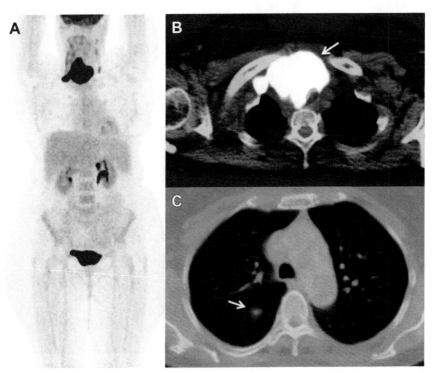

Fig. 3. Staging and prognosis for ATC. Anterior maximal intensity projection (MIP) (*A*) and axial fused PET/CT (*B, C*) images of a 65-year-old woman with a newly diagnosed locally advanced ATC who underwent a staging FDG-PET/CT study. The study showed an intensely FDG-avid (SUV_{max}, 27.6), locally advanced thyroid lesion with metastatic supraclavicular with SUV_{max}, 20.6 (*arrow,* panel B) and pulmonary (SUV_{max}, 1.9) lesions (*arrow,* panel C). Despite aggressive chemotherapy, the disease progressed, resulting in death 8 months after the study.

In a meta-analysis of 24 studies comprising 538 patients with suspected recurrent MTC, the detection rate of FDG-PET or PET/CT in suspected recurrent MTC on a per patient–based analysis was 59% (95% confidence interval [CI], 54%–63%).[65] A separate meta-analysis revealed that the pooled sensitivities of FDG-PET and PET/CT were 0.68 (95% CI, 0.64–0.72) and 0.69 (95% CI, 0.64–0.74), respectively.[66] Ong and colleagues[67] (2007) demonstrated that the sensitivity of FDG PET increases with serum calcitonin. Levels exceeding 1000 pg/mL resulted in improved sensitivity when compared to calcitonin levels below 500 pg/mL (**Fig. 4**). Oudoux and colleagues[68] (2007) reported that SUV significantly correlated with calcitonin doubling times.

Rubello and colleagues[69] (2008) prospectively studied 19 consecutive patients with suspected recurrent MTC (14 sporadic, 5 multiple endocrine neoplasia [MEN] syndrome) presenting with increased calcitonin levels (58–1350 pg/mL). All patients had extrathyroidal extension at initial diagnosis. FDG-PET/CT was the most sensitive imaging modality for detecting metastases. FDG-PET/CT depicted a total of 26 metastatic deposits in 15 patients, a result that was superior to 111In-pentetreotide, contrast-enhanced CT, and ultrasonography.

De Groot and colleagues[70] (2004) prospectively studied 26 patients with biochemical evidence of recurrent or residual MTC. FDG-PET detected disease foci in 50% of patients with a lesion-based sensitivity of 96%. Similar to Rubello and colleagues[69] (2008), this result was superior to 111In-octreotide, 99mTc-Dimercaptosuccinic acid (V) scintigraphy, CT, MR imaging, and ultrasonography. Positive FDG-PET findings led to surgical intervention in 9 patients (35%) who underwent surgery for removal of residual tumor or metastases. Following surgery, serum calcitonin levels were reduced by an average of 58% ± 31%. One patient achieved disease-free status.

Verbeek and colleagues[71] (2012) retrospectively reviewed 47 patients with MTC with detectable

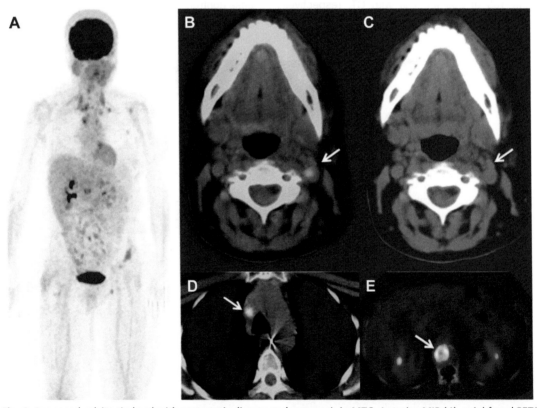

Fig. 4. Increased calcitonin level with metastatic disease and prognosis in MTC. Anterior MIP (*A*), axial fused PET/CT (*B, D, E*), and CT (*C*) images of a 58-year-old woman with a history of metastatic MTC, after thyroidectomy, neck dissection, radioiodine ablation, and radiation therapy who presented for a follow-up with a calcitonin level of 15,300 ng/mL. The restaging FDG-PET/CT study shows multiple hypermetabolic, metastatic lesions in the neck with SUV$_{max}$, 3.4 (*arrow*, panels B and C), mediastinum with SUV$_{max}$, 4.8 (*arrow*, panel D), and vertebra with SUV$_{max}$, 5.6 (*arrow*, panel E). Despite treatment, the patient had disease progression, resulting in death 1 year and 8 months after the study.

calcitonin levels who underwent FDG and/or 18F-DOPA PET/CT for detection of residual or metastatic disease. 18F-DOPA PET detected significantly more lesions (75%, 56 of 75) than FDG-PET (47%, 35 of 75). However, FDG-PET positivity was a better indicator of survival. In the 42 patients for whom follow-up data were available, median follow-up was 63.8 months (range, 2.3–114 months). In 37 patients with sufficient follow-up, survival was significantly lower in FDG-positive patients than in FDG-negative patients. In the univariate analysis of 22 patients who underwent both FDG-PET and 18F-DOPA PET, the survival in FDG-positive patients was lower and independent of the 18F-DOPA PET outcome, whereas survival in 18F-DOPA–positive patients depended on FDG-PET outcome. These data are corroborated by Bogsrud and colleagues[72] (2010), who retrospectively reviewed 29 patients with MTC. After an average follow-up of 37 months, they reported lower survival in FDG-positive cases, of which 6 of 11 patients died (45% survival), whereas no deaths were observed in the FDG-negative cases after an

average of 44 months, even though 1 patient developed recurrent disease.

INCIDENTAL FLUORODEOXYGLUCOSE THYROID UPTAKE

Incidental FDG uptake within the thyroid gland has been observed in up to 4% of patients who undergo FDG-PET imaging for other indications.[73,74] Focal FDG uptake is associated with malignancy with an incidence ranging from 24% to 36% (Fig. 5). The most commonly associated histopathologic subtype is PTC.[75–79] A meta-analysis by Treglia and colleagues[77] of 34 studies evaluating the malignancy risk in incidental focal thyroid uptake revealed a malignancy risk of 36.2% (95% CI, 33.8%–38.6%). In contrast, incidental diffuse FDG uptake has been observed in up to 3% of patients and is most often related to a benign disease process such as thyroiditis (Fig. 6).[80–82] A study by Karantanis and colleagues[81] evaluating 4732 patients who underwent FDG-PET/CT for other indications showed that 59.4% of patients with incidental diffuse

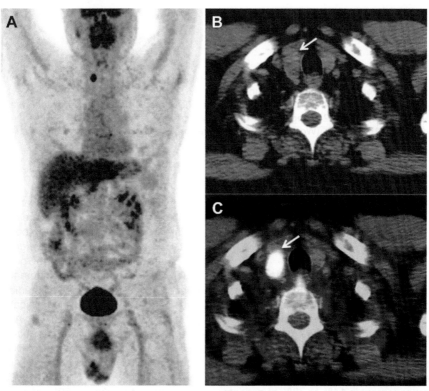

Fig. 5. Incidental focal thyroid uptake. Anterior MIP (A), axial CT (B), and fused PET/CT (C) images of a 57-year-old man who underwent an FDG-PET/CT study for evaluation of pulmonary nodules. The PET/CT images show an incidental focal thyroid uptake with SUV$_{max}$, 8.1 (arrow, panels B and C). Biopsy of the lesion revealed papillary thyroid carcinoma. The patient underwent thyroidectomy and radioiodine ablation following the study.

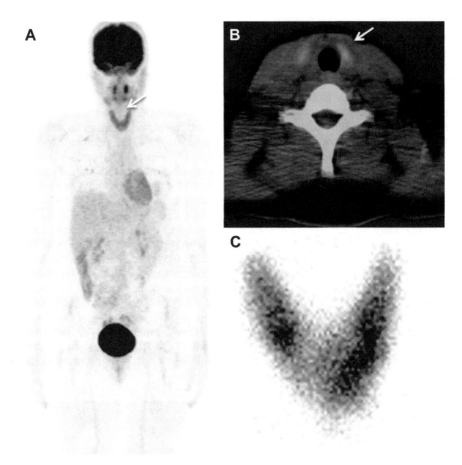

Fig. 6. Incidental diffuse thyroid uptake. Anterior MIP (*A*), axial fused PET/CT (*B*), and I-123 uptake planar (*C*) images of a 23-year-old woman who underwent a restaging FDG-PET/CT study for evaluation of a known stage IV melanoma. The PET/CT images show an incidental diffuse thyroid uptake with SUV_{max}, 5.6 (*arrow*, panels A and B). The I-123 images show uniformly increased radiotracer uptake. Her thyroid peroxidase antibody level was 1633 WHO (World Health Organization) units. These features support a diagnosis of thyroiditis.

thyroid uptake had chronic lymphocytic thyroiditis on further evaluation.

SUMMARY

The utility of FDG-PET/CT in differentiated thyroid cancer is greatest in iodine-refractory cases. It has been shown that the likelihood of a positive scan increases when the serum thyroglobulin level is greater than 10 ng/mL. However, the reported sensitivity and specificity vary widely, which may be the result of a combination of extrinsic and intrinsic factors. FDG-PET/CT has changed the course of management in 14% to 78% of patients with differentiated thyroid cancer; however, this includes both iodine-avid and refractory disease as well as varying degrees of thyroglobulin levels, histologic subtypes and staging, TSH preparation,

and PET technology. Even fewer PET data are available on survival and there are no prospective trials to date. Nevertheless, outcome is consistently poorer in the FDG-positive group.

Anaplastic and medullary thyroid cancers are much less common than differentiated thyroid cancer. Consequently, fewer studies have been performed to evaluate the clinical impact and prognostication of FDG-PET/CT. ATC is aggressive, with high sensitivity and specificity on FDG-PET/CT because of intense FDG uptake. In contrast, MTC has variable FDG uptake. From the available data, FDG-PET/CT changed management in 25% to 50% of cases and FDG-positive cases also had poorer outcomes.

Incidental focal thyroid FDG uptake is associated with a considerable risk of malignancy and should be further evaluated.

REFERENCES

1. Dibble EH, Karantanis D, Mercier G, et al. PET/CT of cancer patients: part 1, pancreatic neoplasms. AJR Am J Roentgenol 2012;199:952–67.

2. Davison J, Mercier G, Russo G, et al. PET-based primary tumor volumetric parameters and survival of patients with non-small cell lung carcinoma. AJR Am J Roentgenol 2013;200:635–40.

3. Hadiprodjo D, Ryan T, Truong MT, et al. Parotid gland tumors: preliminary data for the value of FDG PET/CT diagnostic parameters. AJR Am J Roentgenol 2012;198:W185–90.

4. Jackson T, Chung MK, Mercier G, et al. FDG PET/CT interobserver agreement in head and neck cancer: FDG and CT measurements of the primary tumor site. Nucl Med Commun 2012;33:305–12.

5. Davison JM, Subramaniam RM, Surasi DS, et al. FDG PET/CT in patients with HIV. AJR Am J Roentgenol 2011;197:284–94.

6. Agarwal A, Chirindel A, Shah BA, et al. Evolving role of FDG PET/CT in multiple myeloma imaging and management. AJR Am J Roentgenol 2013;200:884–90.

7. Shah B, Srivastava N, Hirsch AE, et al. Intra-reader reliability of FDG PET volumetric tumor parameters: effects of primary tumor size and segmentation methods. Ann Nucl Med 2012;26(9):707–14.

8. Tahari AK, Alluri KC, Quon H, et al. FDG PET/CT imaging of oropharyngeal squamous cell carcinoma: characteristics of human papillomavirus-positive and -negative tumors. Clin Nucl Med 2014;39:225–31.

9. Paidpally V, Chirindel A, Lam S, et al. FDG-PET/CT imaging biomarkers in head and neck squamous cell carcinoma. Imaging Med 2012;4:633–47.

10. Antoniou AJ, Marcus C, Tahari AK, et al. Follow-up or surveillance 18F-FDG PET/CT and survival outcome in lung cancer patients. J Nucl Med 2014;55(7):1062–8.

11. Schreinemakers JM, Vriens MR, Munoz-Perez N, et al. Fluorodeoxyglucose-positron emission tomography scan-positive recurrent papillary thyroid cancer and the prognosis and implications for surgical management. World J Surg Oncol 2012;10:192.

12. Treglia G, Annunziata S, Muoio B, et al. The role of fluorine-18-fluorodeoxyglucose positron emission tomography in aggressive histological subtypes of thyroid cancer: an overview. Int J Endocrinol 2013;2013:856189.

13. Wong KK, Laird AM, Moubayed A, et al. How has the management of medullary thyroid carcinoma changed with the advent of 18F-FDG and non-18F-FDG PET radiopharmaceuticals. Nucl Med Commun 2012;33:679–88.

14. Hundahl SA, Fleming ID, Fremgen AM, et al. A National cancer data base report on 53,856 cases of thyroid carcinoma treated in the U.S., 1985–1995 [see comments]. Cancer 1998;83:2638–48.

15. Mazzaferri EL, Kloos RT. Clinical review 128: current approaches to primary therapy for papillary and follicular thyroid cancer. J Clin Endocrinol Metab 2001;86:1447–63.

16. Van Nostrand D, Wartofsky L. Radioiodine in the treatment of thyroid cancer. Endocrinol Metab Clin North Am 2007;36:807–22, vii–viii.

17. Cooper DS, Doherty GM, Haugen BR, et al. Revised American Thyroid Association management guidelines for patients with thyroid nodules and differentiated thyroid cancer. Thyroid 2009;19:1167–214.

18. Pacini F, Schlumberger M, Dralle H, et al. European consensus for the management of patients with differentiated thyroid carcinoma of the follicular epithelium. Eur J Endocrinol 2006;154:787–803.

19. Grebe SK, Hay ID. Thyroid cancer nodal metastases: biologic significance and therapeutic considerations. Surg Oncol Clin N Am 1996;5:43–63.

20. Hay ID, Bergstralh EJ, Goellner JR, et al. Predicting outcome in papillary thyroid carcinoma: development of a reliable prognostic scoring system in a cohort of 1779 patients surgically treated at one institution during 1940 through 1989. Surgery 1993;114:1050–7 [discussion: 1057–58].

21. Tubiana M, Schlumberger M, Rougier P, et al. Long-term results and prognostic factors in patients with differentiated thyroid carcinoma. Cancer 1985;55:794–804.

22. Dinneen SF, Valimaki MJ, Bergstralh EJ, et al. Distant metastases in papillary thyroid carcinoma: 100 cases observed at one institution during 5 decades. J Clin Endocrinol Metab 1995;80:2041–5.

23. Schlumberger M, Challeton C, De Vathaire F, et al. Radioactive iodine treatment and external radiotherapy for lung and bone metastases from thyroid carcinoma. J Nucl Med 1996;37:598–605.

24. Sherman SI. Thyroid carcinoma. Lancet 2003;361:501–11.

25. Frilling A, Gorges R, Tecklenborg K, et al. Value of preoperative diagnostic modalities in patients with recurrent thyroid carcinoma. Surgery 2000;128:1067–74.

26. Schlumberger MJ. Diagnostic follow-up of well-differentiated thyroid carcinoma: historical perspective and current status. J Endocrinol Invest 1999;22:3–7.

27. Rouxel A, Hejblum G, Bernier MO, et al. Prognostic factors associated with the survival of patients developing loco-regional recurrences of differentiated thyroid carcinomas. J Clin Endocrinol Metab 2004;89:5362–8.

28. Ashcraft MW, Van Herle AJ. The comparative value of serum thyroglobulin measurements and iodine 131 total body scans in the follow-up study of patients with treated differentiated thyroid cancer. Am J Med 1981;71:806–14.

29. Schlumberger M, Arcangioli O, Piekarski JD, et al. Detection and treatment of lung metastases of differentiated thyroid carcinoma in patients with normal chest X-rays. J Nucl Med 1988;29:1790–4.

30. Ma C, Xie J, Kuang A. Is empiric 131I therapy justified for patients with positive thyroglobulin and negative 131I whole-body scanning results? J Nucl Med 2005;46:1164–70.

31. Koh JM, Kim ES, Ryu JS, et al. Effects of therapeutic doses of 131I in thyroid papillary carcinoma patients with elevated thyroglobulin level and negative 131I whole-body scan: comparative study. Clin Endocrinol (Oxf) 2003;58:421–7.

32. Pacini F, Agate L, Elisei R, et al. Outcome of differentiated thyroid cancer with detectable serum Tg and negative diagnostic (131)I whole body scan: comparison of patients treated with high (131)I activities versus untreated patients. J Clin Endocrinol Metab 2001;86:4092–7.

33. Alzahrani AS, Mohamed G, Al Shammary A, et al. Long-term course and predictive factors of elevated serum thyroglobulin and negative diagnostic radioiodine whole body scan in differentiated thyroid cancer. J Endocrinol Invest 2005;28:540–6.

34. Schonberger J, Ruschoff J, Grimm D, et al. Glucose transporter 1 gene expression is related to thyroid neoplasms with an unfavorable prognosis: an immunohistochemical study. Thyroid 2002;12:747–54.

35. Feine U, Lietzenmayer R, Hanke JP, et al. [18FDG whole-body PET in differentiated thyroid carcinoma. Flipflop in uptake patterns of 18FDG and 131I]. Nuklearmedizin 1995;34:127–34.

36. Piccardo A, Foppiani L, Morbelli S, et al. Could [18] F-fluorodeoxyglucose PET/CT change the therapeutic management of stage IV thyroid cancer with positive (131)I whole body scan? Q J Nucl Med Mol Imaging 2011;55:57–65.

37. Leboulleux S, Schroeder PR, Schlumberger M, et al. The role of PET in follow-up of patients treated for differentiated epithelial thyroid cancers. Nat Clin Pract Endocrinol Metab 2007;3:112–21.

38. Bannas P, Derlin T, Groth M, et al. Can (18)F-FDG-PET/CT be generally recommended in patients with differentiated thyroid carcinoma and elevated thyroglobulin levels but negative I-131 whole body scan? Ann Nucl Med 2012;26:77–85.

39. Giammarile F, Hafdi Z, Bournaud C, et al. Is [18F]-2-fluoro-2-deoxy-d-glucose (FDG) scintigraphy with non-dedicated positron emission tomography useful in the diagnostic management of suspected metastatic thyroid carcinoma in patients with no detectable radioiodine uptake? Eur J Endocrinol 2003; 149:293–300.

40. Helal BO, Merlet P, Toubert ME, et al. Clinical impact of (18)F-FDG PET in thyroid carcinoma patients with elevated thyroglobulin levels and negative (131)I scanning results after therapy. J Nucl Med 2001;42:1464–9.

41. Leboulleux S, Schroeder PR, Busaidy NL, et al. Assessment of the incremental value of recombinant thyrotropin stimulation before 2-[18F]-fluoro-2-deoxy-D-glucose positron emission tomography/computed tomography imaging to localize residual differentiated thyroid cancer. J Clin Endocrinol Metab 2009;94:1310–6.

42. Nahas Z, Goldenberg D, Fakhry C, et al. The role of positron emission tomography/computed tomography in the management of recurrent papillary thyroid carcinoma. Laryngoscope 2005;115:237–43.

43. Palmedo H, Bucerius J, Joe A, et al. Integrated PET/CT in differentiated thyroid cancer: diagnostic accuracy and impact on patient management. J Nucl Med 2006;47:616–24.

44. Rosenbaum-Krumme SJ, Gorges R, Bockisch A, et al. 18F-FDG PET/CT changes therapy management in high-risk DTC after first radioiodine therapy. Eur J Nucl Med Mol Imaging 2012;39: 1373–80.

45. Schluter B, Bohuslavizki KH, Beyer W, et al. Impact of FDG PET on patients with differentiated thyroid cancer who present with elevated thyroglobulin and negative 131I scan. J Nucl Med 2001; 42:71–6.

46. van Dijk D, Plukker JT, Phan HT, et al. 18-Fluorodeoxyglucose positron emission tomography in the early diagnostic workup of differentiated thyroid cancer patients with a negative post-therapeutic iodine scan and detectable thyroglobulin. Thyroid 2013;23:1003–9.

47. Zoller M, Kohlfuerst S, Igerc I, et al. Combined PET/CT in the follow-up of differentiated thyroid carcinoma: what is the impact of each modality? Eur J Nucl Med Mol Imaging 2007;34:487–95.

48. Frilling A, Tecklenborg K, Gorges R, et al. Preoperative diagnostic value of [(18)F] fluorodeoxyglucose positron emission tomography in patients with radioiodine-negative recurrent well-differentiated thyroid carcinoma. Ann Surg 2001;234:804–11.

49. Goshen E, Cohen O, Rotenberg G, et al. The clinical impact of 18F-FDG gamma PET in patients with recurrent well differentiated thyroid carcinoma. Nucl Med Commun 2003;24:959–61.

50. Zuijdwijk MD, Vogel WV, Corstens FH, et al. Utility of fluorodeoxyglucose-PET in patients with differentiated thyroid carcinoma. Nucl Med Commun 2008; 29:636–41.

51. Inoue T, Yutani K, Taguchi T, et al. Preoperative evaluation of prognosis in breast cancer patients by [(18)F]2-deoxy-2-fluoro-D-glucose-positron emission tomography. J Cancer Res Clin Oncol 2004; 130:273–8.

52. Mochiki E, Kuwano H, Katoh H, et al. Evaluation of 18F-2-deoxy-2-fluoro-D-glucose positron emission tomography for gastric cancer. World J Surg 2004; 28:247–53.

53. Padma MV, Said S, Jacobs M, et al. Prediction of pathology and survival by FDG PET in gliomas. J Neurooncol 2003;64:227–37.

54. Oyama N, Akino H, Suzuki Y, et al. Prognostic value of 2-deoxy-2-[F-18]fluoro-D-glucose positron emission tomography imaging for patients with prostate cancer. Mol Imaging Biol 2002;4:99–104.

55. Choi JY, Jang HJ, Shim YM, et al. 18F-FDG PET in patients with esophageal squamous cell carcinoma undergoing curative surgery: prognostic implications. J Nucl Med 2004;45:1843–50.

56. Weber WA, Petersen V, Schmidt B, et al. Positron emission tomography in non-small-cell lung cancer: prediction of response to chemotherapy by quantitative assessment of glucose use. J Clin Oncol 2003; 21:2651–7.

57. Robbins RJ, Wan Q, Grewal RK, et al. Real-time prognosis for metastatic thyroid carcinoma based on 2-[18F]fluoro-2-deoxy-D-glucose-positron emission tomography scanning. J Clin Endocrinol Metab 2006;91:498–505.

58. Creach KM, Nussenbaum B, Siegel BA, et al. Thyroid carcinoma uptake of 18F-fluorodeoxyglucose in patients with elevated serum thyroglobulin and negative 131I scintigraphy. Am J Otolaryngol 2013; 34:51–6.

59. Smallridge RC, Ain KB, Asa SL, et al. American Thyroid Association guidelines for management of patients with anaplastic thyroid cancer. Thyroid 2012;22:1104–39.

60. Poisson T, Deandreis D, Leboulleux S, et al. 18F-fluorodeoxyglucose positron emission tomography and computed tomography in anaplastic thyroid cancer. Eur J Nucl Med Mol Imaging 2010;37: 2277–85.

61. Bogsrud TV, Karantanis D, Nathan MA, et al. 18F-FDG PET in the management of patients with anaplastic thyroid carcinoma. Thyroid 2008;18: 713–9.

62. Roman S, Lin R, Sosa JA. Prognosis of medullary thyroid carcinoma: demographic, clinical, and pathologic predictors of survival in 1252 cases. Cancer 2006;107:2134–42.

63. You YN, Lakhani V, Wells SA Jr, et al. Medullary thyroid cancer. Surg Oncol Clin N Am 2006;15: 639–60.

64. Al-Rawi M, Wheeler MH. Medullary thyroid carcinoma—update and present management controversies. Ann R Coll Surg Engl 2006;88:433–8.

65. Treglia G, Villani MF, Giordano A, et al. Detection rate of recurrent medullary thyroid carcinoma using fluorine-18 fluorodeoxyglucose positron emission tomography: a meta-analysis. Endocrine 2012;42: 535–45.

66. Cheng X, Bao L, Xu Z, et al. 18F-FDG-PET and (1)(8)F-FDG-PET/CT in the detection of recurrent or metastatic medullary thyroid carcinoma: a systematic review and meta-analysis. J Med Imaging Radiat Oncol 2012;56:136–42.

67. Ong SC, Schoder H, Patel SG, et al. Diagnostic accuracy of 18F-FDG PET in restaging patients with medullary thyroid carcinoma and elevated calcitonin levels. J Nucl Med 2007;48:501–7.

68. Oudoux A, Salaun PY, Bournaud C, et al. Sensitivity and prognostic value of positron emission tomography with F-18-fluorodeoxyglucose and sensitivity of immunoscintigraphy in patients with medullary thyroid carcinoma treated with anticarcinoembryonic antigen-targeted radioimmunotherapy. J Clin Endocrinol Metab 2007;92:4590–7.

69. Rubello D, Rampin L, Nanni C, et al. The role of 18F-FDG PET/CT in detecting metastatic deposits of recurrent medullary thyroid carcinoma: a prospective study. Eur J Surg Oncol 2008;34:581–6.

70. de Groot JW, Links TP, Jager PL, et al. Impact of 18F-fluoro-2-deoxy-D-glucose positron emission tomography (FDG-PET) in patients with biochemical evidence of recurrent or residual medullary thyroid cancer. Ann Surg Oncol 2004;11:786–94.

71. Verbeek HH, Plukker JT, Koopmans KP, et al. Clinical relevance of 18F-FDG PET and 18F-DOPA PET in recurrent medullary thyroid carcinoma. J Nucl Med 2012;53:1863–71.

72. Bogsrud TV, Karantanis D, Nathan MA, et al. The prognostic value of 2-deoxy-2-[18F]fluoro-D-glucose positron emission tomography in patients with suspected residual or recurrent medullary thyroid carcinoma. Mol Imaging Biol 2010;12: 547–53.

73. Pagano L, Sama MT, Morani F, et al. Thyroid incidentaloma identified by 18F-fluorodeoxyglucose positron emission tomography with CT (FDG-PET/CT): clinical and pathological relevance. Clin Endocrinol (Oxf) 2011;75:528–34.

74. Nishimori H, Tabah R, Hickeson M, et al. Incidental thyroid "PETomas": clinical significance and novel description of the self-resolving variant of focal FDG-PET thyroid uptake. Can J Surg 2011;54:83–8.

75. Yi JG, Marom EM, Munden RF, et al. Focal uptake of fluorodeoxyglucose by the thyroid in patients undergoing initial disease staging with combined PET/CT for non-small cell lung cancer. Radiology 2005;236: 271–5.

76. Choi JY, Lee KS, Kim HJ, et al. Focal thyroid lesions incidentally identified by integrated 18F-FDG PET/CT: clinical significance and improved characterization. J Nucl Med 2006;47:609–15.

77. Treglia G, Bertagna F, Sadeghi R, et al. Focal thyroid incidental uptake detected by 18F-fluorodeoxyglucose positron emission tomography. Meta-analysis on prevalence and malignancy risk. Nuklearmedizin 2013;52:130–6.

78. Kim H, Kim SJ, Kim IJ, et al. Thyroid incidentalomas on FDG PET/CT in patients with non-thyroid

cancer - a large retrospective monocentric study. Onkologie 2013;36:260–4.

79. Bertagna F, Treglia G, Piccardo A, et al. F18-FDG-PET/CT thyroid incidentalomas: a wide retrospective analysis in three Italian centres on the significance of focal uptake and SUV value. Endocrine 2013;43:678–85.

80. Kurata S, Ishibashi M, Hiromatsu Y, et al. Diffuse and diffuse-plus-focal uptake in the thyroid gland identified by using FDG-PET: prevalence of thyroid cancer and Hashimoto's thyroiditis. Ann Nucl Med 2007;21:325–30.

81. Karantanis D, Bogsrud TV, Wiseman GA, et al. Clinical significance of diffusely increased 18F-FDG uptake in the thyroid gland. J Nucl Med 2007;48:896–901.

82. Chen W, Parsons M, Torigian DA, et al. Evaluation of thyroid FDG uptake incidentally identified on FDG-PET/CT imaging. Nucl Med Commun 2009;30:240–4.

Radiotherapy Planning

Minh Tam Truong, MD*, Nataliya Kovalchuk, PhD

KEYWORDS

- PET/CT • Radiotherapy planning • Intensity-modulated radiotherapy • Deformable registration
- Image guided therapy • Cone beam computed tomography

KEY POINTS

- PET/computed tomography (CT) is a functional imaging tool which may improve the accuracy of target volume delineation for radiotherapy planning by defining a metabolic tumor volume in addition to morphologic imaging and clinical examination findings.
- Conformal radiotherapy techniques rely on accurate delineation of the target volume to ensure coverage of the tumor with the prescribed radiation dose, while sparing adjacent normal tissue.
- PET/CT is used in conjunction with other advanced imaging techniques, and image registration methods assist in target volume delineation.
- Pathologic correlative studies demonstrate that PET/CT-based tumor volumes are more accurate than CT alone for numerous sites.
- Optimal autosegmentation methods for radiotherapy planning remain to be determined.

INTRODUCTION

Over the past decade, there has been increasing integration of fluorine-18-flurodeoxyglucose (F18-FDG)-PET into computed tomography (CT)-based radiotherapy planning alongside 3-dimensional conformal radiotherapy (3DCRT) and intensity-modulated radiotherapy (IMRT). PET/CT has provided the radiation oncologist with a functional imaging tool to accurately define the metabolic tumor volume in addition to anatomic imaging and clinical examination to improve the accuracy of contouring the tumor. Both 3DCRT and IMRT rely on accurate delineation of the tumor volume to ensure coverage of the tumor with the prescribed radiation dose, while sparing adjacent normal tissue. The goal of radiotherapy planning is to ensure reproducible and accurate delivery of radiation dose for the duration of fractionated treatment, while sparing the normal organs at risk from acute and late radiation injury. As radiation planning and treatment delivery have advanced to allow improved conformity of radiation dose to the target and improved accuracy of treatment set up with image-guided therapy, these innovations have allowed potential reduction in treatment margins and sharper dose gradients between the target and adjacent normal tissue. Therefore, accurate target definition of the gross tumor has become a critically important step in the treatment planning process. Integrating PET/CT into oncologic management includes assisting accurate diagnosis and staging to determine the tumor extent, regional lymphadenopathy, and detection of distant metastases or second primary tumors. PET/CT imaging also plays an important role in radiotherapy planning and has been rapidly adopted into routine clinical practice over the past decade. A survey study of 1600 radiation oncologists in the United States, with 386 respondents, showed that utilization of advanced imaging technologies including PET/CT, MRI, 4-dimensional CT, and functional MRI by physicians using any form of advanced technology for target volume delineation in their practice was 94.3%. The most common imaging modalities used were FDG-PET in 78.3% and MRI in 73.1%. FDG-PET was used most commonly in lung and head (89.0%) and neck malignancies (88.3%). In

The author has nothing to disclose.
Department of Radiation Oncology, Boston Medical Center, Boston University School of Medicine, Moakley Building, LL238, 830 Harrison Avenue, Boston, MA 02445, USA
* Corresponding author.
E-mail address: Minh-tam.truong@bmc.org

this study, it was shown that the percentage of respondents using both modalities was 90.9%. Among the physicians surveyed, 14.5% reported using such imaging in more than 50% of their cases, and 8.3% used it routinely in more than 75% of their patients.[1] Many studies have demonstrated improved target volume delineation using PET/CT for radiotherapy planning over PET or CT alone across multiple sites. However, many different registration and segmentation methods exist and controversy still lies in determining which method is superior. This article outlines the integration of PET/CT into multiple cancer sites for radiotherapy planning.

RADIOTHERAPY TECHNIQUES: 3-DIMENSIONAL CONFORMAL RADIOTHERAPY, INTENSITY-MODULATED RADIOTHERAPY, AND STEREOTACTIC BODY RADIOTHERAPY

Over the past 2 decades 3DCRT techniques and IMRT have become standard radiation techniques since the widespread integration of CT into treatment planning. In 3DCRT, treatment planning is performed by choosing radiation beam directions that would best target the tumor and spare the normal structures and shaping each beam with multileaf collimator (MLC) to fit the profile of the target with margin on the digitally reconstructed radiographs. IMRT is a next generation 3DCRT, which allows multiple static or dynamic MLC segments during radiation delivery. These segments shape the intensity of radiation creating sharp dose gradients to deliver uniform and conformal dose to the tumor while sparing adjacent normal tissues which was previously not possible with 3DCRT. For IMRT, beam optimization is done by inverse planning whereby the computer performs hundreds to thousands of computerized iterations.[2] A course of conventional external beam radiotherapy uses small daily fractionated doses of 1.8 to 2 Gy delivered to the tumor with margin, typically over 5 to 7 weeks of treatment. Stereotactic body radiotherapy (SBRT) is another specialized form of conformal radiotherapy using the principles of stereotactic radiosurgery (applied extracranially). SBRT is delivered in a single high dose of radiation or short course of radiotherapy in 5 fractions or less. Primary applications for SBRT include inoperable early stage lung cancers, oligometastases of the spine and liver, and pancreatic and recurrent head and neck cancer.[3] The advantage of SBRT is the ability to escalate radiation dose to the tumor, while maintaining maximal normal tissue sparing to minimize toxicity. SBRT relies on real-time imaged guidance systems to ensure accurate localization and may also compensate for patient external motion and internal tumor motion, and delivers high precision beams without the use of an invasive stereotactic frame.[4]

SIMULATION

To deliver an optimal radiotherapy treatment, a process of simulation and radiotherapy planning takes place before starting treatment. CT scanners used for radiotherapy are modified to contain flat table top for modeling the flat table in treatment room, large bore for the ability to scan the patient with the immobilization devices and lasers for the placement of the treatment isocenter. During simulation the patient is immobilized in the treatment position and then a CT is acquired. Various immobilization devices may be used, such as a custom thermoplastic mask for patients with head and neck cancer (**Fig. 1**); in the chest or abdomen, a custom polystyrene bead vacuum mold may be used to immobilize the patient during simulation and treatment. An isocenter is a reference point defined on planning CT set at the time of simulation and used to set up the patient for each daily treatment. Three-dimensional coordinates of CT-defined isocenter are sent from CT scanner to the wall and ceiling lasers in CT room to mark the lasers intersections with patient surface. Tattoos are usually permanently marked on the patient's skin to allow reproducibility of the patient on a daily basis. Alternatively, the isocenter may also be marked on a custom aquaplast mask for head and neck patients. Lasers are mounted on the walls of the treatment room, simulator, and PET/CT suite and calibrated so that patients may be aligned to an isocenter reference point that is used to reproduce the treatment set up on a daily basis.

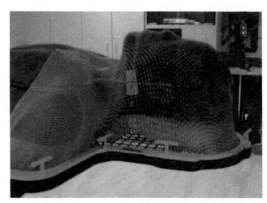

Fig. 1. Immobilization for head and neck intensity-modulated radiotherapy using a thermoplastic head and neck mask. Lasers are used for daily alignment.

PET/COMPUTED TOMOGRAPHY SIMULATION

Ideally, a PET/CT performed in the planning position ensures the greatest accuracy in terms of registration of PET/CT images with the radiotherapy planning CT. Using a PET/CT for radiotherapy planning requires full commissioning of the PET/CT unit and quality assurance tests similar to those applied to radiotherapy CT simulators and adjustments to the PET/CT unit, including lasers for alignment and a flatbed table top. Quality assurance tests are performed to ensure data integrity of the whole pathway of data acquisition and transfer from the PET/CT unit to the radiotherapy treatment planning unit.[5]

At our institution, a dedicated PET/CT performed for radiation treatment planning is performed on a flat bed with the same immobilization devices intended for the treatment set up. The scan may be performed in conjunction with a diagnostic whole body scan or as a separate, limited examination of the intended treatment region. An initial noncontrast CT simulation for isocenter placement and fabrication of any custom immobilization is performed before undergoing the planning PET/CT scan. The patients then undergo a dedicated PET/CT scan with a diagnostic quality, contrast-enhanced CT of the region of interest. Patients are fasted and are injected with a standard dose of 15 to 20 mCi of 18-FDG. A dedicated PET/CT radiation planning scan is then performed with CT images using a slice thickness of 1.25 mm, a 256 PET matrix, and 60 mL of noniodinated intravenous contrast agent.[6] In a study evaluating PET/CT for radiotherapy planning, increased set up time of approximately 7 minutes is required for both lung cancer and head and neck patients, and also affects the workflow of a nuclear medicine and radiotherapy department in terms of scheduling.[7]

IMAGE REGISTRATION METHODS

The CT simulation scan is the primary image set used for treatment planning and dose calculation. The PET, PET/CT, or MRI scans are secondary image sets that are fused or registered to the radiation planning CT. The secondary image sets are used to improve visualization of the target and the normal tissues to aid target definition and accurately contour avoidance structures. Two or more image sets are fused or co-registered to the planning CT. The accuracy of the registration is usually checked visually or evaluated by the physicist and radiation oncologist, and contours can be drawn on either image set. Image registration may be done by either rigid or deformable registration. Rigid registration uses 6 degrees of freedom (3 translations and 3 rotations). Deformable registration is a more comprehensive image registration method to solve the problem of significant temporal and anatomic differences between the imaging studies by estimating the spatial nonuniform and nonlinear relationships between the volume elements of corresponding structures across the imaging data. **Fig. 2** provides an example of deformable registration of the PET/CT to the planning CT and rigid registration of the MRI images with the planning CT. As a result, slight variation exists between the contouring of the gross tumor volume (GTV) on different image sets. Deformable registration uses algorithms to compute a deformation map of vector fields that connect the voxels in diagnostic CT images "hard-wired" to PET images with the corresponding voxels in treatment planning CT images, a process that accounts for nonlinear and nonuniform relationships between the image sets. Deformable registration techniques can be categorized as point based or intensity based.[8,9] Point-based techniques require user-provided identification and matching of image landmarks, such as points, curves, or surfaces of corresponding anatomic structures. Moreover, point-based methods are based on physical models to follow the changes in anatomy. This requires knowledge of material properties and demands heavy computational power.[10] Deformable registration may overcome positional and anatomic variation of 2 image sets of the same patient by deforming 1 scan to match the primary image set and may greatly improve the utility of a diagnostic PET scan which was not performed in treatment position and where repeating the PET/CT scan may not be feasible. In this setting, many commercially available deformable registration engines provide the option of region-of-interest based alignment to increase registration accuracy in the area of interest and save computation time. **Fig. 3** provides an example of deformable registration, whereby a bite block or intraoral stent was placed for CT simulation and the PET/CT scan is deformably registered to the planning CT scan to account for differences in position, particularly the tongue. As a result, the planning target volumes (PTVs) are slightly larger to account for potential differences in imaging and daily set up. Hwang and colleagues[11] demonstrated in a study of 12 head and neck cancer patients that it was possible to co-register a PET or PET/CT acquired in diagnostic position using rigid registration, although they cautioned its use in the neck for nodal target volumes. They found PET/CT more accurate than PET alone. The manual rigid registration error was measured at 3.2 mm for brain and 8.4 mm

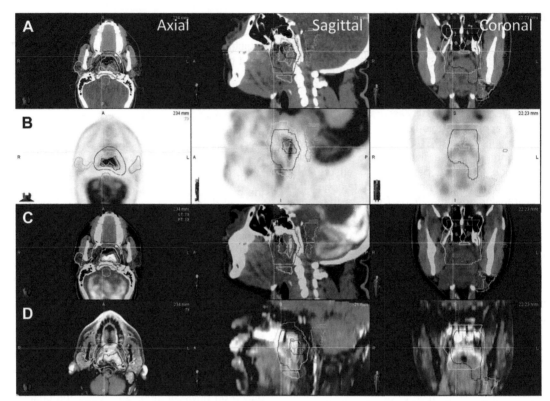

Fig. 2. Fusion of the radiotherapy planning CT with the positron emission tomography (PET)/CT and MRI to assist with target volume delineation. (*A*) Planning CT. (*B*) PET scan. (*C*) PET/CT. (*D*) MRI. The gross tumor volume (GTV) is contoured on all scans and a composite GTV is created based on imaging and clinical information. Adjacent normal organs, such as the bilateral parotid glands, are contoured.

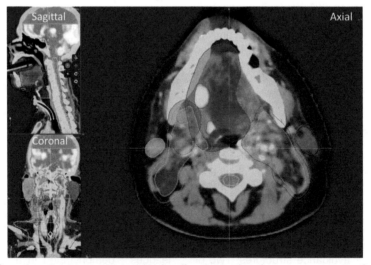

Fig. 3. Deformable registration in a patient with a locally advanced oral tongue cancer. On the treatment planning scan the patient has an intraoral stent or bite block (best seen on the sagittal plane) to assist in normal tissue sparing. The diagnostic positron emission tomography (PET)/CT is deformably registered to the planning CT. The gross tumor volume of the primary tumor is shown in red contour, and ipsilateral lymph node is outlined in light blue. The red colorwash represents the high-dose planning target volume (PTV). The light blue colorwash on the right neck represents the right elective nodal clinical target volume (CTV), and the left colorwash lilac volume represents the left nodal CTV. The bilateral parotids are also contoured (*yellow colorwash* [*left*], *purple colorwash* [*right*]).

for spinal cord using a diagnostic PET/CT. Deformable registration improved the accuracy with errors ranging from 1.1 to 5.4 mm.

In a study by Ireland and colleagues,[12] PET/CT was acquired in 5 head and neck cancer patients in both diagnostic and treatment planning positions and co-registered with the planning CT using both rigid and nonrigid (deformable) registration. They found significantly greater registration errors for rigid registration when using the treatment position PET/CT of 4.96 mm compared with 2.77 mm for deformable registration ($P = .001$). When using the diagnostic planning PET/CT, they found greater accuracy using deformable registration compared with the treatment position PET/CT using rigid registration. This study suggests that deformable registration of the PET/CT was more accurate for treatment planning, even when the PET/CT is acquired in diagnostic position. Deformable registration is also useful in the postoperative setting for head and neck cancer, where the preoperative PET/CT may be fused to the postoperative CT scan used for treatment planning. Because of the significant variations in patient positioning and alteration in anatomy after surgery, deformable registration of the preoperative PET/CT may assist in identifying the location of original primary and nodal disease in conjunction with pathologic information. When performing deformable registration of preoperative and postoperative imaging in the presence of large deformations, intensity-based deformable registration techniques based on voxel similarity measures (ie, sum of square gray value differences, cross-correlation, local correlation, or mutual information) are more suitable than point-based deformable registration techniques.[8]

Deformable registration may also assist in delineating prechemotherapy tumor volumes based on PET/CT scans before neoadjuvant chemotherapy for radiotherapy planning where significant changes in patient anatomy from weight loss and tumor shrinkage may occur after chemotherapy.[9]

Deformable registration methods require validation and continue to evolve so that PET/CT and PET/MRI data may be incorporated into radiotherapy treatment planning to improve the accuracy of tumor volume delineation.[13]

TREATMENT PLANNING

PET/CT data and CT simulation data are transferred to a treatment planning system. The image sets are registered either by rigid or deformable registration. The radiation oncologist defines the GTV using all the available diagnostic information including clinical examination and diagnostic imaging (PET/CT, MR, CT) to accurately define the tumor

on the CT simulation scan. Based on the GTV, volumetric expansions of 5 to 15 mm are usually created from the GTV to form a clinical target volume (CTV) to account for microscopic tumor spread and to ensure coverage of subclinical or suspected disease sites. In lung and gastrointestinal tumors, an internal target volume[14,15] may also be defined to account for internal physiologic movement, such as breathing, which can alter the position, shape, and size of the CTV. A final additional 3- to 5-mm expansion to CTV creates the PTV. The PTV accounts for treatment set up errors and tumor motion both during each treatment (intrafraction) and between treatments (interfraction).[16] The radiation oncologist also defines the adjacent organs at risk, such as the brainstem, spinal cord and parotid glands (see **Figs. 2** and **3**) by contouring these organs and defining dose limits based on published guidelines and literature on tolerance doses for normal tissue. Usually, 5 to 9 beams are arranged for IMRT planning, with the intensities of each beam being modulated during delivery to maximize coverage of the tumor while minimizing radiation to adjacent normal tissue. **Fig. 4** demonstrates an IMRT plan for a nasopharyngeal cancer patient with isodoses overlaid on the planning CT scan in the axial, coronal, and sagittal planes, as well as dose volume histograms, which summarize the radiation dose to the targets and normal tissues. Daily treatments are verified by image guidance before beam delivery. Image guidance systems include electronic portal imaging with both megavoltage and kilovoltage x-rays, and cone beam CT. **Fig. 5** demonstrates comparing the cone beam CT with the radiation plan, which is done before delivering the treatment.

EFFECT OF PET/COMPUTED TOMOGRAPHY ON GROSS TUMOR VOLUME DEFINITION

Over the past decade, there has been an intense interest and rapidly increasing utilization of PET/CT imaging in radiotherapy treatment planning for multiple cancer sites.[1] Many single institutional studies have examined the impact of PET and/or PET/CT on GTV delineation for radiotherapy planning. The majority of studies demonstrate the superiority of PET/CT over PET or CT alone for diagnosis, staging, and consistency of target volume definition in terms of intraobserver and interobserver variability.[17–19]

PET/COMPUTED TOMOGRAPHY PLANNING FOR HEAD AND NECK CANCER

When using PET/CT for head and neck radiotherapy planning, standardization of the procedure

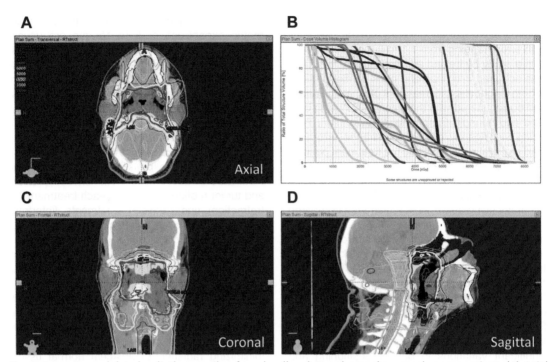

Fig. 4. Intensity-modulated radiotherapy plan for a locally advanced nasopharyngeal cancer patient. (*A*) Axial plane planning CT with overlay of radiation isodose lines. (*C*) Coronal and (*D*) sagittal images. (*B*) Dose volume histogram summarizing the radiation dose coverage to target volumes and normal organs at risk. The red isodose line represents the prescription dose—69.96 Gy. The bilateral parotid glands in blue colorwash are spared with the 26-Gy isodose line wrapping around the medial edge of the bilateral parotid glands. The brainstem, spinal cord, optic structures, oral cavity, larynx, esophagus, pharyngeal constrictors, and other organs at risk are also spared.

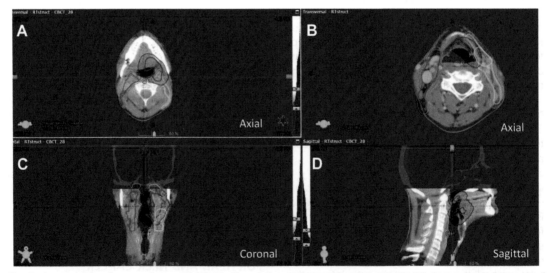

Fig. 5. An example of a cone beam CT (CBCT; *A*) and the radiation planning CT (*B*). (*C*) Coronal and (*D*) sagittal views with the CBCT overlaid on the CT simulation scan. CBCTs are used as part of daily image guidance to verify treatment set up before treatment delivery.

is needed to ensure that the PET/CT unit is modified to accommodate radiotherapy planning in terms of using a flat top couch, external lasers in the PET/CT unit, and using the same immobilization with the custom thermoplastic mask for head and neck cancer patients made during simulation.[5]

PET AND GROSS TUMOR VOLUME DEFINITION FOR HEAD AND NECK CANCER

The accuracy of staging using imaging can alter management in terms of decision making regarding treatment modality and also change target volumes for radiotherapy planning and dose. A study by Abramyuk and colleagues[20] demonstrated alteration in staging in 102 untreated head and neck cancer with respect to TNM staging; PET/CT resulted in downstaging in 36 patients and upstaging in 10 patients for T stage, whereas for N stage, 8 patients were upstaged and 27 patients were downstaged. PET/CT was able to identify metastases in 13 of 102 patients.

Studies have examined the relative value of PET to other imaging modalities, including CT and MRI for target delineation of the GTV. In a study by Daisne and colleagues,[21] diagnostic CT, MRI, and PET/CT were correlated with pathologic surgical specimens in 9 patients with pharyngeal and laryngeal cancer. In this study, the PET/CT tumor volumes were reduced compared to CT- and MRI-based volumes. The PET/CT correlated most accurately with the surgical specimen, although none of the imaging studies were able to determine the superficial extension of the tumor. In a correlation study of PET/CT with pathologic data in 23 head and neck cancer patients, Murakami and colleagues[22] demonstrated that the maximum standardized uptake value (SUV_{max}) overlapped in lymph nodes less than 15 mm diameter for both pathologically positive and negative nodes. Using a sized-based SUV_{max} cutoff of 1.9, 2.5, and 3.0 for lymph nodes less than 10 mm, 10 to 15 mm, and greater than 15 mm, respectively, PET/CT yielded a sensitivity of 79% and specificity of 99% for nodal staging. El-Bassiouni and colleagues[23] found that the CT-based GTVs were greater than the PET-based GTV in 72% of cases, and smaller in 28% of cases in a study of 25 head and neck cancer patients. Few studies demonstrate larger GTVs with PET/CT- than CT-based GTVs,[24,25] although most series generally demonstrating smaller GTVs for the primary tumor when using PET/CT compared with CT alone.[26–30] For delineation of nodal volumes, PET/CT and CT alone demonstrate good correlation with pathologic specimens. PET/CT estimates accurately lymph node volume, but has no added value over CT alone for target delineation.[31]

In a retrospective study of 53 head and neck cancer patients, contrast-enhanced CT alone was compared with PET/CT. The sensitivity of PET-GTV for identifying the primary tumor was 96%; CT-based GTV was 81% (P<.01). In patients with oropharyngeal cancer and tongue cancer, the corresponding sensitivities were 71% and 63%, respectively.[32]

Schinagl and colleagues[33] studied 5 different segmentation methods for FDG-PET target volume definition in 78 head and neck cancer patients, including visual determination, applying a fixed SUV threshold of 2.5, using a fixed threshold of 40% and 50% of the maximum signal intensity, and applying an adaptive threshold based on the signal-to-background ratio. The GTVs were analyzed comparatively. In this study, using an SUV threshold of 2.5 failed to identify the GTV in most of the cases, because the PET-defined GTV was too great compared with the CT-defined GTV. Segmentation methods using 40% and 50% thresholds produced volumes smaller than CT-based GTV. The 50% threshold technique and the adaptive threshold technique seemed to show similar overlapping volumes.

In a series of 8 head and neck cancer patients, Ford and colleagues[34] used an automatic segmentation technique set at progressively greater thresholds and the tumor volumes generated were compared with CT-based GTVs contoured by a physician. The study found that PET-based contours were sensitive to the threshold contouring level and that a 5% change in threshold contour level could translate into a 200% increase in volume.

One of the common methods of PET segmentation used in clinical practice is the threshold value based on SUVs adapted to the signal-to-background ratio described by Daisne and colleagues.[35] In a study by Perez-Romasanta and associates,[36] 19 head and neck cancer patients with 39 lesions underwent contouring using PET/CT done by SUV threshold definition. The threshold value was adapted to the signal-to-background ratio. In this work, the authors determined the relationship between the threshold and the signal-to-background ratio using a phantom study. A discrepancy index was calculated between PET and CT; an overlap fraction and a mismatch fraction were calculated for each lesion and imaging modality. The median discrepancy index for lymph nodes was 2.67 and 1.76 for primary lesions. The overlap factor values were greater for

CT volumes than for PET volumes (P<.001) for primary and lymph node lesions. The mismatch fraction was smaller for CT volumes than for PET volumes (P<.001) for primary and nodal lesions. The overlap factor for PET strongly correlated with lesion volume on CT for lymph nodes. The mismatch factor for PET/CT was negatively correlated with the lesion volume for metastatic lymph nodes. This study noted that PET scan image resolution affects the measured SUV of small lesions secondary to partial volume effects. Hence, for small lesions, inaccuracies may occur in SUV quantification and segmentation methods using threshold value adapted to the signal-to-background ratio.[36]

The discrepancy between studies on whether the PET/CT GTV is larger or smaller than CT-based volumes may depend on multiple factors, including interobserver and intraobserver variability,[18,19] segmentation methods, tumor site, and histology.

In a study by Chatterjee and colleagues,[37] variation of target volume definition when using CT versus PET/CT was studied in 20 oropharyngeal cancer patients in the treatment position. The target volumes were defined on contrast-enhanced CT scans by radiation oncologists who were blinded to the PET/CT scans. Another set of target volumes were outlined on the PET/CT dataset with input from diagnostic radiologists. In 17 of the 20 patients, the TNM stage remained the same when adding the FDG-PET data to the CT. PET prevented geographic miss in 1 patient and identified distant metastases in another patient. PET/CT GTVs were smaller than contrast-enhanced CT GTVs. Nodal targets were similar between PET/CT and CT alone.

The term *metabolic tumor volume* has evolved in the PET/CT literature as a potential surrogate for outcome in head and neck cancer and other solid malignancies.[38–42] Metabolic tumor volumes generally tend to be smaller than GTVs contoured by CT, although both GTV and metabolic tumor volumes are prognostic compared with SUV_{max}, where greater tumor volumes correlated with inferior local control and overall survival in head and neck cancer treated with IMRT.[39]

Although studies have shown that PET/CT can alter target definition, the impact of PET/CT radiotherapy planning on locorgeional control rates after radiotherapy have also been evaluated as PET/CT combined with outcome data become available. Vernon and colleagues[43] demonstrated a high rate of disease control and favorable toxicity profiles in 42 head and neck cancer patients who underwent PET/CT fusion-guided radiotherapy planning.

Evaluation of PET/CT for radiotherapy planning is currently being incorporated into multi-institutional, randomized trials; we await these results to determine the long-term impact of PET/CT in radiotherapy planning.[44]

ROLE OF PET/COMPUTED TOMOGRAPHY IN RECURRENT HEAD AND NECK CANCER FOR STEREOTACTIC BODY RADIOTHERAPY

Target volumes used in SBRT use small margins of 0 to 5 mm on the GTV to create the PTVs compared with 3DCRT and IMRT, because stereotactic localization of the target and real-time imaging minimize set up uncertainties. Hence, target definition for SBRT is critical to avoid marginal tumor miss and to minimize irradiating large volumes of adjacent normal tissue to high dose per fraction. In a retrospective study from the University of Pittsburgh, Wang and colleagues[45] included 96 patients with recurrent head and neck cancer who received previous radiation and were treated with SBRT. PET/CT planning was used for 45 patients (47%). Recurrences were defined in relation to the radiation fields, including in-field (>75% inside PTV), overlap (20%–75% inside PTV), marginal (<20% inside PTV but closest edge within 1 cm of PTV), or regional/distant (>1 cm from PTV). Patients who underwent PET/CT planning versus non-PET/CT planning had a significant improvement in overall failure-free survival (log-rank P = .037) and combined overlap or marginal failure-free survival (log-rank P = .037). Most failures were overlap or marginal failures (61.4%), which underscores the importance of accurate target volume delineation in SBRT treatment planning and highlights the role of PET/CT in facilitating accurate target volume delineation to minimizing near misses. **Fig. 6** provides an example of Cyberknife SBRT in a patient with recurrent head and neck cancer.

ADAPTIVE RADIOTHERAPY

Adaptive radiotherapy in head and neck cancer is of increasing interest because of anatomic and tumor changes in position and shape during radiotherapy which may be seen with image-guided therapy using cone beam CT. Integration of PET/CT into adaptive radiotherapy is of increasing interest, because PET/CT may potentially affect adaptive radiotherapy planning if there are changing areas of metabolic tumor volume during treatment. Biological information from PET assists GTV definition over morphologic imaging from CT and clinical examination findings alone, including defining metabolically active areas with FDG-PET, and alternative radiotracers may also be

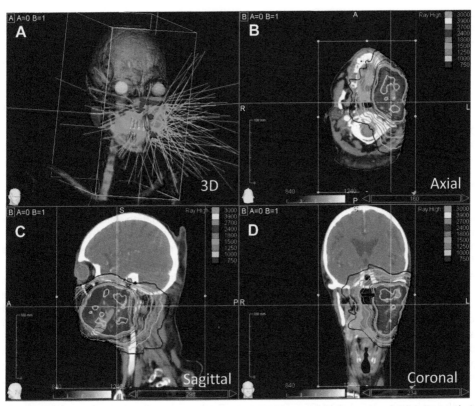

Fig. 6. Example of a Cyberknife stereotactic body radiotherapy plan with 3-dimensional reconstructed view (*A*): axial (*B*), sagittal (*C*), and coronal (*D*) images for a patient with recurrent head and neck cancer. The red colorwash represents the planning target volume with overlay of the radiation isodose lines. The top left panel shows the light blue lines, which represent the entry beams with a total of 139 beams. Normal organs, including the brainstem, spinal cord, oral cavity, optic structures, parotid glands, are also contoured as avoidance structures.

able to hypoxic areas and areas of proliferation. If these areas are identified consistently, potential dose escalation to radiation-resistant areas could be considered using IMRT dose painting techniques. In a comparative study of 10 patients using PET/CT at 3 sequential time points before and twice during radiotherapy, deformable registration was used to co-register the second and third PET/CT scans acquired during treatment.[46] By using serial imaging during radiotherapy, combined with IMRT replanning, it maybe possible to reduce normal tissue dose. Coverage of the target volumes may also improve when using PET/CT to re-plan during radiotherapy. Castadot and colleagues[47] evaluated 10 head and neck cancer patients with FDG-PET/CT before and after a mean dose of 14.2, 24.5, 35.0, and 44.9 Gy and then compared planned dose and delivered dose distributions, which took into account anatomic changes of the patient and tumor during treatment. In this study, there was an increase in delivered dose compared with the planned dose, which correlated with tumor shrinkage. This study demonstrates a novel use of PET/CT in adaptive

radiotherapy to identify changes in GTV during radiotherapy and how planned dose distributions differ from the actual dose delivered.

Finally, PET/CT may also be used to evaluate normal tissue dosimetry during radiotherapy. In a study of 49 patients with head and neck cancer treated with IMRT, FDG-PET imaging performed before and after treatment was used to delineate the parotid glands. It was noted that the parotid glands contracted after treatment, which corresponded with a decline in SUV mean of the glands. At a threshold of 32 Gy mean parotid dose, the SUV_{max} declined rapidly, which corresponds with the tolerance of the parotid gland for development of xerostomia.[48]

ALTERNATIVE TRACERS

Limitations of FDG-PET in being able to distinguish tumor from inflammation or define the radioresistant areas have led investigators to study alternative radiotracers. These include PET with [(18)F]-fluoromisonidazole (FMISO). FMISO characterizes hypoxic volumes in head and neck cancers, such that potential applications for radiotherapy planning include dose escalation to hypoxic regions using IMRT dose painting techniques and potentially improving tumor control probabilities by up to 17% without increasing expected complications.[49,50] However, accurate and reproducible target volume delineation of hypoxic tumor volumes has not been well-defined. In a study of 15 head and neck cancer patients who underwent FMISO PET/CT scans at 2, 3, and 4 hours after FMISO injection, PET segmentation methods were evaluated. In this study, the FMISO volumes were found to be significantly different at the different acquisition periods using fixed threshold, adaptive threshold, and fuzzy locally adaptive Bayesian methods. The hypoxic fraction was calculated using the ratio between the FMISO using the different segmentation methods and CT tumor volumes (which were manually contoured). In this study, there were large discrepancies found between the different segmentation methods. The best contrast was obtained using the FMISO scan 4 hours after injection.[51] Other studies using FMISO have examined the reproducibility of FMISO being able to identify tumor hypoxia quantitatively when images are acquired 4 hours after injection and 48 hours after.[52] In a study of 11 patients with nasopharyngeal carcinoma, 2 FMISO-PET/CT scans were done 48 hours apart and showed high reproducibility between scans in terms of determining the hypoxic volume in the tumor.[53]

Other radiotracers include Cu-diacetyl-bis(N4-methylthiosemicarbazone) [Cu-ATSM], which is a hypoxia-avid positron emitter radiotracer. In a study of 11 head and neck cancer patients, Cu-ATSM and F-FDGPET/CT scans were obtained before and after treatment. In this study, the authors investigated differences between early and late PET/CT scans and biologic tumor volume in radiotherapy treatment planning calculated between Cu-ATSM and F-FDG, There was no significant difference in the SUV_{max} between early and late imaging. F-FDG SUV_{max} before therapy was 15.6 ± 9.4, whereas F-FDG SUV_{max} after therapy was 1.5 ± 1.2. No differences were seen between the biologic tumor volume contoured with Cu-ATSM and F-FDG. According to this study, compared with F-FDG-PET/CT, Cu-ATSM scans were highly sensitive but had low specificity in predicting neoadjuvant chemoradiotherapy response.

Novel use of PET/CT as an in vivo dosimetry tool in radiotherapy delivery as a procedure to give immediate information regarding delivered dose from reconstructed PET images has also been studied. The potential role for PET scanners within the radiotherapy treatment console is currently being evaluated to verify treatment in proton therapy. PET acquisition performed immediately after treatment with shorter lived isotopes such as O15 and N13 may provide improved dosimetric data about actual dose delivered in the patients that were not available previously by other dose calculation algorithms.[33]

PET/COMPUTED TOMOGRAPHY PLANNING FOR LUNG CANCER

In lung cancer, PET/CT is an important tool in the diagnostic workup and staging for both small cell and non–small cell lung cancers.[21,54–56] Radiotherapy advances for non–small cell lung cancer include reduction of treatment volumes by reduction or elimination of elective nodal irradiation, dose escalation of the GTV with IMRT or SBRT. Owing to movement of the tumor with breathing, 4-dimensional CT and respiratory-gated radiotherapy play a role in improving the therapeutic ratio for radiotherapy treatment planning and delivery by improved accuracy in tumor delineation and reducing normal tissue in the radiation field by accounting for respiratory motion. In lung cancer, primary tumor volume delineation can be confounded by adjacent lung collapse or consolidation, where the edge of the tumor cannot be determined by contrast-enhanced CT alone. Furthermore, the volume and dose of normal lung irradiated impacts significantly on lung toxicity, including pneumonitis acutely and/or lung fibrosis in the long term. Radiation oncologists use dose volume histograms to analyze the mean lung dose and volume of lung receiving low doses of radiation at 5 and 20 Gy, because these parameters correlate with toxicity risk. Randomized data have demonstrated the role of FDG/PET in the staging of early stage lung cancer and may significantly change the staging and treatment plan, often upstaging the disease revealing regional lymph node metastases or distant metastases.[54–56] Integrating PET/CT into radiotherapy planning can alter the target volumes when compared with CT-based volumes and also reduce interuser variability of target volume delineation.[57] In a prospective study of 91 consecutive patients, with non–small cell lung carcinoma from 2003 to 2008, undergoing radiation therapy, PET imaging provided additional diagnostic information over CT alone in 20%, leading to upstaging in 17% and alterations in the PTV and subsequent treatment planning in 9%.[58] PET/CT is particularly helpful in distinguishing tumor from lung atelectasis and subsequently reducing the GTV of the primary.[59] PET/CT-assisted tumor volumes also reduces the risk of marginal miss and its use in radiotherapy outcomes demonstrate excellent control outcomes.[60]

However, when PET/CT detects nodal disease, the PTVs are usually increased, which may increase the mean lung dose (V20), esophageal, or cardiac dose.[24,61–72] Repeat PET/CT for radiotherapy planning performed within 120 days of an initial diagnostic PET/CT may upstage disease in up to one-half of cases by detecting nodal and distant metastatic disease, and hence change radiotherapy management significantly. SUV velocity, which is defined as $[(SUV_{scan2} - SUV_{scan1})/$ interscan interval in days, predicts the likelihood of upstaging.[73]

Four-dimensional PET/CT can improve the detection, resolution, and delineation of small lung tumors by controlling for respiratory motion, particularly in tumors located in the lower lobes.[74,75] Respiratory-gated PET/CT scans demonstrate smaller diameter lesions compared with nongated images, and may improve tumor detection because respiratory motion may decrease detection and degrade the quality of the image.[76] Improved delineation of lung tumors by PET/CT or identifying hypoxic regions using FMISO PET may allow the potential to escalate the radiotherapy dose without increasing normal tissue toxicity.[77,78]

Determining which threshold or segmentation method should be used for delineating the PET GTV for accurate target volume definition for lung cancer continues to be debated.[79] In a study by Biehl and colleagues,[80] using thresholds of 40% and 20% underestimated the CT-based GTV for 80% and 70% of lesions, respectively, such that they did not conclude that any single threshold criteria for delineating PET/GTV provided an accurate target volume definition.

Yu and colleagues[81] studied 15 patients with non–small cell lung cancer. Pathologic correlation with PET/CT was studied to determine optimal SUV cutoff criteria. The authors defined the optimal threshold or optimal absolute SUV as the value at which the PET GTV was the same as the pathologic GTV. The optimal threshold SUV was 31% ± 11% and the absolute SUV was 3.0 ± 1.6. The optimal threshold was inversely proportional to the pathologic GTV and tumor diameter. The absolute SUV did not correlate significantly with the pathologic GTV or tumor diameter.

Another study showed that the adaptive 50%, adaptive 41%, threshold-based, and contrast-enhanced delineation methods showed good agreement with pathology, whereas CT delineation showed a significant overestimation compared with pathology.[82]

A prospective, phase II, multicenter trial, the Radiation Therapy Oncology Group (RTOG) trial 0515 evaluated the impact of PET/CT compared with CT alone on radiation treatment plans with the primary endpoint being the impact of PET/CT fusion on treatment plans, and secondary endpoint was regional failure. In 47 evaluable patients of 52 accrued, the GTV was smaller for PET/CT-derived volumes (98.7 vs 86.2 mL; P<.0001) and the mean lung dose for PET/CT plans were slightly lower (19 vs 17.8 Gy; P = .06). There was no difference in the number of involved nodes (2.1 vs 2.4), V20 (32% vs 30.8%), or mean esophageal dose (28.7 vs 27.1 Gy). Nodal contours were altered by PET/CT for 51% of patients. One patient (2%) developed an elective nodal failure. This multicenter study concluded that PET/CT-derived tumor volumes were smaller than those derived by CT alone and changed nodal GTV contours in 51% of patients. The elective nodal failure rate for GTVs derived from PET/CT was low, supporting the RTOG standard of limiting the target volume to the primary tumor and involved nodes.[83]

PET/COMPUTED TOMOGRAPHY PLANNING FOR GASTROINTESTINAL MALIGNANCIES

FDG-PET/CT is part of the standard workup of a number of gastrointestinal malignancies, including esophageal, gastric, rectal, and anal carcinomas. In esophageal carcinoma, using PET/CT for radiotherapy planning seems to improve target volume definition over CT alone, allows better normal tissue sparing of the heart and lungs, and potentially reduces the risk of marginal tumor miss. Studies show modification of treatment plans when using PET/CT compared with CT alone.[84–87] Fig. 7 provides an example of PET/CT used in esophageal cancer radiation treatment planning. In a contrary report, Shimizu and colleagues[88] showed that PET/CT, when correlated with surgical specimens, did not improve the detection of occult subclinical lymph node metastases, and concluded that PET/CT should not be used for CTV definition when 1-cm margins are used. However, typically for definitive radiation therapy, the craniocaudal margins of 3 to 5 cm are still used for defining CTVs, because esophageal cancer has a propensity for submucosal spread and occult periesophageal metastases are still encompassed in the radiotherapy field.

In gastrointestinal malignancies, endoscopic staging is particularly important to determine treatment strategy. In a study by Konski and colleagues,[89] 25 patients with esophageal cancer were evaluated with PET and endoscopic ultrasonography compared with the CT simulation. The length of the tumor measured by endoscopic ultrasound was compared with the CT- and PET-defined tumor length (using a SUV of 2.5). The length of the tumors was significantly longer by

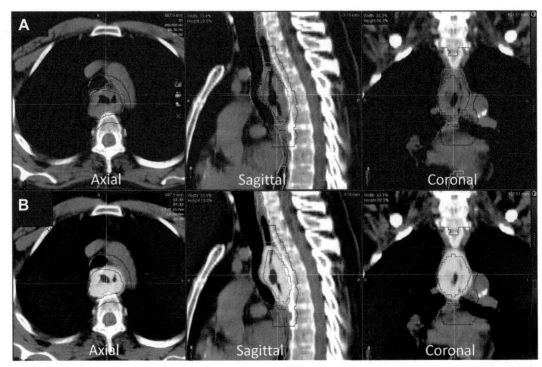

Fig. 7. An example of fusion of the planning CT (*A*) and positron emission tomography (PET)/CT (*B*) for esophageal cancer radiotherapy target volume delineation. The top panel represents the radiotherapy planning scan and the bottom panel is the PET/CT with deformable registration to the planning CT. The blue line represents the CT contoured gross tumor volume, and the pink line represents the 38% SUV threshold autosegmented tumor volume. The brown line represents the planning target volume.

CT compared with PET ($P = .0063$). The length determined by PET correlated better with the endoscopic ultrasonography tumor length. Endoscopic ultrasonography detected more periesophageal and celiac lymphadenopathy compared with PET and CT. The SUV of the esophageal tumors was found to be greater in patients with periesophageal lymphadenopathy identified on PET scans. Based on this study, integration of PET and endoscopic ultrasonography can significantly aid the delineation of the GTV in patients with esophageal carcinoma compared with CT alone.

In a study by Gondi and colleagues,[67] 16 patients with esophageal cancer underwent FDG-PET/CT radiotherapy planning scan. The PET GTV margin was defined by standardizing the liver PET activity in all images. They compared the CT and PET/CT GTVs quantitatively by using a conformality index, defined as the ratio of the 2 GTVs to their union. The mean index of conformality was 0.46 (range, 0.13–0.80). In 62.5% of the patients, FDG-PET data led to the definition of a smaller GTV.

Investigations into alternative molecular markers to FDG are currently being investigated, such as 3-deoxy-3-18F-fluorothymidine (FLT) PET to determine whether improvements in the detection and accuracy of the primary tumor and

regional lymph node metastases can be gained over FDG-PET. In study by Han and colleagues,[90] 22 patients underwent FLT PET and FDG/PET and then correlated it with pathologic examination. The FDG-PET used an SUV of 2.5, and FLT PET used an SUV of 1.4 as the best estimate to determine pathologic length of the tumor. When comparing FLT/PET- with FDG/PET-defined tumor volumes, when using a 7-field IMRT plan, potential improvements in normal tissue dosimetry to the lungs and the heart were demonstrated with the FLT/PET-defined GTVs.

The time between diagnostic PET/CT scans and radiotherapy is critical when using PET/CT to define tumor volumes, because esophageal cancers may progress rapidly such that, if the time interval between diagnostic PET/CT scanning and radiotherapy scanning occurs, then repeat PET/CT should be considered to account for progression of disease. In a study of 45 patients with esophageal cancer, repeat PET/CT was performed for radiotherapy planning with a median scan interval of 22 days; 31% of patients showed tumor length progression of more than 1 cm, and TNM progression was found in 27% of patients, including mediastinal nodal disease (18%) and distant metastases (13%).[91] Four-dimensional

PET/CT is also being applied to esophageal tumors because respiratory motion may also affect the accuracy of tumor volume delineation of esophageal tumors.[92]

GYNECOLOGIC MALIGNANCIES

PET/CT has been incorporated into the staging and radiotherapy planning and management for gynecologic cancers, particularly cervical cancer. PET/CT is a sensitive method to detect nodal metastases and can target volumes for radiotherapy planning. In particular, paraaortic lymph nodes and inguinal lymph nodes, which are not usually encompassed in the traditional elective pelvic nodal fields, can be detected by PET/CT and potentially lead to enlargement of radiotherapy fields. PET/CT detection of involved lymph nodes may also allow dose escalation using IMRT. PET/CT is being used as an imaging tool to assist brachytherapy planning for cervical cancer.[93,94]

GENITOURINARY MALIGNANCIES

PET/CT with (18)F- or (11)C-choline or (18)F- or (11)C-acetate are used as tracers for prostate cancer, reflecting the phospholipid metabolism. These tracers are being studied with PET/CT as emerging tools for localizing prostate cancer.[95] Studies evaluating 11C-choline PET/CT for prostate recurrences associated with prostate-specific antigen biochemical failure are gaining momentum as a restaging tool. Studies are also evaluating its potential role in radiotherapy planning to localize and delineate recurrences.[95,96] In a study of 83 prostate cancer patients with biochemical recurrence after radical primary treatment that demonstrated lesions on 11C-choline PET/CT in regional lymph nodes were treated with simultaneous integrated boost high-dose hypofractionated radiotherapy technique using helical tomotherapy. Metabolic response was evaluated with a repeat 11C-choline PET/CT. In this study, it was demonstrated that it is feasible to use 11C-choline PET/CT to restage, perform radiotherapy planning for regional nodal recurrences, and assess metabolic response to the area treated with radiotherapy.[97] Feasibility studies using choline PET/CT to assess regional nodal disease in intermediate- to high-risk newly diagnosed prostate cancer patients and to aid dose escalation are also being evaluated.[98–101] A study evaluated 61 newly diagnosed intermediate- to high-risk prostate cancer patients with 11C-choline PET/CT. Uptake in the regional lymph nodes with 11C-choline were considered invaded, regardless of their size. Bone lesions were considered positive when they showed greater focal uptake than the surrounding bone. All patients demonstrated prostate gland uptake (20 focal, 8 bifocal, and 33 multifocal). Extraprostatic disease was detected in 24.6%. Patients with locoregional and oligometastatic disease were selected to undergo IMRT with dose escalation based on the PET findings.[99]

SUMMARY

Incorporating PET/CT in radiotherapy planning is becoming part of the standard of care in head and neck, lung, and gastrointestinal malignancies to assist in accurate tumor volume delineation in conjunction with other imaging modalities and clinical examination findings. PET/CT is an emerging imaging tool with applications in gynecologic malignancies and prostate cancer. Overall, PET/CT results in modifications of the GTV when compared with a GTV defined by CT or PET alone. Pathologic correlative studies indicate that PET/CT is more accurate compared with CT alone for numerous sites, although most would advocate the use of PET/CT as a complimentary study in addition to other imaging modalities and clinical examination. Optimal autosegmentation methods for radiotherapy planning remain to be determined. PET/CT is used in conjunction with other advanced imaging techniques, including 4-dimensional CT and deformable registration methods. Novel use of PET/CT as an in-vivo dosimetry tool shows promise, and its use as a replanning tool to redefine changing GTVs during radiotherapy as part of adaptive radiotherapy may become the future standard of integrated PET/CT radiotherapy planning.

REFERENCES

1. Simpson DR, Lawson JD, Nath SK, et al. Utilization of advanced imaging technologies for target delineation in radiation oncology. J Am Coll Radiol 2009;6(12):876–83.
2. Xia P, Amols HI, Ling CC. Three-dimensional conformal radiotherapy and intensity-modulated radiotherapy. In: Leibel SA, editor. Phillips TL textbook of radiation oncology. 2nd edition. , Philadelphia: Elsevier Inc; 2004. p. 163–5.
3. Truong MT, Grillone G, Tschoe C, et al. Emerging applications of stereotactic radiotherapy in head and neck cancer. Neurosurg Focus 2009;27(6):E11.
4. Adler JR Jr, Murphy MJ, Chang SD, et al. Image-guided robotic radiosurgery. Neurosurgery 1999;44(6):1299–306 [discussion: 1306-7].

5. Thomas CM, Pike LC, Hartill CE, et al. Specific recommendations for accurate and direct use of PET-CT in PET guided radiotherapy for head and neck sites. Med Phys 2014;41(4):041710.

6. Subramaniam RM, Truong M, Peller P, et al. Fluorodeoxyglucose-positron-emission tomography imaging of head and neck squamous cell Cancer. AJNR Am J Neuroradiol 2009;31(4):598–604.

7. Sam S, Shon IH, Vinod SK, et al. Workflow and radiation safety implications of (18)F-FDG PET/CT scans for radiotherapy planning. J Nucl Med Technol 2012;40(3):175–7.

8. Kovalchuk N, Jalisi S, Subramaniam RM, et al. Deformable registration of preoperative PET/CT with postoperative radiation therapy planning CT in head and neck cancer. Radiographics 2012; 32(5):1329–41.

9. Schoenfeld JD, Kovalchuk N, Subramaniam RM, et al. PET/CT of cancer patients: part 2, deformable registration imaging before and after chemotherapy for radiation treatment planning in head and neck cancer. AJR Am J Roentgenol 2012; 199(5):968–74.

10. Xing L, Siebers J, Keall P. Computational challenges for image-guided radiation therapy: framework and current research. Semin Radiat Oncol 2007;17(4):245–57.

11. Hwang AB, Bacharach SL, Yom SS, et al. Can positron emission tomography (PET) or PET/Computed Tomography (CT) acquired in a nontreatment position be accurately registered to a head-and-neck radiotherapy planning CT? Int J Radiat Oncol Biol Phys 2009;73(2):578–84.

12. Ireland RH, Dyker KE, Barber DC, et al. Nonrigid image registration for head and neck cancer radiotherapy treatment planning with PET/CT. Int J Radiat Oncol Biol Phys 2007;68(3):952–7.

13. Leibfarth S, Mönnich D, Welz S, et al. A strategy for multimodal deformable image registration to integrate PET/MR into radiotherapy treatment planning. Acta Oncol 2013;52(7):1353–9.

14. Chavaudra J, Bridier A. Definition of volumes in external radiotherapy: ICRU reports 50 and 62. Cancer Radiother 2001;5(5):472–8 [in French].

15. Stroom JC, Heijmen BJ. Geometrical uncertainties, radiotherapy planning margins, and the ICRU-62 report. Radiother Oncol 2002;64(1):75–83.

16. International Commission on Radiation Units & Measurements. Prescribing, recording and reporting photon beam therapy (Supplement to ICRU Report 50), ICRU report 62. Bethesda (MD): ICRU; 1999. ISBN: 0-913394-61-0.

17. Ishikita T, Oriuchi N, Higuchi T, et al. Additional value of integrated PET/CT over PET alone in the initial staging and follow up of head and neck malignancy. Ann Nucl Med 2010;24(2):77–82.

18. Riegel AC, Berson AM, Destian S, et al. Variability of gross tumor volume delineation in head-and-neck cancer using CT and PET/CT fusion. Int J Radiat Oncol Biol Phys 2006;65(3):726–32.

19. Berson AM, Stein NF, Riegel AC, et al. Variability of gross tumor volume delineation in head-and-neck cancer using PET/CT fusion, Part II: the impact of a contouring protocol. Med Dosim 2009;34(1):30–5.

20. Abramyuk A, Appold S, Zöphel K, et al. Modification of staging and treatment of head and neck cancer by FDG-PET/CT prior to radiotherapy. Strahlenther Onkol 2013;189(3):197–201.

21. Daisne JF, Duprez T, Weynand B, et al. Tumor volume in pharyngolaryngeal squamous cell carcinoma: comparison at CT, MR imaging, and FDG PET and validation with surgical specimen. Radiology 2004;233(1):93–100.

22. Murakami R, Uozumi H, Hirai T, et al. Impact of FDG-PET/CT imaging on nodal staging for head-and-neck squamous cell carcinoma. Int J Radiat Oncol Biol Phys 2007;68(2):377–82.

23. El-Bassiouni M, Ciernik IF, Davis JB, et al. [18FDG] PET-CT-based intensity-modulated radiotherapy treatment planning of head and neck cancer. Int J Radiat Oncol Biol Phys 2007;69(1):286–93.

24. Igdem S, Alço G, Ercan T, et al. The application of positron emission tomography/computed tomography in radiation treatment planning: effect on gross target volume definition and treatment management. Clin Oncol (R Coll Radiol) 2010;22(3):173–8.

25. Scarfone C, Lavely WC, Cmelak AJ, et al. Prospective feasibility trial of radiotherapy target definition for head and neck cancer using 3-dimensional PET and CT imaging. J Nucl Med 2004;45(4):543–52.

26. Geets X, Daisne JF, Tomsej M, et al. Impact of the type of imaging modality on target volumes delineation and dose distribution in pharyngo-laryngeal squamous cell carcinoma: comparison between pre- and per-treatment studies. Radiother Oncol 2006;78(3):291–7.

27. Guido A, Fuccio L, Rombi B, et al. Combined 18F-FDG-PET/CT imaging in radiotherapy target delineation for head-and-neck cancer. Int J Radiat Oncol Biol Phys 2009;73(3):759–63.

28. Heron DE, Andrade RS, Flickinger J, et al. Hybrid PET-CT simulation for radiation treatment planning in head-and-neck cancers: a brief technical report. Int J Radiat Oncol Biol Phys 2004;60(5):1419–24.

29. Paulino AC, Koshy M, Howell R, et al. Comparison of CT- and FDG-PET-defined gross tumor volume in intensity-modulated radiotherapy for head-and-neck cancer. Int J Radiat Oncol Biol Phys 2005; 61(5):1385–92.

30. Delouya G, Igidbashian L, Houle A, et al. (1)(8)F-FDG-PET imaging in radiotherapy tumor volume

delineation in treatment of head and neck cancer. Radiother Oncol 2011;101(3):362–8.

31. Schinagl DA, Span PN, van den Hoogen FJ, et al. Pathology-based validation of FDG PET segmentation tools for volume assessment of lymph node metastases from head and neck cancer. Eur J Nucl Med Mol Imaging 2013;40(12):1828–35.

32. Kajitani C, Asakawa I, Uto F, et al. Efficacy of FDG-PET for defining gross tumor volume of head and neck cancer. J Radiat Res 2013;54(4):671–8.

33. Schinagl DA, Vogel WV, Hoffmann AL, et al. Comparison of five segmentation tools for 18F-fluoro-deoxy-glucose-positron emission tomography-based target volume definition in head and neck cancer. Int J Radiat Oncol Biol Phys 2007;69(4):1282–9.

34. Ford EC, Kinahan PE, Hanlon L, et al. Tumor delineation using PET in head and neck cancers: threshold contouring and lesion volumes. Med Phys 2006;33(11):4280–8.

35. Daisne JF, Sibomana M, Bol A, et al. Tri-dimensional automatic segmentation of PET volumes based on measured source-to-background ratios: influence of reconstruction algorithms. Radiother Oncol 2003;69(3):247–50.

36. Perez-Romasanta LA, Bellon-Guardia M, Torres-Donaire J, et al. Tumor volume delineation in head and neck cancer with 18-fluor-fluorodeoxiglu-cose positron emission tomography: adaptive thresholding method applied to primary tumors and metastatic lymph nodes. Clin Transl Oncol 2013;15(4):283–93.

37. Chatterjee S, Frew J, Mott J, et al. Variation in radiotherapy target volume definition, dose to organs at risk and clinical target volumes using anatomic (computed tomography) versus combined anatomic and molecular imaging (positron emission tomography/computed tomography): intensity-modulated radiotherapy delivered using a tomotherapy Hi Art machine: final results of the VortigERN study. Clin Oncol (R Coll Radiol) 2012;24(10): e173–9.

38. Sridhar P, Mercier G, Tan J, et al. FDG PET metabolic tumor volume segmentation and pathologic volume of primary human solid tumors. AJR Am J Roentgenol 2014;202(5):1114–9.

39. Romesser PB, Qureshi MM, Shah BA, et al. Superior prognostic utility of gross and metabolic tumor volume compared to standardized uptake value using PET/CT in head and neck squamous cell carcinoma patients treated with intensity-modulated radiotherapy. Ann Nucl Med 2012;26(7):527–34.

40. Tang C, Murphy JD, Khong B, et al. Validation that metabolic tumor volume predicts outcome in head-and-neck cancer. Int J Radiat Oncol Biol Phys 2012;83(5):1514–20.

41. Murphy JD, La TH, Chu K, et al. Postradiation metabolic tumor volume predicts outcome in head-and-neck cancer. Int J Radiat Oncol Biol Phys 2011;80(2):514–21.

42. Chung MK, Jeong HS, Park SG, et al. Metabolic tumor volume of [18F]-fluorodeoxyglucose positron emission tomography/computed tomography predicts short-term outcome to radiotherapy with or without chemotherapy in pharyngeal cancer. Clin Cancer Res 2009;15(18):5861–8.

43. Vernon MR, Maheshwari M, Schultz CJ, et al. Clinical outcomes of patients receiving integrated PET/CT-guided radiotherapy for head and neck carcinoma. Int J Radiat Oncol Biol Phys 2008;70(3):678–84.

44. Scheibler F, Zumbé P, Janssen I, et al. Randomized controlled trials on PET: a systematic review of topics, design, and quality. J Nucl Med 2012; 53(7):1016–25.

45. Wang K, Heron DE, Clump DA, et al. Target delineation in stereotactic body radiation therapy for recurrent head and neck cancer: a retrospective analysis of the impact of margins and automated PET-CT segmentation. Radiother Oncol 2013; 106(1):90–5.

46. Olteanu LA, Madani I, De Neve W, et al. Evaluation of deformable image coregistration in adaptive dose painting by numbers for head-and-neck cancer. Int J Radiat Oncol Biol Phys 2012;83(2): 696–703.

47. Castadot P, Geets X, Lee JA, et al. Adaptive functional image-guided IMRT in pharyngo-laryngeal squamous cell carcinoma: is the gain in dose distribution worth the effort? Radiother Oncol 2011; 101(3):343–50.

48. Roach MC, Turkington TG, Higgins KA, et al. FDG-PET assessment of the effect of head and neck radiotherapy on parotid gland glucose metabolism. Int J Radiat Oncol Biol Phys 2012;82(1):321–6.

49. Hendrickson K, Phillips M, Smith W, et al. Hypoxia imaging with [F-18] FMISO-PET in head and neck cancer: potential for guiding intensity modulated radiation therapy in overcoming hypoxia-induced treatment resistance. Radiother Oncol 2011; 101(3):369–75.

50. Choi W, Lee SW, Park SH, et al. Planning study for available dose of hypoxic tumor volume using fluorine-18-labeled fluoromisonidazole positron emission tomography for treatment of the head and neck cancer. Radiother Oncol 2010;97(2):176–82.

51. Henriques de Figueiredo B, Merlin T, de Clermont-Gallerande H, et al. Potential of [18F]-fluoromisonidazole positron-emission tomography for radiotherapy planning in head and neck squamous cell carcinomas. Strahlenther Onkol 2013; 189(12):1015–9.

52. Okamoto S, Shiga T, Yasuda K, et al. High reproducibility of tumor hypoxia evaluated by 18F-fluoromisonidazole PET for head and neck cancer. J Nucl Med 2013;54(2):201–7.

53. Yasuda K, Onimaru R, Okamoto S, et al. [18F]fluoromisonidazole and a new PET system with semiconductor detectors and a depth of interaction system for intensity modulated radiation therapy for nasopharyngeal cancer. Int J Radiat Oncol Biol Phys 2013;85(1):142–7.

54. Chatterjee A, Suzuki TM, Takahashi Y, et al. A density functional study to choose the best fluorophore for photon-induced electron-transfer (PET) sensors. Chemistry 2003;9(16):3920–9.

55. Huang Y, Hwang DR, Narendran R, et al. Comparative evaluation in nonhuman primates of five PET radiotracers for imaging the serotonin transporters: [11C]McN 5652, [11C]ADAM, [11C]DASB, [11C]DAPA, and [11C]AFM. J Cereb Blood Flow Metab 2002;22(11):1377–98.

56. Kelley C, Lu S, Parhi A, et al. Antimicrobial activity of various 4- and 5-substituted 1-phenylnaphthalenes. Eur J Med Chem 2013;60:395–409.

57. Morarji K, Fowler A, Vinod SK, et al. Impact of FDG-PET on lung cancer delineation for radiotherapy. J Med Imaging Radiat Oncol 2012;56(2):195–203.

58. Nawara C, Rendl G, Wurstbauer K, et al. The impact of PET and PET/CT on treatment planning and prognosis of patients with NSCLC treated with radiation therapy. Q J Nucl Med Mol Imaging 2012;56(2):191–201.

59. Yin LJ, Yu XB, Ren YG, et al. Utilization of PET-CT in target volume delineation for three-dimensional conformal radiotherapy in patients with non-small cell lung cancer and atelectasis. Multidiscip Respir Med 2013;8(1):21.

60. Mac Manus MP, Everitt S, Bayne M, et al. The use of fused PET/CT images for patient selection and radical radiotherapy target volume definition in patients with non-small cell lung cancer: results of a prospective study with mature survival data. Radiother Oncol 2013;106(3):292–8.

61. Bradley JD, Perez CA, Dehdashti F, et al. Implementing biologic target volumes in radiation treatment planning for non-small cell lung cancer. J Nucl Med 2004;45(Suppl 1):96S–101S.

62. Erdi YE, Rosenzweig K, Erdi AK, et al. Radiotherapy treatment planning for patients with non-small cell lung cancer using positron emission tomography (PET). Radiother Oncol 2002;62(1):51–60.

63. Deniaud-Alexandre E, Touboul E, Lerouge D, et al. Impact of computed tomography and 18F-deoxyglucose coincidence detection emission tomography image fusion for optimization of conformal radiotherapy in non-small-cell lung cancer. Int J Radiat Oncol Biol Phys 2005;63(5):1432–41.

64. De Ruysscher D, Wanders S, Minken A, et al. Effects of radiotherapy planning with a dedicated combined PET-CT-simulator of patients with non-small cell lung cancer on dose limiting normal tissues and radiation dose-escalation: a planning study. Radiother Oncol 2005;77(1):5–10.

65. Ciernik IF, Dizendorf E, Baumert BG, et al. Radiation treatment planning with an integrated positron emission and computer tomography (PET/CT): a feasibility study. Int J Radiat Oncol Biol Phys 2003;57(3):853–63.

66. Ceresoli GL, Cattaneo GM, Castellone P, et al. Role of computed tomography and [18F] fluorodeoxyglucose positron emission tomography image fusion in conformal radiotherapy of non-small cell lung cancer: a comparison with standard techniques with and without elective nodal irradiation. Tumori 2007;93(1):88–96.

67. Gondi V, Bradley K, Mehta M, et al. Impact of hybrid fluorodeoxyglucose positron-emission tomography/computed tomography on radiotherapy planning in esophageal and non-small-cell lung cancer. Int J Radiat Oncol Biol Phys 2007;67(1):187–95.

68. Grills IS, Yan D, Black QC, et al. Clinical implications of defining the gross tumor volume with combination of CT and 18FDG-positron emission tomography in non-small-cell lung cancer. Int J Radiat Oncol Biol Phys 2007;67(3):709–19.

69. Kalff V, Hicks RJ, MacManus MP, et al. Clinical impact of (18)F fluorodeoxyglucose positron emission tomography in patients with non-small-cell lung cancer: a prospective study. J Clin Oncol 2001;19(1):111–8.

70. Mac Manus MP, Hicks RJ, Ball DL, et al. F-18 fluorodeoxyglucose positron emission tomography staging in radical radiotherapy candidates with nonsmall cell lung carcinoma: powerful correlation with survival and high impact on treatment. Cancer 2001;92(4):886–95.

71. Mah K, Caldwell CB, Ung YC, et al. The impact of (18) FDG-PET on target and critical organs in CT-based treatment planning of patients with poorly defined non-small-cell lung carcinoma: a prospective study. Int J Radiat Oncol Biol Phys 2002;52(2):339–50.

72. Messa C, Ceresoli GL, Rizzo G, et al. Feasibility of [18F]FDG-PET and coregistered CT on clinical target volume definition of advanced non-small cell lung cancer. Q J Nucl Med Mol Imaging 2005;49(3):259–66.

73. Geiger GA, Kim MB, Xanthopoulos EP, et al. Stage migration in planning PET/CT scans in patients due to receive radiotherapy for non-small-cell lung cancer. Clin Lung Cancer 2014;15(1):79–85.

74. Wang YC, Tseng HL, Lin YH, et al. Improvement of internal tumor volumes of non-small cell lung cancer patients for radiation treatment planning using interpolated average CT in PET/CT. PLoS One 2013;8(5):e64665.

75. Kruis MF, van de Kamer JB, Houweling AC, et al. PET motion compensation for radiation therapy

using a CT-based mid-position motion model: methodology and clinical evaluation. Int J Radiat Oncol Biol Phys 2013;87(2):394–400.

76. Larson SM, Nehmeh SA, Erdi YE, et al. PET/CT in non-small-cell lung cancer: value of respiratory-gated PET. Chang Gung Med J 2005;28(5):306–14.

77. Moller DS, Khalil AA, Knap MM, et al. A planning study of radiotherapy dose escalation of PET-active tumour volumes in non-small cell lung cancer patients. Acta Oncol 2011;50(6):883–8.

78. Askoxylakis V, Dinkel J, Eichinger M, et al. Multimodal hypoxia imaging and intensity modulated radiation therapy for unresectable non-small-cell lung cancer: the HIL trial. Radiat Oncol 2012;7: 157.

79. Moussallem M, Valette PJ, Traverse-Glehen A, et al. New strategy for automatic tumor segmentation by adaptive thresholding on PET/CT images. J Appl Clin Med Phys 2012;13(5):3875.

80. Biehl KJ, Kong FM, Dehdashti F, et al. 18F-FDG PET definition of gross tumor volume for radiotherapy of non-small cell lung cancer: is a single standardized uptake value threshold approach appropriate? J Nucl Med 2006;47(11):1808–12.

81. Yu J, Li X, Xing L, et al. Comparison of tumor volumes as determined by pathologic examination and FDG-PET/CT images of non-small-cell lung cancer: a pilot study. Int J Radiat Oncol Biol Phys 2009;75(5):1468–74.

82. Cheebsumon P, Boellaard R, de Ruysscher D, et al. Assessment of tumour size in PET/CT lung cancer studies: PET- and CT-based methods compared to pathology. EJNMMI Res 2012;2(1):56.

83. Bradley J, Bae K, Choi N, et al. A phase II comparative study of gross tumor volume definition with or without PET/CT fusion in dosimetric planning for non-small-cell lung cancer (NSCLC): primary analysis of Radiation Therapy Oncology Group (RTOG) 0515. Int J Radiat Oncol Biol Phys 2012;82(1):435–41.e1.

84. Moureau-Zabotto L, Touboul E, Lerouge D, et al. Impact of CT and 18F-deoxyglucose positron emission tomography image fusion for conformal radiotherapy in esophageal carcinoma. Int J Radiat Oncol Biol Phys 2005;63(2):340–5.

85. Muijs CT, Schreurs LM, Busz DM, et al. Consequences of additional use of PET information for target volume delineation and radiotherapy dose distribution for esophageal cancer. Radiother Oncol 2009;93(3):447–53.

86. Leong T, Everitt C, Yuen K, et al. A prospective study to evaluate the impact of FDG-PET on CT-based radiotherapy treatment planning for oesophageal cancer. Radiother Oncol 2006;78(3):254–61.

87. Schreurs LM, Busz DM, Paardekooper GM, et al. Impact of 18-fluorodeoxyglucose positron emission tomography on computed tomography defined target volumes in radiation treatment planning of

esophageal cancer: reduction in geographic misses with equal inter-observer variability. Dis Esophagus 2010;23(6):493–501.

88. Shimizu S, Hosokawa M, Itoh K, et al. Can hybrid FDG-PET/CT detect subclinical lymph node metastasis of esophageal cancer appropriately and contribute to radiation treatment planning? A comparison of image-based and pathological findings. Int J Clin Oncol 2009;14(5):421–5.

89. Konski A, Doss M, Milestone B, et al. The integration of 18-fluoro-deoxy-glucose positron emission tomography and endoscopic ultrasound in the treatment-planning process for esophageal carcinoma. Int J Radiat Oncol Biol Phys 2005;61(4): 1123–8.

90. Han D, Yu J, Yu Y, et al. Comparison of (18)F-fluorothymidine and (18)F-fluorodeoxyglucose PET/CT in delineating gross tumor volume by optimal threshold in patients with squamous cell carcinoma of thoracic esophagus. Int J Radiat Oncol Biol Phys 2010;76(4):1235–41.

91. Muijs CT, Pruim J, Beukema JC, et al. Oesophageal tumour progression between the diagnostic (1)(8) F-FDG-PET and the (1)(8)F-FDG-PET for radiotherapy treatment planning. Radiother Oncol 2013;106(3):283–7.

92. Wang YC, Hsieh TC, Yu CY, et al. The clinical application of 4D 18F-FDG PET/CT on gross tumor volume delineation for radiotherapy planning in esophageal squamous cell cancer. J Radiat Res 2012;53(4):594–600.

93. Salem A, Salem AF, Al-Ibraheem A, et al. Evidence for the use PET for radiation therapy planning in patients with cervical cancer: a systematic review. Hematol Oncol Stem Cell Ther 2011;4(4):173–81.

94. Upasani MN, Mahantshetty UM, Rangarajan V, et al. 18-fluoro-deoxy-glucose positron emission tomography with computed tomography-based gross tumor volume estimation and validation with magnetic resonance imaging for locally advanced cervical cancers. Int J Gynecol Cancer 2012; 22(6):1031–6.

95. Pinkawa M, Eble MJ, Mottaghy FM. PET and PET/CT in radiation treatment planning for prostate cancer. Expert Rev Anticancer Ther 2011;11(7): 1033–9.

96. Souvatzoglou M, Krause BJ, Pürschel A, et al. Influence of (11)C-choline PET/CT on the treatment planning for salvage radiation therapy in patients with biochemical recurrence of prostate cancer. Radiother Oncol 2011;99(2):193–200.

97. Picchio M, Berardi G, Fodor A, et al. C-Choline PET/CT as a guide to radiation treatment planning of lymph-node relapses in prostate cancer patients. Eur J Nucl Med Mol Imaging 2014;41(7):1270–9.

98. Pinkawa M, Piroth MD, Holy R, et al. Dose-escalation using intensity-modulated radiotherapy for

prostate cancer - evaluation of quality of life with and without (18)F-choline PET-CT detected simultaneous integrated boost. Radiat Oncol 2012;7:14.

99. Garcia JR, Jorcano S, Soler M, et al. 11C-Choline PET/CT in the primary diagnosis of prostate cancer: impact on treatment planning. Q J Nucl Med Mol Imaging 2014. PMID: 24844254. [Epub ahead of print].

100. Schwarzenbock SM, Kurth J, Gocke Ch, et al. Role of choline PET/CT in guiding target volume delineation for irradiation of prostate cancer. Eur J Nucl Med Mol Imaging 2013;40(Suppl 1):S28–35.

101. Pinkawa M, Holy R, Piroth MD, et al. Intensity-modulated radiotherapy for prostate cancer implementing molecular imaging with 18F-choline PET-CT to define a simultaneous integrated boost. Strahlenther Onkol 2010;186(11):600–6.

Printed and bound by CPI Group (UK) Ltd, Croydon, CR0 4YY

03/10/2024

01040377-0016